# Advanced Radiographic and Angiographic Procedures
## With an Introduction to Specialized Imaging

**MARIANNE R. TORTORICI, EdD, ARRT(R)**
Professor
Department of Radiological Sciences
University of Nevada, Las Vegas

**PATRICK J. APFEL, MEd, ARRT(R)**
Assistant Professor
Department of Radiological Sciences
University of Nevada, Las Vegas

F. A. DAVIS COMPANY • Philadelphia

F. A. Davis Company
1915 Arch Street
Philadelphia, PA 19103

Printed in the United States of America

Last digit indicates print number: 10  9  8  7  6  5  4  3

*Publisher:* Jean-François Vilain
*Editor:* Lynn Borders Caldwell
*Production Editors:* Marianne Fithian, Jessica Howie Martin, Roberta Massey
*Cover Design:* Louis J. Forgione

As new scientific information becomes available through basic and clinical research, recommended treatments and drug therapies undergo changes. The author(s) and publisher have done everything possible to make this book accurate, up to date, and in accord with accepted standards at the time of publication. The authors, editors, and publisher are not responsible for errors or omissions or for consequences from application of the book, and make no warranty, expressed or implied, in regard to the contents of the book. Any practice described in this book should be applied by the reader in accordance with professional standards of care used in regard to the unique circumstances that may apply in each situation. The reader is advised always to check product information (package inserts) for changes and new information regarding dose and contraindications before administering any drug. Caution is especially urged when using new or infrequently ordered drugs.

**Library of Congress Cataloging-in-Publication Data**

Tortorici, Marianne R.
    Advanced radiographic and angiographic procedures with an introduction to specialized imaging / Marianne R. Totorici, Patrick J. Apfel.
        p.      cm.
    Includes bibliographical references and index.
    ISBN 0-8036-8571-8 (hard)
    1. Radiography, Medical.  2. Angiography.  3. Contrast media.  I. Apfel, Patrick A.  II. Title.
    [DNLM: 1. Diagnostic Imagimg—methods.  2. Radiography—methods.  3. Angiography—methods.  WM 180 T712a 1995]
RC78.T6848  1995
616.07′54—dc20
DNLM/DLC
for Library of Congress                                                                                            95-13456

# Dedication

This text is dedicated to Carol, Sallie, and the memory of William (Bill) Apfel, who always encouraged and supported us in the pursuit of our ideas and dreams. Their motivation inspired us to believe in ourselves. It was their confidence and reassurance that allowed us to take risks without fear of failure. Through their efforts, we learned that it was better to take a risk and lose than never to try at all.

# Preface

Although there have been many advancements in radiology from the time Roentgen first discovered x-rays on November 8, 1895, most areas of improvement for the first 70 years were in the conventional imaging area. In the last 20 years, with the advent of computer technology, changes have occurred in the types of imaging procedures performed in radiology. The growth has been so rapid that, to meet employer needs, the training of technologists in the new modalities has primarily been a concentrated on-the-job training process.

As the field expanded, new terminology evolved. Operators of conventional x-ray machines, once identified as technicians, became known as technologists and then radiographers. Nonionizing imaging modalities such as ultrasound have motivated department name changes from x-ray to radiology to diagnostic imaging.

With the evolution of the imaging field, procedures once considered "special" became routine. Originally, the phrase "special procedures" was reserved for angiography and advanced contrast media studies such as myelography. As the advanced procedures became more commonplace and angiography began to include interventional techniques, the phrase "special procedures" came to refer to angiographic and interventional procedures. The technologists working in these areas are usually called cardiovascular interventional technologists (CIT).

Although many texts have been written for the technologist, few include advanced procedures. This book was written to reduce the gap between current clinical practice and the limited resources in these areas.

When this book was first being planned, we asked various professionals in the United States for their opinions on the content of a text describing advanced radiographic and angiographic imaging procedures. There was no consensus as to which procedures should be identified as "advanced" or which angiographic procedures should be included. This made the planning of the content very difficult. In an attempt to provide a text that would be comprehensive enough to meet the majority of needs, we designed its content to:

1. Provide education in advanced procedures for radiographers who are certified or nearing certification and are familiar with conventional radiography;
2. Provide a reference for imaging departments, including those in small rural areas that do not have the luxury of CT, MR, or other specialized scanners;
3. Concentrate on the procedures rather than the physics of examination;
4. Provide an introduction to specialized imaging modalities for all health care professionals.

Diagnostic medical sonography (ultrasound) and nuclear medicine were omitted from this text because these disciplines have their own training criteria and registry, and are well established in the imaging field.

We are always interested in new ideas, and encourage readers to write to us with any comments or suggestions for future editions of this text:

Marianne R. Tortorici and Patrick Joseph Apfel
c/o Lynn Borders Caldwell, Editor
F. A. Davis Company
1915 Arch Street
Philadelphia, PA 19103

# Acknowledgments

Hundreds of students and colleagues whom we have encountered over the years helped and supported us with this textbook. Although we cannot mention each person individually, we want to express our deepest gratitude for their support.

We would also like to express our gratitude to our immediate families and friends, who served as our greatest advocates. It was their "words of wisdom" and belief in us and the project that encouraged us to continue working during times of frustration and doubt.

Special thanks go to Mary Klein, Vicki Gooss, and William O'Donnell from Sunrise Hospital and Medical Center and Sunrise Children's Hospital, Las Vegas, Nevada, who assisted us in the clinical photography used throughout the text. We are grateful for their patience and time in ensuring that our needs were met.

We express appreciation to Nancy Sedin, RN, and Minnie Dunn, LPN, also from Sunrise Hospital and Medical Center and Sunrise Children's Hospital; and Dr. Frank Nemec, gastroenterologist, for sharing their knowledge of ERCP procedures.

Many thanks to Brandy Johnson for her invaluable assistance in editing some of the specialized imaging chapters. Her suggestions helped to ensure the accuracy of the text.

We are especially thankful to Joseph Tortorici, who did the illustrations. He dedicated hundreds of hours to developing them on computer and ensuring their accuracy. We appreciate his visits to Nevada, computer and all in tow, to work with us.

Many talented educators and radiographers reviewed various portions of the developing manuscript and offered valuable suggestions for improvement. We would also like to thank them for their time and expertise:

Those who reviewed the entire manuscript:

Dennis A. Bair, AS, ARRT(R)(CV)
Supervisor of Angiography
United Regional Medical Services Inc.
Milwaukee, Wisconsin

Joseph R. Bittengle, MEd, ARRT(R)
Chairman and Assistant Professor
Department of Radiologic Technology
University of Arkansas for Medical
  Sciences
Little Rock, Arkansas

William F. O'Donnell, Jr., AS, ARRT(R)
Supervisor Special Procedures
Department of Diagnostic Imaging
Sunrise Hospital and Medical Center
and Sunrise Children's Hospital
Las Vegas, Nevada

Sandra D. Ostresh, MEd, ARRT(R)
Program Director
Radiologic Technology Program
Quinsigamond Community College
Worcester, Massachusetts

Wanda Wesolowski, ARRT(R)MAEd
Professor/Chairperson
Department of Radiologic Technology
Community College of Philadelphia
Philadelphia, Pennsylvania

Those who reviewed the original
  proposal or individual chapters:

Patricia A. Bynum, MAEd,
  ARRT(R)(N)CNT
Staff Nuclear Medicine Technologist
Department of Nuclear Medicine
Sibley Memorial Hospital
Washington, DC

Mary Jane Clarke, MS, ARRT(R)
Program Director
Radiography Department
Quinnipiac College
Hamden, Connecticut

Steven B. Dowd, MA, ARRT(R)
Program Director
Radiography Program
University of Alabama at Birmingham
Birmingham, Alabama

Michael Drafke, MS, ARRT(R)
Professor
College of DuPage
Glen Ellyn, Illinois

Patricia Duffy, MPS, ARRT(R)
Assistant Director/Clinical Coordinator
Radiologic Technology
State University of New York
Syracuse, New York

Joseph S. Field, DO
Director
Southwest Imaging Center
Kingman, Arizona

Bruce Foreman, ARRT(R)(CV)
Radiographer-Angiographic Imaging
University of Arkansas Hospital
Little Rock, Arkansas

Angeline B. Golden, MS, JD
Appellant Attorney
Special Fund
Commonwealth of Kentucky
Louisville, Kentucky

Janice D. Hall, MAEd, ARRT(R)
Associate Professor
Radiography Program
University of Alabama at Birmingham
Birmingham, Alabama

Kay Kisner, ARRT(CR)(M)
Staff Mammographer
Department of Diagnostic Imaging
Sunrise Hospital and Medical Center
and Sunrise Children's Hospital
Las Vegas, Nevada

Katherine Mauri, ARRT(R)(M)
Staff Mammographer
Department of Diagnostic Imaging
Sunrise Hospital and Medical Center
and Sunrise Children's Hospital
Las Vegas, Nevada

Suzanne M. McNutt, ARRT(R)(M)
Mammography Supervisor
Department of Diagnostic Imaging
Sunrise Hospital and Medical Center
and Sunrise Children's Hospital
Las Vegas, Nevada

Jeanne L. Neuman, ARRT(R)(CV)
Lead Cardiovascular/Interventional
  Technologist
Department of Cardiovascular/
  Interventional Technology
McKee Medical Center
Loveland, Colorado

Milton Schwartzberg, JD
Attorney at Law
Boston, Massachusetts

Brien Vokits, MS, ARRT(R)
Assistant Director
Sunrise Diagnostic Center
Las Vegas, Nevada

Many of the photographs and some of the illustrations are supplied through the
courtesy of medical supply and book publishing companies. All were very helpful in providing us with the items we needed. We'd like to thank (in alphabetical order):

Abbott Laboratories
AGFA Corporation
B. Braun Vena Tech and B. Braun Celsa
Cook Incorporated

Cordis Corporation
Elema-Schonander
F. A. Davis Company
General Electric Medical Systems
Imatron Inc.
ISG Technologies Inc.
Johnson & Johnson Interventional Systems Co.
Little, Brown and Company
Lea & Febiger (Williams & Wilkins)
Mallinckrodt Medical, Inc.
Medcom Trainex
Medi-tech (Boston Scientific Corporation)
Medrad, Inc.
Microvena Corporation
Mosby Year Book
Nitinal Medical Technologies, Inc.
Pfizer Hospital Products Group, Schneider (USA) Inc.
Sanofi Winthrop Pharmaceuticals
Siemens Medical Systems, Inc.
Squibb Diagnostics (Bristol Myers Squibb)
Target Therapeutics
W. B. Saunders Company

# Contributors

**Angie Alford, AS, ARRT(R)(M)**
Computed Tomography Supervisor
Department of Radiology
Desert Springs Hospital
Las Vegas, Nevada

**Patrick J. Apfel, MEd, ARRT(R)**
Assistant Professor
Department of Radiological Sciences
University of Nevada, Las Vegas
Las Vegas, Nevada

**Dennis A. Bair, AS, ARRT(R)(CV)**
Supervisor of Angiography
United Regional Medical Services Inc.
Milwaukee, Wisconsin

**Joseph R. Bittengle, MEd, ARRT(R)**
Chairman and Assistant Professor
Department of Radiologic Technology
University of Arkansas for Medical
  Sciences
Little Rock, Arkansas

**Kathi A. Clark, BSBA, ARRT(R)(CV)**
Special Procedures Technologist
St. Joseph Hospital
Denver, Colorado

**Donna C. Davis, MEd, ARRT(R)(CV)**
Instructor
Department of Radiologic Technology
University of Arkansas for Medical
  Sciences
Little Rock, Arkansas

**Janice C. De'Ath, ARRT(R)(M)**
Mammography Coordinator
Department of Radiology
Desert Springs Hospital
Las Vegas, Nevada

**Joan K. MacDonald, MS, ARRT(N)**
Assistant Professor
Department of Radiological Sciences
University of Nevada, Las Vegas
Las Vegas, Nevada

**Carol A. Mascioli, AS, ARRT(R)(CV)**
Director of Business Services
Miami Vascular Institute at Baptist
  Hospital
Miami, Florida

**Patricia A. Messmer, RN, CCRN**
Radiology Nurse
McKee Medical Center
Loveland, Colorado

**Jeanne L. Neuman, ARRT(R)(CV)**
Lead Cardiovascular Interventional
  Technologist
Department of Cardiovascular/
  Interventional Technology
McKee Medical Center
Loveland, Colorado

**Ann M. Obergfell, JD, ARRT(R)**
Associate Professor
Radiography Program
University of Louisville
Louisville, Kentucky

**William F. O'Donnell, Jr., AS, ARRT(R)**
Supervisor Special Procedures
Department of Diagnostic Imaging
Sunrise Hospital and Medical Center
and Sunrise Children's Hospital
Las Vegas, Nevada

**Marianne R. Tortorici, EdD, ARRT(R)**
Professor
Department of Radiological Sciences
University of Nevada, Las Vegas
Las Vegas, Nevada

**Kenneth M. Wintch, MA, ARRT(R)(N),**
 **RN**
Associate Professor
Department of Radiological Sciences
University of Nevada, Las Vegas
Las Vegas, Nevada

# Contents

# PART ONE

# INTRODUCTION

# CHAPTER 1

# Radiology in Motion

*Marianne R. Tortorici, EdD, ARRT(R)*

In 1895, Wilhelm Conrad Roentgen discovered a new kind of radiant energy. He named the new radiation x ray, using the letter "x" for the mathematical representation of an unknown. Roentgen realized almost immediately that x rays had major application in medical diagnosis. With the aid of this new energy, it was possible to "see" pathologies within the human body without the trauma of surgery. This advancement in medicine greatly enhanced the therapeutic treatment and prognosis of patients.

This discovery led to an ever-increasing demand for x-ray machines. Early equipment had no provisions for the protection of the operator or patient. The long-term effects of radiation began to unfold after about 20 years. The lack of proper radiation protection practices and devices meant that many early pioneers absorbed an excessive amount of radiation and subsequently died of cancer. Thus, the first 50 to 60 years of x-ray use were associated with the improvement of radiographic equipment designed to decrease radiation exposure to the patient and operator as well as increase the quality of the image.

In the last 20 years, the field of radiology has moved so rapidly that the training of technologists has not caught up with the advancements in technology. As the field has expanded, so has the terminology. Operators of x-ray machines, once identified as technicians, next became known as technologists, and are now called "radiographers." New imaging modalities that do not employ radiation, for example, ultrasound, have also led to changing first the designation "x-ray department" to "radiology department" and now to "imaging department."

As the imaging field changed, so did the type of procedures performed in departments. Originally, the term "special procedures" was reserved for angiographic procedures and advanced contrast media studies, for example, myelography. As advanced procedures became more commonplace and as angiographic procedures began to include interventional techniques, the term "special procedures" was replaced by other terms. Today special procedure technologists are now referred to as "cardiovascular interventional technologists."

3

Often the public is so involved with the benefits of technologic developments that the pioneers responsible for developing the technology are forgotten. It is not unusual for the physician who orders an angiographic procedure to know little, if anything, about the complexity of the equipment, the technology involved, or the individuals responsible for the development of the procedures. The events and individuals that are responsible for the present-day equipment and procedures are often taken for granted.

The intent of this chapter is to acknowledge the major events and individuals responsible for current practices of the procedures in this text. As time passes, new technologies evolve. Because these new technologies are unknown to us today, the content of this chapter is limited by the date of publication.

## EVENTS PRIOR TO THE DISCOVERY OF X RAYS

Prior to the nineteenth century, the human body was studied through autopsy. Scientists would dissect human bodies, study the organs, and attempt to explain each organ's function.

The heart in particular has always intrigued scientists. It was considered the pulse of life and was the primary organ studied in early medical history. The first recorded injection into the heart took place in ancient Greece when Hippocrates injected both air and water into the heart chambers.

The first recorded attempt to provide controlled medical research and training was between 300 and 200 BC. During this time, the medical library of Alexandria was built. The library housed autopsy rooms, lecture halls, and more than 1 million scrolls of medical information and data. Unfortunately, political unrest led to the downfall of Alexander the Great's empire and the burning of the library. The destruction of the library set medicine back many years. It was not until the Renaissance that science and medicine saw a revival.

Leonardo da Vinci, a scientist as well as an artist, helped to advance medicine through his meticulous drawings of dissected organs of the body, including precise pictures of the heart. His drawings of the heart valves were perfect; in fact, many of his diagrams are still used in today's anatomy and physiology texts.

An improved method for demonstrating blood vessels was developed by English architect and professor of astronomy, Christopher Wren, in the midseventeenth century. Wren used a hollow reed to inject colored dyes into the blood vessels of corpses. The colors outlined the vessels and facilitated the recording of their location in the body. By the end of the seventeenth century, the injection of various materials into vessels became a common practice, not only in corpses but also in live humans.

During the late nineteenth century, French physiologist Claude Bernard inserted catheters into the jugular veins, the inferior vena cava, and the femoral arteries of living patients to obtain blood samples for the cardiac chambers. A modification of Bernard's approach serves as the basis for today's vascular catheterization technique.

Sixteen years after Bernard's catheterization techniques were developed, German physicist Wilhelm Conrad Roentgen discovered x rays, which revolutionized medicine by making it possible to visualize pathologic conditions. This new discovery, coupled with the results of further experimentation with injection of various materials into the bloodstream, represents the birth of angiography.

## 1896 TO 1929

In 1896, Edward Hascheck and Otto Lindenthal injected chalk ($CaCO_3$) into the brachial artery of a corpse. After injection, a radiograph was taken with an exposure time of 57 minutes. Angiography in live patients did not occur until a later date, when contrast agents were developed and equipment was improved to allow for optimal exposure times, injection rates, and filming.

From 1896 to 1912, poor radiographic equipment hampered progress in radiology. One of the major problems was the "gassy" x-ray tube. Once a tube became gassy, it was no longer functional. In 1913, American physical chemist W.D. Coolidge invented and patented the tungsten filament x-ray tube. One characteristic of tungsten is that it can be heated without emitting gas ions. Coolidge's use of a tungsten filament extended the life of the tube and represents the first milestone in the construction of modern x-ray tubes. This tube also improved radiographic image quality and substantially decreased exposure time.

The next milestone in imaging was reached in 1919, when Carlos Heuser used sodium iodide as a contrast medium for urologic studies. Sodium iodide was also used by Barney Brooks for femoral arteriography in 1924, Egas Moniz for carotid angiography in 1927, and Raybaldo dos Santos in 1928 for percutaneous aortography. Unfortunately, the merit of using iodine salts as a contrast medium was not recognized immediately, and their widespread use did not occur until the 1930s. Also in 1919, Jacobaeus, a Swedish internist, performed the first air myelography. In 1921, Lipiodol, a positive oil-based medium, was developed and became the first popular positive contrast agent for myelography.

Cardiac catheterization saw a milestone in 1929, when Werner Forssmann performed a cutdown on his own artery, inserted a catheter, and with the aid of a nurse and another physician, performed the first heart catheterization on himself.

## 1930 TO 1949

In 1931, the first general arteriography and aortography text, written by Raynaldo dos Santos, Augusto Lamas, and Jose Caldas, was published. The text contained hundreds of examples of arteriograms. The number and type of examinations performed by these authors that were documented in the text far exceeded those of any other experimental group.

In 1932, Moniz and Pereira Caldas developed a manual rapid film changer, which solved the problem of imaging contrast medium in a blood vessel before it was washed away by the rapid blood flow. Previous to Moniz's film changer introduction, attempts to keep the contrast medium in the vessels included ligation or clamping of arteries, compression of the extremities, and multiple injections of the contrast medium. Moniz's changer took three films, or exposures, in rapid succession that demonstrated the arterial, capillary, and venous phases of the blood vessels.

At the same time Moniz was developing the film changer, Stafford Warren improved mammography diagnosis when he discovered that by using an anterior oblique position of a patient's breast and moving the opposite breast out of the imaging field, the radiograph demonstrated the breast and axillary fossa. Using a stereoscopic filming technique with this position, he was able to accurately diagnose 93 percent of the mammography cases he performed. However, as Warren himself noted, many of the patients x-rayed had advanced cancer, which may have attributed to his high accuracy rate. Even with the new mammography position, the image quality was so poor that little attention or research occurred in this area for many years. It was not until the 1950s that an interest in mammography was revived.

Venography was introduced by dos Santos in 1938, when he injected contrast medium into a superficial vein behind the lateral malleolus. His technique was improved with the addition of applying a tourniquet above the ankle to prevent the contrast medium from entering the superficial veins. The early years of venography required "blind" filming. It was not until the development of the image intensifier that venography increased in popularity.

The 1940s saw the manual rapid film changer modified by Jesus Sanchez-Perez, who developed a motor-driven film changer. Cater further improved the film changer in 1943.

Another event occurred in the area of myelography when, in 1944, Ramsy and Strain substituted Pantopaque for Lipiodol while performing a myelogram. Pantopaque proved safer than Lipiodol and soon became the contrast medium of choice for myelography.

## THE 1950s

Around 1950, film changers were further improved. The rapid automatic roll film changer was developed by Scott and Moore in 1949, and the biplane automatic cassette changer was developed by Fredzell and his colleagues in 1950. As rapid film changers were being improved, other important events were occurring in the field.

In the early 1950s, Jacob Gershon-Cohen, a radiologist, and Helen Insleby, a pathologist, worked together to improve mammography imaging. They determined that by using high contrast filming, collimation, and compression, mammographic image quality increased.

The years from 1949 to 1952 saw the preliminary development of image intensifiers. The image intensifier permitted the physician to visualize the actual movement of the heart, lungs, and other organs. The original intensifiers allowed for the visualization of the image directly or through the use of a mirror, but viewing was limited to one person. Further refinement of the intensification systems permitted group viewing of the image on a television monitor. Image intensification also proved useful in angiography for catheter placement in vessels.

During the development of image intensifiers, angiography advanced with the evolution of three-phase generators. The use of generators and tubes, which allowed high milliamperage stations of 1000 mA and greater, decreased the exposure time to a fraction of a second, making rapid film exposure possible.

As angiographic equipment improved, it became evident that to visualize vessels a need existed to deliver a large bolus of contrast medium in a short period of time. Hand injections were too slow and the bolus too small. In 1956, Gidlund constructed the first reliable automatic injector, which operated by the use of compressed gas. Contrast medium was injected under a constant, preset pressure.

The development and improvement of the major pieces of equipment necessitated new accessory equipment and new catheter techniques. Seldinger is credited with the use of the guide wire for catheterization (see Chap. 19, Catheterization Methods and Patient Management). Seldinger's technique was simple and reduced patient complications that were caused by catheter manipulation within the body.

Also occurring in the 1950s was the development of lymphography. In 1952, Kinmonth developed a method of cannulating the lymphatic vessels of the foot. He used an injection of blue dye between the toes to visualize the lymphatic vessels. A cutdown on the dorsum of the foot was used to cannulate the lymphatic vessel.

## THE 1960s

The 1960s saw the fabrication of new materials for vascular catheters. These materials were less toxic to the body, permitted better control of the catheter during placement in the vessel, and decreased the possibility of blood clotting.

Also, mammography continued to improve when Robert L. Egan used Gershon-Cohen and Insleby's recommendation and produced a high-quality mammogram using a high milliampere, low kilovoltage peak technique and industrial film in 1960. Charles M. Gros used a molybdenum focal spot to increase image contrast in mammography. Also, CGR Company introduced the first dedicated mammography unit with a

0.7-mm molybdenum focal spot size and a built-in compression device. The late 1960s saw the introduction of xeroradiography for mammography. There has been much debate over whether xeroradiography or film produces the better mammogram. Currently, film appears to have essentially replaced xeroradiography.

Another event of the 1960s involved the continual improvement of automatic injectors. Gidlund's injector was refined in 1967 by Viamonte and Hobbs, who developed an electric injector with mechanical safety features. Their injector allowed for a slow rise in the pressure of the injection. Today's advanced injectors include electrocardiograph monitors that permit the physician to inject contrast medium in correlation with the heartbeat.

Also, in 1961, a great advancement occurred in cardiac catheterization, when Ricketts and Abrams performed the first transfemoral selective coronary angiography. Melvin Judkins developed preshaped catheters for coronary angiography in 1967. These techniques provided a means to record pressures and take blood samples to increase the accuracy of diagnosing cardiac disease.

Probably the greatest milestone of the 1960s is the introduction of interventional angiography. This specialty of radiology included percutaneous transluminal angioplasty (PTA), thrombolysis, embolization, and biopsy. Charles Dotter and Melvin Judkins performed the first PTA of the right common iliac artery in 1964. This procedure was performed by using tapered coaxial Teflon dilators to open the lumen of the vessel. These dilators were limited to small vessel use. The development of a double-lumen polyvinyl chloride balloon catheter by Andreas Gruntzig made PTA safer and increased its popularity. Besides PTA, thrombolysis was introduced in the early 1970s as a means of relieving vascular occlusion. Thrombolysis employs the injection of thrombolytic agent(s), such as streptokinase, in a vessel to help open an occluded artery.

Embolization, which is the opposite of thrombolysis and PTA, is designed to occlude a vessel. In 1967, Nusbaum and Baum used embolization by injecting a vasoconstrictor into the superior mesenteric artery to decrease portal hypertension. This began the era of pharmacoangiography. The popularity of embolization increased during the 1970s as a result of the development of new long- and short-term embolization materials. Currently, embolization is used in the treatment of bleeding, arteriovenous (A-V) malformations, A-V fistulas, and hemorrhage.

## THE 1970s

In the 1970s the first successful myelographic study employing a nonionic water-soluble contrast medium, metrizamide (Amipaque), was performed in the United States. This contrast medium mixed well with the cerebrospinal fluid (CSF) and, unlike Pantopaque, did not have to be removed from the patient. The more recent, less toxic, nonionic contrast media used today for myelography are Omnipaque and Isovue.

The 1970s also saw another improvement in mammography when DuPont introduced a single-emulsion film in combination with a high-resolution intensifying screen. The film and screen were sealed in an air-evacuated plastic bag.

The advent of computer technology in the 1970s led the way for the birth of new imaging modalities including computed tomography (CT) and magnetic imaging. Computerized axial tomography (CAT) was introduced in 1972 by Godfrey Hounsfield. CAT employed the concept of using a computer to reconstruct an image taken at various angles. The images were limited to axial views. However, as image reconstruction improved, the images produced were of transverse planes, coronal planes, multiple planes, and three dimensions. This prompted the name to change in the mid-1980s from CAT to CT. The first-generation images required long scanning times, up to 5 months. Early CAT units employed a gantry with a stationary x-ray tube and two side-by-side detectors that moved over the patient. After the detector moved over the patient, the gantry would move 1 degree. This translate-rotate method would be repeated for 180 degrees.

The second-generation CT scanners used a 10-degree x-ray beam fan that spread over an array of 8 to 30 detectors. The translate-rotate method was used, which limited the passes to 18 at 10-degree increments for 180 degrees. This substantially decreased average scanning time to about 1 minute.

The third generation of CT scanners used a rotation, rather than a translate-rotate, system. In this method, the tube and detector are mounted opposite one another and move around the patient, compared with the back-and-forth movement of the early scanners.

In the fourth generation of CT scanners, the detectors are stationary and the tube rotates around the patient. This produces an image in 2 to 3 seconds.

The other recent imaging modality, nuclear magnetic resonance (NMR), was applied to medicine in the 1970s. NMR was adapted from its use in chemistry in which it proved successful as a means of analyzing chemical compounds. In 1974, an NMR of a mouse was performed at the University of Aberdeen. It was not until 1977 that Raymond Damadian obtained an NMR cross-sectional image of a human. This image was obtained using a field focusing (FONAR) technique and was extremely time consuming. Researchers at the University of Nottingham and the University of Aberdeen, experimenting with a planar (versus point) technique and using a constant duration radiofrequency (spin-warp) to stimulate the cells, improved the visibility of the image.

## 1980 TO PRESENT

In 1980, the quality obtainable with NMR continued to improve, and NMR rapidly became a popular imaging technique. It was in 1980 that the first high-quality human images, of the brain, were obtained by Moore and Hinshaw. NMR became popular because it was nonionizing, noninvasive, and capable of visualizing vascularity without the use of a contrast medium. Around 1985, the term "nuclear" was dropped because of the negative connotation it had with the public. Thus, NMR became known as magnetic resonance imaging (MRI). Although MRI was popular and produced quality images, a need existed to develop a magnet that was lightweight, produced a strong magnetic field, and had minimal power loss. Currently, the superconducting magnet is the magnet of choice. It is able to provide high magnetic fields (up to 2 tesla [T]) with little power loss. However, the magnet is expensive and must be surrounded by liquid helium, which is surrounded by liquid nitrogen. The current construction of an MRI room prevents interference of the magnetic field from outside influences. This further enhances the usefulness and popularity of MRI. As the 1980s came to a close, MRI researchers began to introduce the use of contrast agents, for example, gadolinium, to produce a higher-quality image and improve diagnosis.

## TODAY'S STATUS

New equipment, catheters, imaging modalities, and catheterization methods influence the role of the technologist. Today's imaging technologist performs both selective diagnostic radiographs and interventional procedures. Computers are continuing to make a rapid and significant impact on our lives in general and radiology specifically. The advent of nonionizing imaging, three-dimensional imaging, and virtual reality are leading radiology in a new direction. Imaging departments are beginning to implement computed radiography, with the hope of eliminating the need for films and making images available to anyone in the world by using a computer internet. Like so many fields that grow swiftly, the technical advances of radiology seem to occur more rapidly than the educational system's ability to provide technologists with the knowledge and skills necessary to understand and operate the new equipment.

There seems to be a dearth of instructional information and curriculum in the new modalities, especially at the technological level. The intent of this text is to provide an in-depth presentation of angiography, a comprehensive discussion on selected advanced radiographic procedures, and an introduction to new imaging modalities. We hope this information will assist in providing the knowledge needed to produce a more competent radiographer and will serve as an incentive for the reader to pursue further knowledge and education in the specialized areas.

## REVIEW QUESTIONS

1. The organ most often studied in early medical history was the _____.
   A. brain
   B. heart
   C. lung
   D. kidney

2. The first recorded attempt to provide controlled medical research and training was during _____.
   A. the nineteenth century
   B. the Renaissance
   C. the seventeenth century
   D. 300 to 200 BC

3. _____ helped advance medicine through his meticulous drawings of dissected organs.
   A. Leonardo da Vinci
   B. Alexander the Great
   C. Claude Bernard
   D. Christopher Wren

4. In _____, W.D. Coolidge invented the tungsten filament x-ray tube.
   A. 1898
   B. 1913
   C. 1929
   D. 1933

5. _____ was first used for urologic studies in 1919.
   A. Chalk
   B. Ethiodal
   C. Sodium iodine
   D. Barium

6. _____ developed the first manual rapid film changer.
   A. Gidlund
   B. Dos Santos
   C. Lamas and Caldas
   D. Moniz and Caldas

7. Forssmann performed the first cardiac catheterization on _____.
   A. himself
   B. a volunteer prisoner
   C. a corpse
   D. his colleague

8. The development of _____ was helpful in decreasing exposure time.
   A. image intensification
   B. three-phase generators
   C. automatic injectors
   D. rapid film changers

9. The first automatic injector operated by use of (a) _____.
   A. electricity
   B. battery
   C. compressed gas
   D. manual power

10. A valuable development that occurred because of computer technology is _____.
    A. computed tomography
    B. three-phase generators
    C. video recording
    D. rapid film changers

11. The first popular oil-based contrast medium for myelography was _____.
    A. Pantopaque
    B. Lipiodol

C. Amipaque
D. sodium iodide

12. Stafford Warren improved mammography by _____.
    A. developing the molybdenum focal spot
    B. using an anterior oblique position
    C. using a dedicated mammography unit
    D. employing compression

13. Venography increased in popularity when _____.
    A. the image intensifier was developed
    B. a tourniquet was added to the technique
    C. rapid film changers evolved
    D. the automatic injector was introduced

14. Kinmonth employed a cut-down of the _____ to cannulate a lymphatic vessel.
    A. hand
    B. axillary
    C. foot
    D. brachial

15. In 1967, _____ developed preshaped catheters for coronary angiography.
    A. Ricketts
    B. Abrams
    C. Hobbs
    D. Judkins

16. _____ is a useful interventional technique to occlude a vessel.
    A. embolization
    B. PTA

C. thrombolysis
D. biopsy

17. _____ introduced CAT scanning in 1972.
    A. Moore
    B. Damadian
    C. Hinshaw
    D. Hounsfield

18. The third-generation CT scanner used a _____ system of imaging.
    A. translate-rotate
    B. rotation
    C. stationary
    D. rotation-rotation

19. The most popular magnet for MRI is the _____.
    A. ferromagnetic
    B. permanent
    C. superconductive
    D. horseshoe

## BIBLIOGRAPHY

Abrams, H: Angiography, Vol 1, ed 3. Little, Brown & Co, Boston, 1983.

Baltaxe, H, Amplatz, K, and Levin, D: Coronary Angiography. Charles C Thomas, St Louis, 1975.

Doby, T: Development of Angiography and Cardiovascular Catheterization. Publishing Sciences Group, New York, 1976.

Eisenberg, RL: Radiology: An Illustrated History. Mosby-Year Book, St Louis, 1992.

# CHAPTER 2

# Medical Legal Implications

*Ann M. Obergfell, JD, ARRT(R)*

Angiographic and interventional procedures use invasive techniques that require the introduction of both foreign objects (guidewires and catheters) and foreign substances (contrast media or other medications) into the body. During the procedure the possibility of adverse reaction from the foreign materials may arise. The type of reaction may range from a simple hematoma to contrast-related respiratory distress to the occasional possibility of death. Therefore, the invasive nature of the procedure coupled with the possibility of complications mandates that the patient be given adequate information to allow for an informed consent. Additionally, it is important that the hospital personnel complete the appropriate documentation for each procedure.

This chapter discusses the recommended forms for angiographic and interventional procedures. Also included in the chapter is a brief summary of legal liability.

## INFORMED CONSENT

Every person of adult years and sound mind has the right to determine what will happen to his or her own body; this includes the right to determine the course of medical diagnosis and treatment. While current medical technology is so complex that the layperson may have a difficult time determining an appropriate course of diagnosis and treatment, it is imperative that the patient be given enough information to make decisions and give consent.

The amount of information necessary for a person to make an informed consent may vary from patient to patient. Generally, the physician should give information based on a knowledge of the patient's reasoning ability and personal sensitivities. However, a minimum amount of information must be given to each patient.

## Requirements of Informed Consent

One of the requirements the patient is entitled to is advisement of the nature of the procedure, including

**9**

the techniques to be used and the anticipated outcome (i.e., diagnosis of condition). The information should be explained to the patient in such a way that a basic understanding of the procedure by the patient can be ascertained by the physician. Also, the patient must be informed of the risks and benefits of the specific procedure and any alternative procedures that may be performed that could offer the same or similar result. It is also necessary to explain the risks and benefits of the alternatives and the rationale for the physician's recommendation of one option over another.

It is possible for a patient to have difficulty understanding the complex medical terms but be reluctant to ask questions. Therefore, it is important that the individuals who acquire consent and perform the procedure assess the patient's reactions to information and respond accordingly.

After the information has been clearly explained to the patient and an opportunity for questions not only permitted but also encouraged, the consent should be authorized in writing on a form that documents the information relayed to the patient. The signature of the patient on the consent form should then be witnessed by one or two individuals who have no specific interest in the outcome of the procedure. Such individuals may include a ward clerk, a chaplain, or an individual not directly involved with the case. Technologists should not be witnesses as they are part of the procedure and department and therefore have a direct interest in the outcome of the procedure; the same may be true for a family member of the patient.

### The Consent Form

A written consent form should be acquired for every person who is to undergo a diagnostic or therapeutic angiographic procedure. The form should contain an authorization clause, disclosure statement, and a statement acknowledging that the patient understands the explanation (Fig. 2–1), all written in a language the patient understands. Departments located in areas with large populations of non–English-speaking people should have consent forms written and available in the language of the patient, and an individual fluent in the language should be available to assist the patient in reading and signing the form. Information contained in the form should flow logically and should not be ambiguous as to content or meaning. An authorization clause describes the facility as well as the individuals who will be participating in the procedure. The disclosure statement explains the nature, purpose, benefits, risks, and alternatives of the specific procedure. While every risk cannot possibly be disclosed in this statement, it is clear that those risks a reasonable person would find important for decision making must be included. The last statement of the form should explain that the information contained in the form was discussed with the patient and that the patient consents to the procedure. This should be followed by the signature of the patient and the disinterested witnesses.

The requirements for informed consent and the language required for the consent form vary from state to state depending on state statutes or regulations that may govern informed consent or by the case law of a specific jurisdiction. Some facilities may require disclosures that are institution-specific; for example, a teaching institution may have to disclose that students will be observing or participating in the procedure. The specific requirements for the consent form should be determined by input from the institution's legal counsel, the risk management personnel, and the professionals involved in the procedures, such as the cardiovascular interventional technologist, the radiologist, and, if applicable, the radiology nurse.

The consent is to be obtained by the physician who will be performing the procedure; however, the cardiovascular interventional technologist may be required to establish that the consent has been signed and included in the patient's medical record.

## DOCUMENTATION

Record keeping in a special procedures suite is important not only for continuity of patient care, but also to help assist the hospital in determining the course of treatment if there is a claim of improper or negligent care. Often such claims arise an extended period of time after the performance of the procedure; therefore, the personnel may not be able to remember the specifics of the procedure without referring to documentation written at the time of the procedure, which may be used to refresh their memory. The types of forms and amount of documentation vary with the institution, but standard forms such as procedure data and incident reports should be kept by every facility.

### Procedure Data Form

A standardized procedure data form should be used by the facility and completed by the cardiovascular interventional technologist during the procedure. Information in the form should include but not necessarily be limited to (Fig. 2–2):

Basic patient data
Vital signs (before, during, and after the procedure)
List of personnel in the room during the procedure
Type and amount of contrast media used
Other medications used during the procedure
Fluoroscopy time
The size and number of films and the exposures for each series or run
An area for notes and comments

The completed form should become a part of the patient's permanent medical record.

### Complication or Incident Report

If complications arise during the procedure, the health care professionals involved in the procedure

ST. ELSEWHERE HOSPITAL
CONSENT TO PERFORM INVASIVE PROCEDURES

Name _____

Medical Record # _____

I, _____ , hereby authorize Dr. _____

to perform the following procedure _____

at _____

I have been informed that during this procedure a small incision will be made in the groin or arm. A small tube (catheter) will be placed in one or more blood vessels and a medication (contrast media) will be injected through the catheter that will help visualize the blood vessels.
The possibilities of complications from catheter insertion include an accumulation of blood in the tissue at the site of insertion (hematoma) or a less likely complication is the formation of blood clots that would need to be treated by certain medications to dissolve the clot or by surgery to remove the clot. Although this risk is very small, clotting the blood supply to an organ can result in loss of that organ and in a very rare case the loss of life.
The injection of contrast media may also have rare adverse reactions ranging from hives or shortness of breath, to temporary or permanent paralysis. In a very rare case death may occur.
The benefits of the procedure as well as alternative procedures that could be used have been clearly explained to me, and I acknowledge that no guarantee or assurance has been made as to the results that may be obtained.
If the use of anesthesia is necessary, I authorize Dr. _____ to administer those medications that he/she deems necessary and I have been informed of the risks, benefits, and alternatives for the administration of the anesthetic agents.

**I certify that I have read and fully understand the above consent to perform an invasive procedure, that the explanations referred to were made, and that all questions were answered to my satisfaction. All blanks and statements requiring the insertion of information were filled in and the inapplicable paragraphs, if any, were crossed out before I signed.**

Date _____    _____

Time _____    Signature of Patient/Legal Guardian

When patient is a minor or incompetent to give consent the authorized legal guardian must sign.

_____    _____

Witness                    Date        Witness                    Date

**Figure 2–1.** Example consent form.

should complete a complication or incident report. This form should include data concerning the type of complication or incident that occurred, what treatment or course of action was taken, and what follow-up procedures were conducted (Fig. 2–3).

The complication or incident report form should be forwarded to the risk management department, where it is analyzed and the appropriate action taken. In some cases, the form may not be considered a document that the courts will permit both sides to have during the evidence discovery process; therefore, it is generally not included in the medical record.

Facilities may develop other forms of documentation that may be useful before, during, and following the angiographic procedure. One such form is a risk management survey that is used to determine the effectiveness of follow-up procedures after a complication or incident (Fig. 2–4).

## Protocol and Procedure Manual

Each department should develop a policy and procedure manual for each area. The manual ensures that all personnel in the department perform procedures in a consistent manner and that each is familiar with the workings of the department and area of concentration. The manual should include protocols for each process, from scheduling to dismissal of patients. The protocols should have a policy statement followed by a step-by-step analysis of the procedure. The manual should be readily accessible in the department, and new employees should be required to familiarize themselves with the procedures before they are permitted to begin work with patients. A mechanism should be implemented that allows for regular review of the manual and, if any revisions are made, ensures that each employee is notified of the changes.

**ST. ELSEWHERE HOSPITAL: RADIOLOGY DEPARTMENT**

Name _____ Age _____ Sex _____ DOB _____

Medical Record No._____ Date _____ Location _____

Procedure _____ Requesting Dr _____ Date of order _____

**SPECIAL INSTRUCTIONS**

1. _____

2. _____

3. _____

**ALLERGIES**

_____

| RADIOLOGY CHECKLIST | YES | NO | N/A | STATISTICS | | FILM COUNT | | |
|---|---|---|---|---|---|---|---|---|
| Patient identified | ___ | ___ | ___ | Time in | _____ | 14x17 ___ | **DIGITAL** | |
| Procedure identified | ___ | ___ | ___ | Exam time | _____ | 10x12 ___ | 11x14 ___ | |
| Pregnancy status | ___ | ___ | ___ | Time out | _____ | 8x10 ___ | 8x10 ___ | |
| Informed consent | ___ | ___ | ___ | Fluoro time | _____ | 11x14 ___ | ___ | |
| Exam completion | ___ | ___ | ___ | Radiologist | _____ | 9x9 ___ | **DUPLICATING** | |
| Exam rescheduled | ___ | ___ | ___ | Technologist | _____ | 7x17 ___ | 14x17 ___ | |
| Discharge instructions | ___ | ___ | ___ | Technologist | _____ | 14x14 ___ | 10x12 ___ | |
| Condition unchanged | ___ | ___ | ___ | Other | _____ | ___ | ___ | |

| DISPOSITION | | | SKIN PREP | | ANESTHETIC | |
|---|---|---|---|---|---|---|
| LOCATION | TO | FROM | Area | | Type | |
| Inpatient | ___ | ___ | Shave prep | ___ | Method of adm. | ___ |
| Outpatient | ___ | ___ | Antiseptic scrub | ___ | Adm. by | ___ |

Figure 2–2. Example procedure data form.

## LEGAL LIABILITY

### Negligence or Failure to Acquire Informed Consent

Patients who feel they have suffered some type of injury during a procedure in the vascular suite may make a claim for damages based on any number of theories. In most cases the patient must prove that the health care personnel have not met the standard of care recognized in the medical community. In cases of medical negligence or failure to acquire informed consent, the burden of proof is placed on the patient and requires the use of expert testimony. In the case of negligence, the patient must prove four elements. These include showing proof (1) that the technologist has a duty to the patient, such as performing the procedure; (2) that the technologist in some way breached this duty by his or her acts or failure to act in an appropriate manner; (3) that the patient was injured; and (4) that the injury was caused by the technologist's breach of duty.

These elements are often difficult to prove and require the use of an elaborate investigative process in preparation for displaying evidence at trial. Expert witnesses are needed to define the standard of care that would be used under the same or similar circumstances. Another expert may be needed to explain how the act or the failure to act by the defendant caused the injury to the patient.

Failure to acquire informed consent also requires the use of an expert who will testify as to what is the generally accepted practice of disclosure under the same or similar circumstances as the case in question.

Outpatient surgery _____ _____        By _____

ER        _____ _____

ICU        _____ _____        **METHOD OF APPROACH**        **INTRAVENOUS**

Surgery _____ _____        Side _____        Size _____

Other        _____ _____        Type _____        Location _____

Vessel _____        Solution _____

**MODE OF TRANSPORTATION**        **VITAL SIGNS**

| | TO | FROM |
| --- | --- | --- |
| | | |

| PULSE | PRE | POST |
| --- | --- | --- |
| Brachial | _____ | _____ |
| Radial | _____ | _____ |

**LAB RESULTS**

Creatinine _____

BUN _____

| | TO | FROM |
| --- | --- | --- |
| Ambulatory | _____ | _____ |
| Wheelchair | _____ | _____ |
| Stretcher/litter | _____ | _____ |

| | PRE | POST |
| --- | --- | --- |
| Carotid | _____ | _____ |
| Femoral | _____ | _____ |
| Pedial | _____ | _____ |
| Blood pressure | _____ | _____ |
| Respiration | _____ | _____ |

Other _____

**PATIENT STATUS**

| | YES | NO |
| --- | --- | --- |
| Alert | _____ | _____ |
| Oriented | _____ | _____ |
| Confused | _____ | _____ |
| Agitated | _____ | _____ |
| Lethargic | _____ | _____ |
| Non-responsive | _____ | _____ |
| Other | _____ | _____ |

**CONTRAST MEDIA**

| | INJECTION | TYPE | AMOUNT | TIME ADMINISTERED |
| --- | --- | --- | --- | --- |
| 1. | _____ | _____ | _____ | _____ |
| 2. | _____ | _____ | _____ | _____ |
| 3. | _____ | _____ | _____ | _____ |
| | | | TOTAL | _____ |

**ALLERGY HISTORY**

Source: _____ Patient _____ Records _____ Other

Type _____

**MEDICINE ADMINISTRATION RECORD**        **INSTRUCTIONS/COMMENTS**

Type _____        _____

Route _____        _____

Amount _____        _____

Time _____        _____

By _____        _____

_____

_____

RADIOLOGIST _____

**Figure 2–2** *Continued.*

# Assault, Battery, and False Imprisonment

There are three types of claims that do not require expert testimony, but still place the burden of proof on the patient. These claims are assault, battery, and false imprisonment.

In the case of assault, an intentional, generally ver-bal, threat of imminent harm to a patient may occur during the course of a procedure, and the patient must feel that the person has the ability to immediately follow through with the threat. Such threats occur when a patient is not as cooperative as the technologists would like, so a threat of injury may be used to obtain cooperation.

**COMPLICATION OR INCIDENT REPORT**

Patient _____ Date of emergency _____

Date of evaluation _____

Personnel present and evaluating:

_____

_____

_____

_____

1. Briefly describe the complication or incident that occurred.

2. Summarize the treatment that was administered.

3. Summarize the follow-up treatment that occurred.

4. Additional remarks:

**Figure 2-3.** Complication or incident report.

---

**RISK MANAGEMENT SURVEY**

Patient _____ Date of emergency _____

Date of evaluation _____

Personnel present and evaluating:

_____

_____

_____

_____

1. Was needed equipment readily available? If not, what was missing?

2. Did personnel present do what was required of them? Did they initiate treatment of their own?

3. Did auxiliary personnel (ECG, respiratory, etc.) respond promptly?

4. What could have been done differently for a more effective and efficient emergency procedure?

5. Additional remarks:

**Figure 2-4.** Risk management survey.

For a claim of battery, the patient must show an unlawful touching. Whereas the concept of unlawful touching seems rather ominous, it may be as simple as performing a procedure on the wrong patient or touching a patient without permission. For example, "Patient alleging physician battery need only prove that treatment rendered was unauthorized. . . ." (*Kenner v. Northern Illinois Medical Center*, 517 NE2 1137, 1991.) Likewise, "evidence that a patient was subjected (without consent) to a medical procedure and emergency situation did not require procedure clearly supported finding of battery."

Use of any restraint requires permission from the patient or from an individual authorized to give consent. Failure to acquire such permission may promote a claim of false imprisonment. Although the cardiovascular interventional technologist may have a defense of privilege—such as he or she is privileged to threaten, restrain, or touch within the scope of his or her practice—the privilege is not absolute and requires that the technologist use good judgment in touching or using restraint without consent. The general exception to this rule is if a patient is going to hurt him- or herself or another. For example, "Holding of the patient's head and suturing of laceration did not constitute independent acts of confinement beyond that authorized by privilege to confine a patient in the emergency room in order to prevent further harm to herself or others." (Blackmun for *Blackmun v. Rifkin*, 759 P2 54, 1989.)

Regardless of the claim, the burden of proof is always on the patient, except in the case where the theory of *res ipsa loquitur* is invoked. Loosely translated, this means "the thing speaks for itself." In these instances the burden of proof shifts from the patient (plaintiff) to the hospital, doctor, or cardiovascular interventional technologist (defendant). Such a theory is raised when the plaintiff is under the complete control of the defendant and, through no fault of the plaintiff's, an injury, which would not have happened but for the negligent acts of the defendant, is sustained. In the health care setting, such a situation may arise when the patient is anesthetized, as may happen in an angiographic suite. Therefore, it is imperative that the cardiovascular interventional technologist follow the established protocols, abide by the standard of care established for the discipline, and ensure that the patient is comfortable and understands the techniques to be used during the procedure.

## CONCLUSIONS

Avoiding liability for injury to a patient during an angiographic procedure is not a certainty. However, cardiovascular interventional technologists may be able to insulate themselves by following five steps:
1. Be familiar with established facility protocols.
2. Know and follow the appropriate standard of care for cardiovascular-interventional technologists.
3. Determine that an informed consent has been obtained from each patient who is scheduled for an angiographic procedure.

4. Assess each patient to ascertain information that may aid in diagnosis or will decrease the chances of injuring a patient (i.e., a patient behaves as if sedated, which may make the patient unstable on his or her feet).
5. Maintain communication with the patient so that a relationship of trust and mutual respect can be established.

## REVIEW QUESTIONS

1. It is recommended that a(n) _____ should witness an informed consent.
    A. technologist
    B. ward clerk
    C. radiologist
    D. individual over the age of 21 years

2. The _____ of an informed consent describes the facility and individuals performing the procedure.
    A. disclosure statement
    B. introduction
    C. authorization clause
    D. physical clause

3. The language of a consent form should be in _____.
    A. English
    B. medical terms
    C. patient's language
    D. radiology terms

4. A consent form should be obtained by _____.
    A. the physician performing the procedure
    B. the technologist performing the procedure
    C. the floor nurse
    D. an uninterested medical party

5. List at least three items that should be on a procedure data form.

6. A risk management survey is used to _____.
    A. identify the type of complication
    B. determine the effectiveness of follow-up procedures
    C. document the treatment used for the complication
    D. determine liability of the complication

7. One objective of a procedure manual is to ensure that _____.
    A. all personnel perform procedures in a consistent manner
    B. the same exposure factor is used for all procedures
    C. the ratio of technologists to procedures is consistent
    D. errors are documented properly

8. The burden of proof for medical negligence rests with the _____.
    A. physician
    B. patient
    C. technologist
    D. hospital

9. Select the type of claim below that requires an expert witness.
   A. assault
   B. battery
   C. false imprisonment
   D. negligence

## BIBLIOGRAPHY

Anderson, GR and Glesnes-Anderson, V: Health Care Ethics: A Guide for Decision Makers. Aspen Publishers, Rockville, MD, 1987.

Furrow, BR, et al: Liability and Quality Issues in Health Care. West Publishing, St Paul, 1991.

Katz, J: Physicians and patients: A history of silence. In Beauchamp, TL and Walters, L (eds): Contemporary Issues in Bioethics. Wadsworth Publishing, Belmont, CA, 1989.

Miller, RD: Problems in Hospital Law. Aspen Publishers, Rockville, MD, 1986.

Tortorici, MR: Fundamentals of Angiography. CV Mosby, St Louis, 1982.

# CHAPTER 3

# Contrast Media

*Marianne R. Tortorici, EdD, ARRT(R)*

The human body is made up of organs and tissues of differing composition and density. In some instances, the density differences between adjacent organs or tissues are very minor. In these cases, the organs or tissues have a similar appearance when imaged, making it very difficult to differentiate between them. Consequently, the primary method used to distinguish an organ from surrounding tissues is by the introduction of a pharmaceutical agent (contrast medium) into the body.

The contrast medium is directed to a specific organ based on the type of medium and method of introduction. The major characteristic of a contrast medium that makes it effective is its ability to alter the density of an organ in relation to the surrounding tissues. A positive medium (radiopaque) temporarily increases the organ's density, absorbing more radiation, which creates a decrease in the radiographic density of the organ (i.e., the area appears lighter on the radiograph). When a negative (radiolucent) medium is introduced, it temporarily decreases the density of the organ, allowing more radiation to penetrate the object, which creates an increase in the radiographic density of the organ (i.e., the area appears darker on the radiograph). Utilization of either type of medium results in a higher radiographic contrast image of the organ than if it were radiographed without contrast medium.

Often, sole use of the contrast medium in the vessels is inadequate to visualize pathology. Thus, it is common to use vasoconstrictors or vasodilators in association with contrast medium. Because normal anatomy responds differently to these medications than vessel pathology, they are useful in distinguishing the normal anatomy from pathology.

When introducing any type of foreign substance, such as contrast medium, into the body, there is a risk that the body will react to the material. The reaction may result in minor (non–life-threatening) complications or, in the worst case, may result in death. Reaction rates tend to be very low. The most common type of reaction is minor and occurs in approximately 5 percent of patients. Severe (life-threatening) reactions tend to occur at a rate of 0.1 percent. Thus, in the vast majority of patients, contrast media increase radiographic quality, providing a more accurate diagnosis, which outweighs the risk of possible reaction. However, the use of contrast media must be determined by individual assessment of the patient.

This chapter presents the basic characteristics of contrast media, their physiologic effects on various organs, and their pharmacoangiography. Also included is a brief discussion of emergency treatment in the event of a contrast medium reaction. Discussion of the specific uses and quantities of contrast media is presented in the appropriate procedural chapter.

## METHODS OF INTRODUCING CONTRAST MEDIA

There are several ways to introduce a contrast medium into the body. The four most common methods employed are:
1. ingestion
2. retrograde administration
3. intrathecal administration
4. parenteral administration

Ingestion involves drinking the contrast medium, for example, barium. The retrograde method pertains to administration of the contrast medium against the normal body flow. A common example of the retrograde method is cystography, in which the contrast agent is instilled through an external catheter into the urinary bladder via the urethra and against the normal direction of movement of urine. Intrathecal administration involves introducing the medium into a sheath. Myelography is an example. Parenteral administration of contrast medium involves injecting the agent into the bloodstream. The type of injection most commonly used in imaging an organ or an organ system is intravenous or intra-arterial.

The method of contrast medium introduction varies from procedure to procedure. It is also possible for there to be more than one method of introduction for a procedure; for example, a contrast medium for cholecystography may be administered orally or intravenously. The actual method(s) of administration of a contrast medium for specific examinations is covered in detail in the procedural chapters.

## CONTRAST MEDIA CLASSIFICATION

Contrast media may be classified as positive or negative. Positive media are radiopaque (i.e., they absorb x rays). Negative media are radiolucent (i.e., they are easily penetrated by x rays). Examples of positive media are barium sulfate and water-soluble iodines. Radiolucent media are gases, such as air or oxygen.

Radiopaque media appear light or white on a radiograph, whereas radiolucent media appear dark or black. The decision to use a radiopaque medium instead of radiolucent medium depends on the organ and the type of pathology. For example, if the area of interest is the interior part of a vessel, a radiopaque medium is the agent of choice, for example, to demonstrate an obstruction.

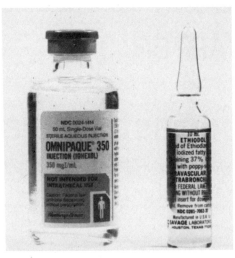

**Figure 3–1.** Water-soluble or organic-salt contrast media (left) and oil-based contrast media (right).

Radiopaque media are distributed in a variety of forms. These include water-soluble or organic salts, pills (Oragrafin), suspensions (barium sulfate), and oil-based (fat-soluble) contrast agents (Fig. 3–1). Water-soluble media can be used for intravenous or intra-arterial injections, whereas oil-based contrast agents are not injected into the bloodstream but are used to fill hollow organs. Examples of water-soluble media are diatrizoate meglumine (Hypaque), diatrizoate sodium and meglumine (Renografin), and iothalamate sodium (Conray). The most common oil-based contrast agents are propyliodone (Dionosil), ethiodized oil (Ethiodol), and iodized oil (Lipiodol). Water-soluble agents may be ionic or nonionic in composition. The primary difference between the ionic and nonionic solutions rests with the physiologic interaction within the body. Current research indicates there is a significant decrease in the number and intensity of patient reactions when nonionic agents are employed. This decrease is attributed to the low osmolality of the nonionic agent.

Nonionic solutions are more complex to produce than ionic solutions; therefore, the cost for a nonionic agent is substantially higher than for an ionic agent. This cost may be 10 to 20 times higher than ionic agents. Steinberg and coworkers suggest that the annual cost to use only nonionic media in the United States would increase from $40 million to between $400 and $800 million. In these times of cost-effectiveness and accountability, the price for nonionic media becomes a major factor in the decision of when to use nonionic media.

## CHEMICAL PROPERTIES OF RADIOPAQUE CONTRAST MEDIA

Modern contrast media are triiodinated compounds based on the benzoic acid ring structure. The three iodine atoms represent the opacifying portion of the structure and are located on carbon numbers 2, 4, and

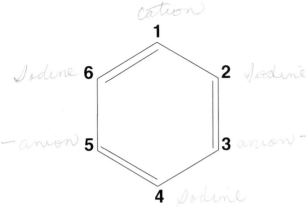

**Figure 3-2.** Benzyl ring.

6 of the ring (Fig. 3-2). Iodine is used because of its high atomic number, thus providing a high absorption of radiation. The anions (negatively charged ions) are located in the number 3 and 5 positions (Fig. 3-2). The three primary anions employed are diatrizoate, iothalamate, and metrizoate. The anions are responsible for stabilizing and detoxifying the contrast medium. The cation (positively charged ion), carboxyl group, or salt is located at carbon position number 1 (Fig. 3-2). The salts most commonly used are derivatives of sodium, calcium, magnesium, and meglumine. The cations are responsible for increasing the solubility of the medium.

Low osmolality ionic contrast media link two benzoic acid rings together. This process also alters one of the carboxyl groups to a nonionizing amide. The result is six iodine atoms, four anions, and one cation.

Nonionic contrast media (iopromide, iohexol, iopamidol, ioversol, iodixonol, and ioxilan) differ in composition from the ionic media by the substitution of one or more of the noniodine portions of the benzoic ring with a nonionizing side chain. This reduces the osmolality (see "Osmolality or Hypertonicity of Radiopaque Contrast Media" section of this chapter) of the medium, which decreases the rate and severity of reactions.

## CONTRAST MEDIA NOMENCLATURE

Contrast media tend to be labeled by either their generic name or their product name. The generic name is the class or type of chemical compound for the medium. It is derived from the cation and anion. The preferred order of the generic name is anion-cation, for example, diatrizoate sodium. However, it is also possible to transpose the terms so that they are arranged cation-anion, for example, sodium diatrizoate. The product name is the trade name given to the contrast medium by the manufacturer. The name refers to a specific product and is easier to remember than the generic name. Product names usually have suffixes or prefixes that correspond to the anatomic area in which they may be employed. For example, *Cardio*grafin is used for studies of the heart. Product names may also have a number after the name, which may refer to the

percentage of concentration or to the milligrams of iodine per milliliter. A list of various contrast media and their generic names can be found in Table 3-1.

Care should be taken when selecting and using contrast media because of similarities in both product names and visual appearance. A nonchalant attitude when selecting contrast media increases the possibility of selecting the incorrect medium, which may result in improper use and an increase in the probability of a reaction. Name modifications, commonly found when the same agent is used in different countries, may also contribute to the potential to select the wrong contrast medium. The standards for a contrast medium vary from one nation to the next, and although attempts have been made to standardize the nomenclature for generic names, differences in spelling do occur. For example, some terms in the United States use the letters "ph," while the World Health Organization uses "f." Another common difference in spelling is the shortening of terms, for example, methylglucamine to meglumine. Last, problems may occur when the same product is known under a certain name in one country and labeled under a different name in another country.

## CONCENTRATION

Concentration of a medium represents the amount of salt in the solution. The concentration level can be found on the label of the medium. Contrast media often have a number following the name to represent the concentration of the medium. The number may define the concentration in several ways.

One method indicates the percentage of salt(s) in the solution. For example, Hypaque 60 percent may be read as a 60 percent concentration of meglumine in the solution.

Concentration may also be expressed by the weight, usually in grams, of the salt per 100 milliliters (ml) of solvent (liquid). This method is better known as weight (W) per volume (V) or W/V. Again using the Hypaque 60 percent example, the W/V indicates 60 grams of meglumine per 100 ml of solvent.

Suspensions, such as barium sulfate, often express concentration in terms of weight per weight (W/W) or specific gravity. The W/W indicates the weight of the medium compared with the weight of the solution. Because barium is not used in angiography, it is mentioned here only as a reference.

## AMOUNT OF IODINE IN RADIOPAQUE CONTRAST MEDIA

Iodine is selected as an opacifying agent because it has a high atomic number (protons) and a low toxicity, is easily excreted by the body, and forms stable compounds that do not break down or react in the body. The high atomic number of iodine (53) allows iodine to absorb five times the radiation as soft tissue and three times more radiation than bone. Thus, the amount of iodine in the medium determines the opacity of the medium. The higher the iodine content, the greater opac-

Table 3–1. **Some Common Generic and Product Names of Contrast Media**

| Generic Name | Product Name | Manufacturer |
|---|---|---|
| *Ionic Media* | | |
| Diatrizoate meglumine | Angiovist 282 | Berlex Laboratories |
| Diatrizoate meglumine | Hypaque, 60% | Sanofi-Winthrop |
| Diatrizoate meglumine | Reno-M-DIP | Bristol-Myers Squibb |
| Diatrizoate sodium (25%) and meglumine (50%) | Hypaque-M, 75% | Sanofi-Winthrop |
| Diatrizoate sodium (10%) and meglumine (66%) | Renografin-76 | Bristol-Myers Squibb |
| Iothalamate meglumine | Conray 43 | Mallinckrodt |
| Iothalamate sodium | Conray 400 | Mallinckrodt |
| Iothalamate sodium | Angio-Conray | Mallinckrodt |
| Iothalamate sodium (26%) and meglumine (52%) | Vascoray | Mallinckrodt |
| *Low Osmolality Ionic Media* | | |
| Ioxaglate meglumine and ioxaglate sodium | Hexabrix | Mallinckrodt |
| *Nonionic Media* | | |
| Metrizamide | Amipaque | Sanofi-Winthrop |
| Iopamidol 61.2% | Isovue 300 | Bristol-Myers Squibb |
| Iohexol | Omnipaque | Sanofi-Winthrop |

ity of the contrast medium. A medium having a high opacity results in a higher radiographic contrast on the film. The amount of iodine in the medium is stated on the label of the drug.

The quantity of iodine is stated as weight per volume (W/V) in grams per milliliter (g/ml) or milligrams per milliliter (mg/ml). For example, Conray 400 has 40 g/ml or 400 mg/ml of solvent. In general, in conventional radiography, the amount of iodine needed to produce an image is about 180 to 200 mg of iodine per milliliter (mg I/ml). For digital subtraction angiography (DSA), the amount is 15 to 65 mg I/ml, and for computed tomography (CT), it is 3 to 5 mg I/ml. Thus, a high iodine content in the contrast medium plays a more important role in conventional radiography than in DSA or CT.

## VISCOSITY OF RADIOPAQUE CONTRAST MEDIA

Viscosity is the resistance of a fluid to movement and is measured by the amount of force required to move the liquid under specific conditions. One standard used is the force needed to move water at 20°C or at 68°F and is measured in centipoise (cP). For example, the viscosity of Conray 400 at 25°C is 7.9. Therefore, to move Conray 400 at 25°C the same distance as water at 20°C would require a force 7.9 times greater than the force to move water.

Viscosity is inversely proportional to temperature; that is, as temperature increases, viscosity decreases. Thus, warming contrast medium makes the medium less viscous and easier to inject. This is important in bolus injections into small lumen catheters that may need to be administered rapidly.

Viscosity may also be expressed relative to density. This is called kinematic viscosity. Kinematic viscosity (expressed in centistokes [cSt]) is calculated by dividing the absolute viscosity (in centipoise) by the density. The following represents the kinematic viscosity formula:

$$\text{Kinematic viscosity} = \frac{\text{absolute viscosity}}{\text{fluid density}}$$

Based on the kinematic viscosity formula, if two contrast media have comparable excretory properties, toxicity, and absolute viscosity, then the contrast agent with the lower kinematic viscosity is preferred. This is because the lower kinematic viscosity has more density per volume, resulting in higher radiographic contrast. The following table is an example of two similar contrast agents and their respective density:

| | Absolute Viscosity | Kinematic Viscosity | Fluid Density |
|---|---|---|---|
| Contrast A | 10 | 5 | x |
| Contrast B | 10 | 2 | x |

Using the kinematic viscosity formula above, the calculations for the fluid density for both media are

| Contrast A | Contrast B |
|---|---|
| 5 = 10/x | 2 = 10/x |
| 5x = 10 | 2x = 10 |
| x = 2 | x = 5 |

Thus, contrast B is more desirable because it has a higher density, resulting in a higher radiographic contrast.

## OSMOLALITY OR HYPERTONICITY OF RADIOPAQUE CONTRAST MEDIA

The osmolality or hypertonicity of the contrast medium represents the number of dissolved ions (anions and cations) in a liter (1 liter = 1000 ml) of solution. This is expressed as the number of milliosmoles per kilogram (mOsm/kg) of water. Contrast media may have hundreds of anions and cations per milliliter; hence, contrast media are considered to have high hypertonicity. The osmolality of ionic contrast agents ranges from 1000 to 2400 mOsm/kg. The average osmolality of nonionic media is 750 mOsm/kg. Both types of media are well above the human osmolality of about 300 mOsm/kg. Because the osmolality of contrast media is higher than the body, it can penetrate blood cells.

Osmolality has been identified by researchers as a primary factor in causing adverse contrast media reactions. It is also thought to be the main cause of pain and heat sensation during injection. The ratio between the number of iodine atoms and the number of particles in solution, that is, cations and anions, can be calculated and is useful in determining the probability of reaction.

Recall that the conventional ionic medium (ionic monomer) contains 3 iodine particles, cations (carboxyl group), and an anion. In solution, the medium disassociates into one cation, one anion, and three iodine particles. Thus, the ratio of iodine atoms and number of particles in solution is 3:2 for a numeric value of 1.5 (3/2 = 1.5). A low osmolality ionic (monacidic dimer) solution links two triiodinated benzoic rings at the cations and changes one of the carboxyl groups to a non-disassociating group (e.g., amide). This results in six iodine particles to two particles in solution for a 6:2 ratio and a numeric value of three. A nonionic medium contains three iodine particles and one ionizing particle. Consequently, the iodine to particle relationship is 3:1 for a numeric value of three. A higher numeric value, usually three or higher, is preferred because the reaction rate and intensity are decreased. Therefore, it is recommended that contrast media with low osmolality be employed. The disadvantage of a low osmolality ionic medium of three is that it tends to have a substantially higher molecular weight and viscosity than most nonionic media.

## EFFECT OF CONTRAST MEDIA ON ORGANS

When introducing a contrast medium into a patient, there is a risk that the patient will have an adverse reaction to the contrast agent. Reactions may be chemotoxic or idiosyncratic. Chemotoxic reactions relate to the various hemodynamic changes that may occur on injection. These are often caused by the properties of the medium, the amount of medium injected, or the speed of the injection. Reactions other than hemodynamic changes are termed idiosyncratic. These reactions may or may not be caused by the medium's

properties, speed of injection, or amount of medium injected. Reactions tend to occur most often to patients between the ages of 20 and 40 years. The incidence of reactions varies with the type of procedure. The incidence is greatest for intravenous pyelography and intravenous cholangiography.

Unfortunately, there are no signs or symptoms that enable a physician to determine which patients will or will not have an adverse reaction. However, research by Written does suggest that certain groups are at a higher risk of having a reaction than others. These groups include patients with asthma, hay fever, urticaria of unknown cause, food allergy, iodine sensitivity, or history of previous reaction to contrast medium. Of these groups, individuals with a history to iodine sensitivity and a previous reaction to contrast medium are three times more apt to have a reaction than the other groups.

Although it is known that contrast media are responsible for causing adverse side effects and sometimes death, the actual reason for these reactions is still unknown. There have been many studies performed to determine what is present in a contrast medium that may cause adverse reactions. The result of these investigations has been to identify many factors about the medium and the methods of injection that increase the possibility of reaction. However, no single factor has been identified as a sole cause of adverse side reactions in patients. The contrast agent factors that relate to reactions include toxicity, iodine content, number of impurities, osmolality, volume, speed of injection, and concentration. An increase in any one of these factors increases the possibility and severity of complications.

Contrast media may cause physiologic changes in some organs of the body. The method and site of contrast medium administration and the type of contrast agent employed determine the organ affected. Organs most proximal to the injection site have the greatest reaction rate. Most commonly affected are the neurologic, respiratory, cardiovascular, gastrointestinal, urinary, and cutaneous systems (Table 3–2).

Reactions of the neurologic system include headache, aphasia, unconsciousness, and, in rare instances, hemiplegia, coma, or convulsions. The severity of the reaction is directly related to the concentration of the contrast agent. As the concentration increases, the severity increases.

Common respiratory physiologic responses include coughing, difficulty in breathing, an increase or decrease in respiration rate, and, the most severe, respiratory arrest. Some respiratory reactions may be related to the central nervous system. For example, injection of contrast medium into the carotid artery has been known to cause respiratory paralysis.

Most cardiac responses occur after injection of a contrast medium into the cerebral or coronary arteries. These responses include depressed ST wave segment, lowering or inversion of the T wave, premature ventricular beats, and sinus arrhythmias. If the blood vessels are affected, most often blood pressure is, too. A slow decrease in blood pressure with a gradual return to normal is associated with a slow injection of a large

Table 3–2. **Effects of Contrast Media on Organs**

| Organ/System | Effect |
| --- | --- |
| Neurologic | Headache |
| | Aphasia |
| | Unconsciousness |
| | Hemiplegia |
| | Coma |
| | Convulsion |
| Respiratory | Coughing |
| | Difficulty in breathing |
| | Increase in respiratory rate |
| | Decrease in respiratory rate |
| | Respiratory arrest |
| Cardiovascular | Depressed ST wave segment |
| | Lowering of T wave |
| | Inversion of T wave |
| | Premature ventricular beats |
| | Sinus arrhythmias |
| | Vasodilation (with slow injection) |
| | Systemic hypotension (with slow injection) |
| | Sudden drop in blood pressure with slow return to normal (with rapid injection) |
| Gastrointestinal | Nausea |
| | Vomiting |
| | Metallic taste in the mouth |
| Kidney | Temporary increase in renal blood flow followed by a decrease in blood flow |
| | Hematuria |
| | Lower nephron nephrosis |
| | Flank pain |
| | Renal failure |
| Cutaneous | Flushed feeling |
| | Sweating |
| | Urticaria |

dose of contrast medium. Slow injections also may produce vasodilation and some systemic hypotension. Rapid injections result in a sudden drop in blood pressure with a slow return to normal.

The majority of reactions associated with the gastrointestinal system are minor. Common responses are nausea, vomiting, and a metallic taste in the mouth. The responses are transient and pass quickly.

Injection of contrast medium into the kidney area causes an initial temporary increase in renal blood flow. This is followed by a decrease in flow, resulting from vasoconstriction that persists for about 15 minutes. Research studies suggest that contrast agents containing iothalamate are more nephrotoxic than agents containing diatrizoate. Other responses of the kidneys include hematuria, lower nephron nephrosis, flank pain, and renal failure.

Cutaneous reactions are usually classified as minor. The most common responses are flushed feeling, sweating, and urticaria (hives). Often these reactions require no treatment other than reassurance and observation of the patient.

## PRECAUTIONS AND PREVENTIVE TECHNIQUES WHEN USING CONTRAST MEDIA

Although it is extremely difficult to predict whether or not a patient is going to have a reaction to the con-

trast medium, there are several steps that should be taken when using any contrast agent to avoid or prepare for a reaction. These steps include obtaining a thorough patient history, possible premedication of the patient, selection of the correct contrast agent, and ensuring availability of emergency equipment.

Research indicates that certain individuals are in a high risk group for reactions to contrast media based on their allergic history. Thus, the most important step for determining the possibility of a reaction is obtaining a history of the patient. When collecting information about the patient's medical history, the following questions should be asked:

1. Do you have asthma?
2. Do you get hay fever?
3. Have you ever broken out in hives? If so, what happened to cause the hives?
4. What, if any, foods are you allergic to?
5. What, if any, type of allergy might you have?
6. Have you ever had this type of x-ray procedure before? If so, what, if any, physical responses do you remember having during the examination?

The manner in which a question is asked affects the answer received. Of primary importance is to design the questions so that they are asked in a layperson's terms. For example, asking a patient if he or she has ever experienced urticaria may only confuse the patient because most people do not know medical terminology. Thus, the response may be less than accurate. However, most people are familiar with the lay word for urticaria — hives. Also, note the phrasing of the second part of question number 6. The question asks, ". . . what, if any, physical responses do you remember having . . .". The question does not ask, "Did you have nausea, vomiting, or hives." The latter question suggests to the patient that he or she will or should expect to have nausea, vomiting, or hives. The former question requires the patient to think back to the previous examination and relate his or her experiences. The decision to ask more direct questions regarding physical response should be based on the patient's response to the standard questions. In addition to asking the patient questions, it is important to review an in-patient's medical chart for information that may place the patient in a high risk category. This would include checking the chart to determine the following: allergies, proper hydration of patient, creatinine level, blood urea nitrogen (BUN), and cardiac status. This information is obtained by reviewing the nurse's or doctor's notes and the laboratory reports.

After the history is taken, any information that indicates increased risk should be reported to the radiologist. There are at least four preventive measures that can be taken for high risk patients:

1. Have the patient undergo a noncontrast diagnostic procedure.
2. Use a nonionic contrast medium.
3. Dispense premedication.
4. Hydrate patients with renal insufficiency.

Sometimes, alternate procedures can be performed that avoid the need to use a contrast agent. These procedures may not produce identical results, but they may provide adequate information. The physician should determine if substitute examinations need to be considered. Nonionic contrast agents have a substantially lower rate of reaction. If a nonionic medium is available, the physician should evaluate the possibility of replacing an ionic medium with a nonionic agent. Steroids and antihistamines have been successfully used as a premedication to reduce the rate and intensity of contrast media reaction. A common premedication regimen might include an intramuscular injection or oral administration of 50 mg of diphenhydramine (Benadryl) 1 hour prior to the examination and three 50-mg intravenous injections of prednisone at 13, 7, and 1 hour prior to contrast medium injection. Another preventive treatment is to administer 32 mg of methylprednisolone (Medrol) orally 12 and 2 hours prior to injecting contrast medium. Patients with renal insufficiency should not be dehydrated. Also, hydrating the patient (e.g., with 50 g mannitol in 180 ml of 5 percent dextrose) during and after the examination helps reduce the possibility of renal failure.

If the decision is to proceed with the examination, then the next step is to select the proper contrast agent. Protocol for contrast media is the responsibility of the radiologist. However, selecting and preparing the medium, for example, drawing up the contrast medium, is usually the task of the technologist. When preparing the medium, it is recommended that the label be checked three times prior to administration to the patient. The first check is performed when removing the medium from the package, a second check occurs when preparing the medium for injection, and the last check is to read the label again just prior to administering the medium. The control number of the medium should be recorded, and the contrast agent container should not be disposed of until the examination is completed. One reason for recording the control number is to determine whether there are any common factors among reactions occurring within the department, for example, whether patients are having reactions to contrast medium having the same control number. Also, control numbers are useful when collecting media that are recalled.

Prior to administering a contrast medium, the technologist should check to ensure that emergency equipment is readily available. This includes checking that syringes, needles, tourniquets, alcohol preps, and the drugs most often used for treating moderate reactions are in the room where the examination is being performed. Also, the department crash cart used for major reactions should be within acceptable proximity to the room. All drugs for both moderate and severe reactions should be checked on a regular basis to ensure that they are stocked and that the expiration date has not lapsed. It is also important to test equipment, such as the electrocardiograph, periodically to ensure that they are in working order. Accessory equipment, such as syringes, needles, and alcohol preps, should be checked to make sure that they are sterile and that there is a sufficient quantity readily available.

Most severe reactions occur within the first 5 minutes of administration. Ninety-five percent of all reactions occur within the first 20 minutes. However, reactions have occurred as long as an hour after administration.

Therefore, it is important that a physician be available until the examination is completed.

There is much controversy over whether or not a sensitivity test dose of the contrast medium should be administered to the patient prior to administration of a contrast agent. Test doses may be administered intradermally, subcutaneously, sublingually, conjunctivally, or intravenously. These types of test doses are usually associated with the parenteral drugs. Currently, there is no evidence to support the practical value of sensitivity testing. A small test dose has been known to cause severe reactions; at other times, it has produced no reaction, yet when additional contrast agent is injected, a reaction occurs. Thus, whether or not to use sensitivity tests is determined by the individual physician or institution.

## PHARMACOANGIOGRAPHY

As mentioned previously, vasoconstrictors and vasodilators are useful in the diagnosis and treatment of disease. Vasoconstrictors are commonly used to distinguish between normal and abnormal vasculatures and to treat bleeding. Epinephrine, angiotensin, and vasopressin are common vasoconstrictors used in angiography. Vasodilators are employed to differentiate between organic and functional vascular changes, alleviate vasospasm, treat nonobstructive intestinal ischemia, stimulate bleeding for diagnosis, and improve image quality of peripheral and venous vessels. Common vasodilators employed in angiography are papaverine, tolazoline, acetylcholine, and glucagon. Table 3–3 summarizes the characteristics of vasoconstrictors and vasodilators.

## CONTRAST MEDIA AND PHARMACOANGIOGRAPHY INCOMPATIBILITY

Sometimes contrast medium is injected through an intravenous tube that is also used to administer other medications. It is possible that the contrast medium may have a chemical reaction to other medications. There are thousands of drugs available on the U.S. market. To assess all drugs relative to their compatibility to the various contrast media is an impossible task. However, there have been several research studies that compare the compatibility of medications commonly employed in imaging with popular contrast agents. The results indicate that some contrast agents are incompatible with select drugs.

Among the research studies conducted is that of Mancini and McGillem, who compared the results of mixing Renografin-76 or Omnipaque (300 mg/ml and 350 mg/ml) with the popular vasodilator papaverine hydrochloride (HCl). Pilla and coworkers mixed Renografin-76, Amipaque, Hexabrix, and Conray 60 with papaverine HCl. Shah and Gerlock mixed Hexabrix with a variety of medications. Irving and Burbridge performed a study that compared six different contrast

Table 3–3. **Characteristics of Vasoconstrictors and Vasodilators**

| Type of Agent | Effect | Application | Dose | Contraindication | Side Effects |
|---|---|---|---|---|---|
| *Vasoconstrictors* | | | | | |
| Epinephrine | Constricts vessels. Constriction varies with vessel area. Generally, diseased arteries do not constrict or constrict to lesser degree than normal vessels. | Used to evaluate kidney, liver, or pancreas. Demonstrate abnormal veins. Adrenal arteriography. | 3–8 $\mu$g | Shock, narrow-angle glaucoma | Headache, anxiety, restlessness, tremor, palpitations |
| Angiotensin | Constricts normal vessels. Abnormal vessels are unaffected. | Used to evaluate hypovascularity of liver, kidney, and extremity neoplasms. | 0.5–10 $\mu$g | None | Flank pain |
| Vasopressin | Decreases blood flow in splenic, gastric, mesenteric arteries. | Gastrointestinal bleeding, vascular redistribution for angiography of the pancreas. | 0.2–1 unit | Angina | Abdominal cramps, nausea, hyperperistalsis of intestines |
| *Vasodilators* | | | | | |
| Papaverine | Operates as smooth muscle relaxant. | Vasodilator of peripheral vascular diseases for vasospastic disorders, nonocclusive mesenteric ischemia. | 20–30 mg bolus | Low cardiac output | Decreased A-V node, intraventricular condition, arrhythmias, tachycardia, drowsiness |
| Acetylcholine | Dilates renal arteries. | Used to evaluate small intrarenal vasculature and tumors; to differentiate between fixed anatomic changes and vasospasm of intrarenal branches. | 30–100 mg/min | Cholinesterase deficiency, bronchial asthma, hyperthyroidism | Decreased blood pressure |
| Tolazoline | Dilates vessels of heart. | Used to assess hemodynamic significance of arterial stenosis, evaluate bone and soft tissue tumors, evaluate hypovascularity of kidney, peripheral vessel angiography. | 25 mg | Coronary arterial disease, arrhythmias, gastritis, peptic ulcer, GI bleeding | Arrythmias, angina |
| Glucagon | Relaxes duodenum; functions as vasodilator. | Vasodilation of splenic and renal arteries, prevent DSA artifacts, stimulate for pancreatic angiography. | 0.5–1 mg | Pheochromocytoma, hyperglycemia | Nausea, vomiting, hyperperistalsis |

media with 12 different medications. All these studies produced similar results (see below).

Pilla and coworkers demonstrated that Hexabrix and papaverine HCl developed a white, amorphous precipitation. Renografin-76 demonstrated a white suspension that disappeared. Conray 60 and Amipaque were able to be mixed, respectively, with papaverine HCl without forming a suspension or precipitating. Mancini and McGillem's study, which was performed after they read Pilla and coworkers' results, showed that with a 6.8 pH, papaverine HCl and Renografin-76 developed a white suspension and did develop a precipitation after 12 hours. Both Omnipaque concentrations showed no response when each was mixed individually with papaverine HCl. Pilla and coworkers attribute the difference in Mancini and McGillem's results to the higher pH value used by Mancini and McGillem.

Shah and Gerlock mixed Hexabrix with saline, epinephrine (1 : 1000), vasopressin, tolazoline, nitroglycerin, lidocaine, heparin (1000 units), Benadryl, and Tagamet, respectively. The results demonstrated that Hexabrix and saline developed a suspension that cleared rapidly. When Hexabrix was mixed with either tolazoline or heparin, the solution resulted in an oil that cleared. Benadryl mixed with Hexabrix resulted in a dense, cloudy precipitation. Tagamet and Hexabrix caused a threadlike precipitation. There was no reaction when Hexabrix was mixed with epinephrine (1 : 1000), vasopressin, nitroglycerin, or lidocaine.

Irving and Burbridge mixed Hexabrix, Hypaque 60, MD 60, Omnipaque, Isovue, and Conray 60 with adrenalin, Benadryl, heparin, protamine, papaverine HCl, ampicillin, Ilotycin, Garamycin, Chloromycetin, Tagamet, Solu-Cortef, and Solu-Medrol. Each medication was put in a test tube and mixed separately with each contrast medium. Of the combinations tested, Hexabrix was found to form a precipitation that lasted at least 2 hours when mixed separately with Benadryl, papaverine HCl, protamine, and Tagamet. Garamycin and Hexabrix formed a transient precipitation that cleared in less than 5 minutes. Hypaque 60 and Benadryl demonstrated both an immediate precipitation, which cleared, and a 1-hour delayed precipitation that persisted. Papaverine HCl and Hypaque 60 showed a transient precipitation. Protamine and Hypaque 60 showed a precipitation for 2 hours. MD 60 mixed with Benadryl and papaverine HCl demonstrated an immediate transient precipitation that lasted for 5 minutes and a delayed persistent precipitation (1 hour for Benadryl and 2 hours for papaverine HCl). There was a persistent precipitation when MD 60 was mixed with protamine. All other contrast media and medication mixtures had no visible effect.

These research studies support the concept of flushing catheters and infusion tubes with saline between injections of contrast medium and medications. Using contrast medium to flush papaverine HCl should be avoided. Administering Benadryl through a tube that contains contrast medium should be avoided.

## EMERGENCY TREATMENT OF CONTRAST MEDIA REACTIONS

Reactions to contrast media are identified according to the severity of the reaction. The three classifications are minor, moderate or intermediate, and severe. Most reactions are minor. Minor reactions are transient and require no treatment other than reassuring the patient. An example of a minor reaction is a metallic taste in the mouth. Moderate or intermediate reactions require some form of treatment for patient comfort and to prevent escalation to a severe reaction; however, generally, moderate reactions are not life threatening. Urti-

**Table 3 – 4. Some Common Types of Contrast Media Reactions**

| Minor | Moderate | Severe |
|---|---|---|
| Nausea | Urticaria (hives) | Convulsions |
| Vomiting | Asthma attack (minor) | Cyanosis |
| Flushing | Erythema | Pulmonary edema |
| Metallic taste | Rhinitis | Shock |
| Coughing (minor) | Facial edema | Cardiac arrest |
| Sweating | | Renal failure |
| Feeling of warmth | | Laryngospasm |
| | | Respiratory arrest |

caria is an example of a moderate reaction. Severe reactions are life threatening and require immediate treatment. An example of a severe reaction is cardiac arrest. Table 3 – 4 lists examples of various types of reactions for each classification.

The following discussion provides suggested treatments for moderate and severe reactions. It should be noted that new drugs are continually being developed. Thus, it is possible that some of the drugs listed are no longer used or new drugs are being substituted. Most moderate reactions in adults are satisfactorily treated with an intramuscular injection of 0.3 ml (1 : 1000) of epinephrine or a 50-mg injection of diphenhydramine hydrochloride (Benadryl).

Severe reactions usually affect the respiratory, neurologic, cardiovascular, or urinary systems. Regardless of the organ(s) affected, it is mandatory to administer 100 percent oxygen, record the blood pressure and pulse, and start an intravenous infusion of normal saline or 5 percent dextrose in water. The specific treatment depends on the type of reaction and may vary from one institution to another or from one physician to another.

There are a variety of respiratory reactions that may occur with contrast media. Minor reactions require the technologist to observe and reassure the patient. More severe reactions require some form of treatment. Epinephrine (1 : 1000), 0.3 to 0.5 ml subcutaneously, is used for bronchospasm. Other drugs that may be employed are 25 to 50 mg intravenously or intramuscularly of diphenhydramine hydrochloride and 100 to 300 mg intravenously of hydrocortisone. An intravenous drip should be started to keep a vein open. Severe laryngospasm results in airway obstruction caused by adduction of the vocal cords. To relieve the obstruction, 10 to 30 mg of succinylcholine chloride (Anectine) is injected intravenously or into the tongue. If adequate ventilation cannot be maintained, a tracheotomy should be performed. Severe asthmatic attack is usually treated by administering 0.5 to 1.0 ml of 1 : 1000 epinephrine subcutaneously. Other drugs that may be employed include a slow intravenous injection of 250 mg of aminophylline in 5 percent dextrose in water over 10 to 20 minutes. Respiratory arrest is the most severe respiratory reaction because a lack of oxygen to the brain for more than 4 minutes may cause permanent brain damage and cardiac arrest. The treatment for respiratory arrest is administration of 100 percent oxygen by intubation and forced ventilation.

The most common severe reaction in the neurologic system is convulsion. The best treatment is an initial intravenous injection of 25 to 50 mg of sodium thiopental (Pentothal). Small doses of the drug may be administered at intervals until the convulsions have stopped.

Cardiovascular reactions often appear in the form of vagal reactions (hypotension and sinus bradycardia) or anaphylactoid shock. The primary treatment for vagal reactions is injection of atropine, 0.75 to 2.0 mg intravenously. Anaphylactoid shock is often experienced with tachycardia. The most important treatment for shock is maintaining adequate ventilation and blood pressure. To maintain adequate ventilation, the patient is intubated and oxygen is administered. Drug therapy is the best treatment for maintaining blood pressure. The drugs include 25 mg of epinephrine administered intravenously (1 : 10,000) or subcutaneously (1 : 1000) and an infusion containing 100 mg of metaraminol (Aramine) per 500 ml of saline solution. Congestive heart failure has a variety of treatments. Some therapeutic drugs include meperidine hydrochloride (Demerol), morphine, and lanatoside C (Cedilanid). An electrocardiogram should be used to monitor the heart for other cardiac problems. The appropriate treatment should be administered for any additional cardiac problems. Arrhythmias are usually treated as a "wait-and-see" situation. If ventricular tachycardia or atrial flutter occurs, an intravenous injection of quinidine should be administered. Ventricular fibrillation requires the use of a defibrillator.

The most severe cardiovascular reaction is cardiac arrest. The initial treatment is administration of basic life support (cardiopulmonary resuscitation [CPR]) techniques. A discussion of CPR is beyond the scope of this text. However, it is recommended that all technologists become CPR-certified and maintain CPR certification. If CPR fails, then advanced life support techniques (e.g., defibrillation) are required and are usually performed by an emergency cardiac team.

Renal reactions may be life threatening. Most severe reactions result in renal failure and should be treated according to the pathology indicated. Examples of treatment for the most severe renal reactions include dialysis and kidney transplant.

All severe reactions require prompt and accurate response for patient survival; thus, a crash cart should be readily available. The contents of the cart will vary from institution to institution. Technologists should familiarize themselves with the contents of their department's emergency cart.

Each individual in the imaging department should be assigned a specific task to perform if a major reaction occurs. An example would be for a given individual to draw up the appropriate drug and record the injection time. This facilitates the speed and accuracy of the treatment. All individuals should be familiar with other technologists' tasks. This is especially useful when a technologist is absent and another technologist must perform the absent individual's tasks. Larger facilities usually have a cardiac team that is made up of personnel from various specialty areas, such as a respiratory therapist, nurse, and so on. Where the institution has a cardiac team, the radiology personnel should be familiar with the emergency codes. In the event of a cardiac emergency, radiology personnel should attempt to sustain the patient until the cardiac team arrives and to work in conjunction with that team according to the interdepartmental policies.

## REVIEW QUESTIONS

1. The major characteristic of a contrast medium that makes it effective is its ability to _____ of an organ in relation to surrounding tissues.
   A. alter the density
   B. decrease the function
   C. change the volume
   D. increase the molecular structure

2. In angiography, vasoconstrictors are useful in distinguishing the _____ from pathology.
   A. density of an organ
   B. normal anatomy
   C. origin of the disease
   D. type of tissue composition

3. List at least four common methods used for administering contrast medium.

4. There is a significant decrease in the number and intensity of patient reactions when _____ contrast agents are used.
   A. ionic
   B. oil-based
   C. nonionic
   D. suspension

5. Iodine is used in radiopaque contrast medium because of its _____.
   A. high atomic number
   B. radiolucent characteristics
   C. solubility
   D. toxifying feature

6. Nonionic contrast medium substitutes one or more of the _____ portion(s) of the benzoic ring with a nonionizing side chain.
   A. opacifying
   B. iodine
   C. position 2
   D. noniodine

7. _____ of a medium represents the amount of salt in the solution.
   A. Osmolality
   B. Concentration
   C. Viscosity
   D. Hypertonicity

8. The amount of _____ in the contrast medium determines the opacity of the medium.
   A. salt
   B. anions
   C. iodine
   D. cation

9. The amount of iodine needed to produce an image in conventional radiography is about _____ mg I/ml.
   A. 140 to 160
   B. 160 to 180
   C. 180 to 200
   D. 200 to 220

10. _____ is the number of dissolved ions in a liter of solution.
    A. Osmolality
    B. Concentration
    C. Salt
    D. Cations

11. _____ contrast medium reactions refer to the various hemodynamic changes that may occur upon injection.
    A. Idiosyncratic
    B. Allergic
    C. Minor
    D. Chemotoxic

12. List at least three preventive measures that may be taken when injecting contrast medium into a high risk patient.

13. Ninety-five percent of all contrast medium reactions occur in the first _____ minutes.
    A. 5
    B. 10
    C. 15
    D. 20

14. List three common vasoconstrictors.

15. Hexabrix and _____ result in precipitation.
    A. tolazoline
    B. papaverine HCl
    C. heparin
    D. epinephrine (1:1000)

16. A _____ reaction is life threatening.
    A. minor
    B. moderate
    C. intermediate
    D. severe

17. _____ is an example of a moderate contrast medium reaction.
    A. Metallic taste
    B. Laryngospasm
    C. Urticaria
    D. Convulsion

18. Severe contrast medium reactions require _____ be administered.
    A. 100 percent oxygen
    B. 0.3 ml (1:1000) epinephrine
    C. 50 mg Benadryl
    D. 100 mg diphenhydramine HCl

## BIBLIOGRAPHY

Abrams, HL: Angiography, Vol 1, ed 3. Little, Brown & Co, Boston, 1983.

Andrews, EJ, Jr: Severe adverse reactions to contrast media: A simplified means of recognition and treatment. South Med J 70(12):140, 1977.

Bettmann, MA: Clinical experience with Ioversol for angiography. Invest Radiol 24(Suppl 1): S61–S66, June 1989.

Bookstein, JJ and Lang, EV: Penile magnification pharmacoarteriography: Details of intrapenile arterial anatomy. AJR 148:883, May 1987.

Bragg, MNJ, Horwitz, TA, and Bester, L: Comparison of patient responses to high and low osmolality contrast agents injected intravenously. AJR 147(1):185, 1986.

Butler, HH: How to read an ECG. Medical Economics Company, Oradell, NJ, 1976.

Cho, KJ and Thornburg, JR: Severe reactions to contrast material by three consecutive routes: Intravenous, subcutaneous and interarterial. AJR 131(3):509, 1978.

Christensen, C: Contrast Media. Multimedia Publishing Corporation (audio tape and slide material), Denver, 1979.

Christensen, C: Reaction to contrast media. Multimedia Publishing Corporation (audio tape and slide material), Denver, 1979.

Cohan, RH and Dunnick, NR: Progress in radiology intravascular contrast media: Adverse reactions. AJR 149:665, October 1987.

Cohan, RH, Dunnick, NR, and Bashore, TM: Treatment of reactions to radiographic contrast material. AJR 151(2):263, August 1988.

Fisher, HW: Choices for intravascular contrast agents. Curr Probl Diagn Radiol 6(3):1, May–June, 1976.

Fisher, HW: Incompatibilities between contrast media and pharmacologic agents. Letter. Radiology 162(3):875, March 1987.

Fisher, HW, Spataro, RF, and Rosenberg, PM: Medical and economic considerations in using a new contrast medium. Arch Intern Med 146(9):1717–1721, September 1986.

Gluck, BS and Mitty, HA: Reactions to iodinated radiographic contrast agents: How to identify and manage patients at risk. Postgrad Med 88(5):187, October 1990.

Greenberger, PA and Patterson, R: The prevention of immediate generalized reactions to radiocontrast media in high-risk patients. J Allergy Clin Immunol 87(4):867–872, April 1991.

Henegham, M: Contrast-induced acute renal failure (editorial). AJR 131(6):1113, December 1978.

Ionic versus nonionic contrast use. Curr Probl Diagn Radiol 20(2):47, March–April 1991.

Irving, HD and Burbridge, BE: Incompatibility of contrast agents with intravascular medications: Work in progress. Radiology 173:91, October 1989.

Johnsrude, IS, Jackson, DC, and Dunnick, NR: Practical Approach to Angiography, ed 2. Little, Brown & Co, Boston, 1987.

Kadir, S: Diagnostic Angiography. WB Saunders, Philadelphia, 1986.

Katayama, H: The contrast media controversy: Implications of a landmark safety study. Admin Radiol 9(11):20, November 1990.

Kelly, JF, et al: Radiographic contrast media studies in high-risk patients. J Allergy Clin Immunol 62(3):181, September 1978.

Krumlowsky, FA, et al: Acute renal failure association with administration of radiographic contrast material. JAMA 239(2):125, January 1978.

Lasser, EC, et al: Pretreatment with corticosteroids to alleviate reactions to intravenous contrast material. N Engl J Med 317(14):845, October 1, 1987.

Levin, D: Nonionic agents: Okay, they're safer—but how much safer and at what cost to society? Admin Radiol 9(11):97, November 1990.

Mancini, GBJ and McGillem, MJ: Letter. AJR 147:1095, November 1986.

McGill, JE, et al: Letter. Radiology 166(2):577, February 1988.

McMahon, KA, Frewin, DB, and Lee, TI: Adverse reactions to radiographic contrast media. Australas Radiol 21(2):195, June 1977.

Miller, K: Advantages of a low-osmolality ionic contrast medium in intra-arterial applications. Radiol Technol 59(1):43, September–October 1987.

Miller, RE and Skucas, J: Radiographic Contrast Agents. University Park Press, Baltimore, 1977.

Ohnesorgen, EG and Yoshino, MT: Selective use of low osmolality contrast agents: Cost and benefits. Radiol Technol 59(6):499, July–August, 1988.

Parvez, Z, Moncada, R, and Sovak, M: Contrast media: Biologic effects and clinical application, Vols I, II, and III. CRC Press, Boca Raton, FL, 1987.

Physician's Desk Reference for Radiology and Nuclear Medicine. Medical Economics Company, Oradell, NJ, 1979–80.

Pilla, TJ, Beshany, SE, and Shields, JB: Incompatibility of Hexabrix and papaverine. AJR 146:1300, June 1986.

Saxton, HM and Strickland, B: Practical Procedures in Diagnostic Radiology. Grune & Stratton, New York, 1972.

Shah, SJ and Gerlock, AJ: Incompatibility of Hexabrix and papaverine in peripheral arteriography. Radiology 162(3):619, March 1987.

Shehadi, WH: Adverse reactions to intravascularly administered contrast media. Scientific exhibit presented at Radiologic Society of North America, Chicago, December 2–5, 1974.

Siegle, RL: Iodinated contrast material reactions: Treatment and prevention. Contemporary Diagn Radiol 9(16):1, 1986.

Skucas, J: Radiographic Contrast Agents, ed 2. Aspen, Rockville, MD, 1989.

Snopek, AM: Fundamentals of Special Radiographic Procedures. WB Saunders, Philadelphia, 1984.

Stafford, CT: Life-threatening allergic reactions, anticipating and preparing are the best defense. Postgrad Med 86(1):235, July 1989.

Steinberg, EP, et al: Use of low-osmolality contrast media in a price-sensitive environment. AJR 151(2):271, August 1988.

Swanson, DP, et al: Product selection criteria for intravascular ionic contrast media. Clin Pharmacy 4(5):527–538, September–October 1985.

von Kaenel, LH and Modic, M: 100% nonionics: Everything added up. Admin Radiol 9(11):100, November 1990.

White, RI: Fundamentals of Vascular Radiology. Lea & Febiger, Philadelphia, 1976.

Wolf, G: Nonionic agents: Okay, they're safer—now what? Admin Radiol 9(11):92, November 1990.

# PART TWO

# Advanced Contrast Media Procedures

# CHAPTER 4

# Knee Arthrography

*Patrick J. Apfel, MEd, ARRT(R)*

Arthrography is a radiographic study of synovial joints of the body. This procedure can be performed on the hip, elbow, ankle, shoulder, wrist, knee, and temporomandibular joints. Of all the joints in the body, the knee is most dependent upon its ligaments and cartilages for its integrity. This explains the high percentage of traumatic injury to these structures, and subsequent arthrography of the knee, as compared to other joints. Injury of the knee joint is often the result of sudden and forceful stress on this area such as occurs during athletic activities. When abnormal stress is applied to the knee, the supporting ligaments and cartilages may compensate by giving way to the stress, resulting in a tear.

Knee arthrography is a safe, reliable, and simple method of demonstrating various knee problems. Cartilages, ligaments, and the joint capsule are the major structures of interest in arthrography; therefore, a contrast medium is required to visualize and delineate these from other, surrounding soft tissues such as muscle.

Since most arthrography is performed on the knee, this chapter is dedicated to that area. It is important to note, however, that the basic technique of arthrography is similar for other joints examined by this procedure.

## ANATOMY

The knee is a hinge joint formed between the distal femur and proximal tibia. The fibula is not considered to be part of the knee joint proper since it articulates proximally with the tibia. In addition to bones, the joint area comprises cartilages, ligaments, and membranes. The knee joint is a synovial joint. This type of joint is diarthrodial (freely movable) and surrounded by a fibrous joint capsule, or bursa. The bursa is internally lined by a synovial membrane. Although the bursa is referred to in the singular, it is actually made up of several smaller bursae, which may or may not communicate with each other (Fig. 4–1*A*, *B*). The joint capsule is surrounded by, and sometimes continuous with, a variety of ligaments and lends support to the knee joint.

**31**

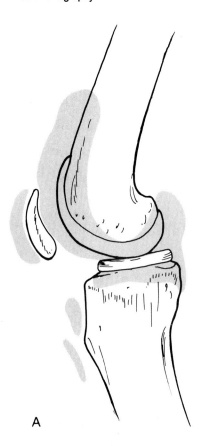

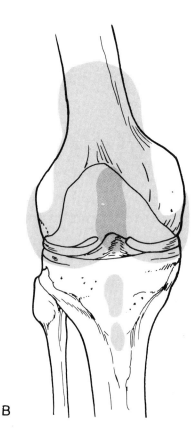

A

B

**Figure 4–1.** (A) Lateral view and (B) anterior view of knee joint bursae. (Adapted from Squibb X-ray Atlas 2: Knee arthrography, with permission.)

The synovial membrane produces synovial fluid, which provides lubrication and nutrition to articular cartilages and aids in cushioning the joint. Within the joint space, the bone ends are covered with a tough, slick hyaline cartilage. Between the bone end cartilages, but outside the joint capsule, lie two accessory cartilages, the lateral and medial menisci. The menisci are cup-shaped cartilages that rest on the tibial plateau and aid in providing a depression for the articular surfaces of the distal femur, thus strengthening the joint (Fig. 4–2). Menisci further provide for slight rotational movements of the joint and serve to absorb shock to the knee during stress. The menisci are similar in that they are both C-shaped with the outer border thicker than the inner border; however, they are not identical. The medial meniscus is almost a semicircle and is narrower anteriorly than it is posteriorly. It is fixed to the tibial intercondylar fossa both anteriorly and posteriorly and accommodates the articular surface of the medial condyle of the femur. The lateral meniscus is more circular, is more uniform in width, and covers a larger area of the tibial plateau than the medial meniscus. It is attached both anteriorly and posteriorly to the area of the intercondylar eminence of the tibia and accommodates the articular surface of the lateral condyle of the femur.

There are many ligaments that maintain the knee as a hinge joint. The major ligaments of interest in arthrography are the anterior and posterior cruciate ligaments and the lateral (fibular) and medial (tibial) collateral ligaments (Fig. 4–3).

The anterior and posterior ligaments are termed "cruciate" because they cross over each other, within the joint, in an X pattern. These ligaments aid in maintaining the anterior-posterior alignment of the femur and tibia. The anterior cruciate ligament is attached to the tibia, anterior to the tibial spine, where it is part of the anterior aspect of the lateral meniscus. The ligament extends posteriorly and laterally to a point where it is fixed to the posterior, medial surface of the lateral condyle of the femur. The posterior cruciate ligament is shorter and stronger than the anterior cruciate. It is fixed to the posterior intercondylar fossa of the tibia and the posterior aspect of the lateral meniscus and extends anteriorly and medially where it attaches to the anterior, medial surface of the medial condyle of the femur.

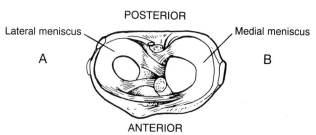

POSTERIOR

Lateral meniscus

Medial meniscus

A

B

ANTERIOR

**Figure 4–2.** Superior view of menisci: (A) Lateral meniscus; (B) medial meniscus. (Adapted from Squibb X-ray Atlas 2: Knee arthrography, with permission.)

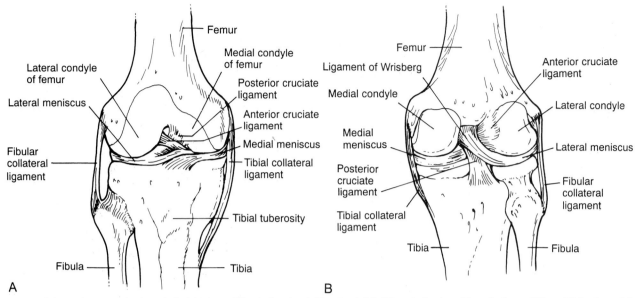

**Figure 4-3.** Major ligaments and menisci of the knee: (*A*) anterior view (without patella); (*B*) posterior view. (From Anthony, CP, and Thibodeau, GA: Textbook of Anatomy and Physiology, ed 10. Mosby-Year Book, St. Louis, 1979, pp 140–141, with permission.)

The collateral ligaments (tibial and fibular) help maintain the alignment of the femur and tibia by preventing lateral or medial movements or flexion. The tibial collateral is a membranous structure that is flat and broad and located at the posterior aspect of the joint. It is fixed to the medial condyle of the femur and extends distally, where it is attached to the medial condyle, and medial aspect, of the tibia. The fibular collateral ligament is a fibrous structure more round in appearance than the tibial collateral ligament. It is fixed to the posterior aspect of the lateral condyle of the femur and extends distally to its attachment on the lateral aspect of the proximal fibula.

## INDICATIONS

Knee arthrography is indicated when symptoms of torn menisci or ligaments, capsular damage, cysts, or loose bodies are evident. The symptoms are usually pain, swelling, or both. "Locking" of the knee joint may occur when loose bodies bind in the joint during movement. Most pathology diagnosed in the knee area is the result of trauma.

## CONTRAINDICATIONS

Contraindications for arthrography include known allergy to contrast agents or local anesthetic. Infection of the joint, or near the joint, would also preclude arthrography.

## PREPROCEDURAL CARE

Prior to knee arthrography, the procedure should be thoroughly explained to the patient and an informed consent signed. If the patient is extremely apprehensive about the procedure, a mild sedative may be administered to reduce the patient's fear. Whether or not to administer a sedative and the type and dose of sedative are the options of the physician performing the examination.

## EQUIPMENT

### Major Equipment

The major equipment for knee arthrography may include a conventional radiographic room or a radiographic and fluoroscopic room. The choice of conventional radiography, fluoroscopy, or a combination of both depends on the radiologist's protocol and the type of contrast medium used. If fluoroscopy is used, the fluoroscopic tube must have a fractional-millimeter (less than 1 mm) focal spot to produce the image quality necessary to visualize the menisci. Most general fluoroscopic tubes have a larger focal spot (in millimeters), which does not produce the necessary image quality. It is helpful if the spot-film device accommodates a 9″ × 9″ cassette and has a 9 on 1 capacity (i.e., nine exposures on one film).

### Accessory Equipment

For this examination, minor equipment can vary significantly based on the method of filming. Typically, filming the lateral and medial meniscus, joint capsule, and major ligaments is included as routine. Filming can be accomplished by vertical beam radiography, horizontal beam radiography, or vertical beam fluoroscopy. The latter two methods of filming are most commonly used and are discussed in the Positioning and Filming section of this chapter.

The preparation and injecting equipment remains the same for all methods of arthrography. A commercially prepared, sterile, disposable tray is generally used for arthrography, or the radiology department may use and maintain items usually found in the tray. The contents of a typical tray include two 10-ml and one 50-ml syringe; 18-, 20-, 21-, and 25-gauge needles; extension tubing; gauze sponges; towels; prep cup; prep sponges; fenestrated drape; local anesthetic; and a bandage. Other equipment needed includes a 3″-wide elastic (Ace) bandage, sterile gloves, an antiseptic solution (e.g., Betadine), a razor, and the contrast medium(ia). Contrast material can include a radiolucent agent, such as room air, oxygen, or carbon dioxide, and/or a water-soluble, radiopaque medium.

For horizontal beam radiography using dual contrast media, additional accessory equipment needed includes a 7″ × 17″ cassette, measured and marked off along its length to accommodate a series of six exposures on one film; a lead diaphragm with an opening to match the area to be exposed on the 7″ × 17″ cassette (reduces scatter radiation and improves film quality); a small, low wooden table used during radiography of the lateral meniscus; a round, firm support (usually a bed sheet rolled to a diameter of approximately 6″); and a 5-lb sandbag. The last two items are used to widen or "open" up the joint space in order to visualize the menisci better.

Vertical beam fluoroscopy uses a single or dual contrast medium(ia). In addition to lead aprons, gloves, and other protective devices normally used during fluoroscopy, a patient restraint (e.g., the type used to support the patient when the table is upright) is used to apply stress to the knee to open up the joint space.

## INJECTION PROCEDURE

Injection of the contrast medium(ia) is directly into the joint capsule. This can be accomplished by a lateral, or medial, retropatellar approach to the capsule. The site of injection is the choice of the physician, based upon circumstances of the examination. The lateral approach facilitates aspiration of joint fluid; however, it is more painful to the patient because the lateral aspect of the joint capsule lies deeper within the tissues than the medial aspect. The medial approach is less painful to the patient because the medial portion of the capsule is closer to the skin; however, it is more difficult to remove joint fluid from this area. Sterile technique must be maintained for this part of the procedure because knee joint infection is the most common complication of this procedure. Therefore, the area of the injection site is prepared by shaving away any body hair; cleansing the area with an antiseptic; and applying a sterile, fenestrated drape.

Once prepared, the site is injected with 2 to 5 ml of a local anesthetic (e.g., Xylocaine), using a 10-ml syringe and a 25- or 21-gauge needle. With the area anesthetized, a 20-gauge needle is introduced into the joint space and more anesthetic may be injected. At this time, all (or as much as possible) of the joint fluid is aspirated using a 10-ml syringe and the 20-gauge needle (which has been left in place). To ensure that the needle is within the joint capsule, the patient's knee may be flexed, which causes additional pressure within the capsule and a backflow of joint fluid through the needle. Normal synovial fluid is tinged yellow and is clear in appearance. If the fluid is cloudy, it is sent to the laboratory for analysis to determine if an infectious process is present. If the fluid appears bloody, it may indicate a possible injury and the preliminary knee radiographs should be re-examined to determine if any trauma was overlooked in the initial evaluation. The radiopaque contrast medium is drawn up in a clean 10-ml syringe and injected into the joint capsule through the 20-gauge needle, via the extension tubing. The 50-ml syringe is used to inject a radiolucent medium, if used in the study. The knee may be flexed and extended or the patient directed to walk for a brief period. This movement of the knee ensures dispersal of the contrast medium throughout the joint and, in the case of a positive medium, provides even coating of the structures to be examined. At this point, an Ace bandage is applied over the distal femur to obliterate the suprapatellar bursae.

## CONTRAST MEDIA

For knee arthrography, a radiolucent or radiopaque medium or a combination of both media may be employed. Radiolucent media include room air, oxygen, or carbon dioxide, and, if used as the sole agent, the dose is from 100 to 120 ml. At its inception, knee arthrography was performed exclusively with radiolucent media. These agents produced very little irritation of the joint capsule; however, they do not accurately define structures, particularly under fluoroscopy.

The radiopaque medium used for knee arthrography is a water-soluble, (relatively) low density agent such as Renografin 60 in the amount of 5 to 15 ml. Although a positive contrast medium tends to define structures better than a negative medium in the knee, it can also obscure small structures (e.g., small bone chips) because of its density. Currently, the method of choice for knee arthrography is a dual contrast study. Generally, 80 to 110 ml of negative medium and 5 ml of positive medium are employed. Based on research over the years, the dual contrast study provides the most accurate diagnostic information. The negative medium provides an excellent enhancement for the thin layer of positive medium coating the pertinent structures of the knee.

## POSITIONING AND FILMING

Arthrography most often demonstrates pathologic conditions of the medial and lateral menisci. Thus, the routine filming and discussion of filming methods in this text are based on the projections that best demonstrate these structures. It should be noted that although the menisci are of interest in the filming sequence, other abnormalities such as ligament tears and loose bodies can also be visualized. Additional views may be needed to better demonstrate these findings and others, such as a Baker's cyst (Fig. 4–4), which is best visualized on a lateral view of the knee (popliteal area).

For arthrography, a routine set of knee films should be obtained and reviewed by the radiologist before the procedure is begun. Imaging for knee arthrography can employ a conventional radiographic tube in a vertical or horizontal position or a fluoroscopic tube in a vertical position. The most popular methods of filming for arthrography today include the horizontal radiographic method and the vertical fluoroscopic method; therefore, only these two filming techniques are discussed. It is important to note that what is presented in this section is a suggested filming routine based on the most commonly accepted techniques. Variations (particularly in equipment, degree of leg rotation during positioning, and so on) are common in knee arthrography.

## Horizontal Beam Radiographic Method

Horizontal beam arthrography produces the best results when dual contrast media are used. For radiography of the medial meniscus, the patient is placed in a semiprone position so that the posterior aspect of the medial meniscus of the affected leg is upward. The joint may be "opened up" on the medial aspect by placing a pillow under the distal femur and a sandbag over the ankle, thus providing the stress needed to widen the joint (Fig. 4–5). The central ray is directed through the area of the medial meniscus, parallel to the tibial plateau. It is helpful if the plateau can be identified

under fluoroscopy and the area marked on the skin to facilitate accurate centering, which is essential to the examination. A film holder with a 7″ × 17″ cassette and diaphragm is placed between the patient's knees. The cassette is adjusted so that the central ray and tibial plateau are aligned in the center of the opening of the diaphragm and are the first (end) portion of the cassette to be exposed. An exposure is made to demonstrate the posterior aspect of the medial meniscus. The cassette is moved so that the second portion of the cassette is aligned with the diaphragm. The patient is rotated 30 degrees toward the supine position (making sure the leg also rotates the same 30 degrees), and the central ray and tibial plateau alignment is adjusted in the same manner as the first exposure. A second exposure is made.

This sequence of cassette adjustment and 30-degree patient rotation and central ray alignment is continued through a series of four more exposures. The leg that is not under examination is positioned so that it does not obscure the area under examination and is comfortable for the patient.

When all six exposures are completed, the resulting film demonstrates the medial meniscus in profile around its circumference, from posterior to anterior aspect, in 30-degree increments (Fig. 4–6). The first exposure should demonstrate the femoral condyles as not quite superimposed, and because the patient is rotated 180 degrees during filming, the last exposure should again demonstrate the femoral condyles, again not quite superimposed. Superimposition of the condyles is avoided, because this would also superimpose the lateral and medial menisci.

Lateral meniscus radiography is performed by placing the patient in the semiprone position with the affected leg on a small wooden table so that the posterior aspect of the lateral meniscus is upward (Fig. 4–7).

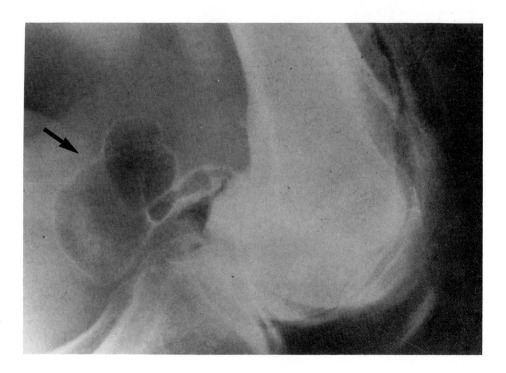

**Figure 4–4.** Baker's cyst. (Courtesy of Medcom Trainex, Garden Grove, CA.)

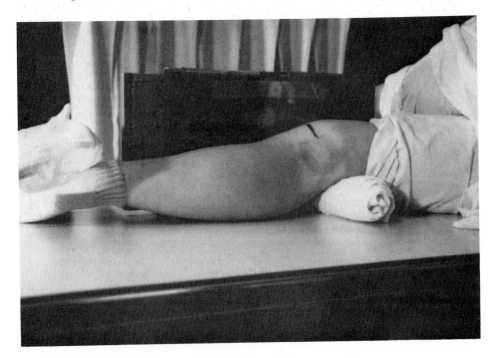

**Figure 4 – 5.** Medial meniscus radiography, horizontal beam method.

From this point the filming technique is similar to that of radiography of the medial meniscus. The cassette holder, the 7″ × 17″ cassette, and the diaphragm are placed on the small table and aligned with the tibial plateau in the same manner as for radiography of the medial meniscus. Again, similar to medial meniscus radiography (starting with the posterior aspect of the lateral meniscus), six consecutive exposures, with a 30-degree rotation of the patient between each exposure, are made. The resulting film demonstrates the lateral meniscus in profile around its circumference, from the posterior to anterior aspect, in 30-degree increments (Fig. 4 – 8). As with radiography of the medial meniscus, the femoral condyles will be almost superimposed on the first and last exposure on the film of the lateral meniscus. Because radiographs of both menisci will be similar in appearance, they should be marked, with small lead markers, as M (for medial) and L (for lateral),

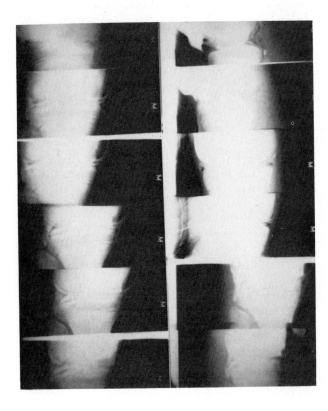

**Figure 4 – 6.** Medial meniscus, horizontal beam method.

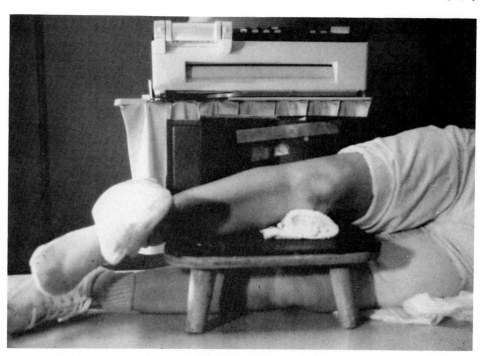

**Figure 4–7.** Lateral meniscus radiography, horizontal beam method.

indicating the meniscus demonstrated. These markers are used in addition to the standard right and left markers. In order to ensure that any pathology identified can be accurately localized, the filming sequence must be strictly followed.

When filming of the menisci is completed, the Ace bandage is removed and an anteroposterior (AP) projection and a lateral view of the knee are taken on 8″ × 10″, or 10″ × 12″, cassettes to demonstrate the entire joint capsule and ligaments (Fig. 4–9). Positioning and centering for these views is the same as for routine views of the knee.

## Vertical Beam Fluoroscopic Method

For fluoroscopic filming, the patient is recumbent, with the knee to be filmed under the fluoroscopic

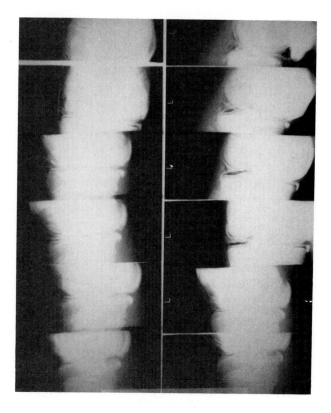

**Figure 4–8.** Lateral meniscus, horizontal beam method.

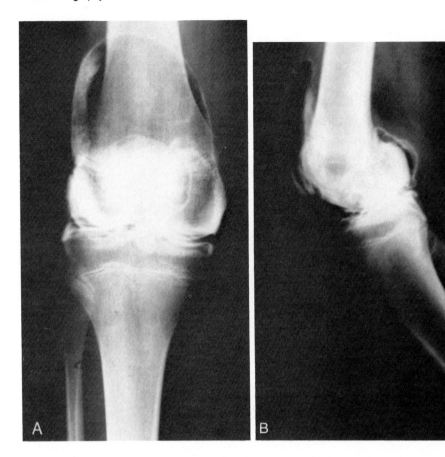

**Figure 4–9.** (*A*) AP projection of entire knee with contrast; (*B*) lateral view of entire knee with contrast.

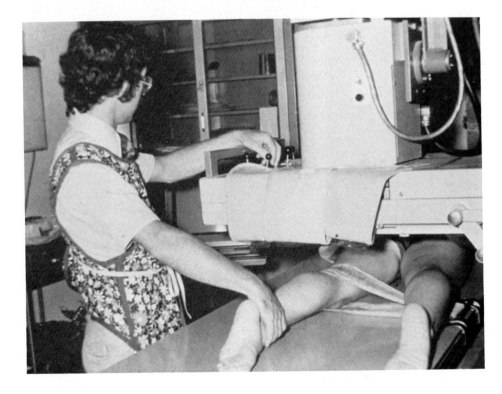

**Figure 4–10.** Medial meniscus radiography, fluoroscopic method. (Courtesy of Medcom Trainex, Garden Grove, CA.)

image intensifier. For the medial meniscus, the patient is semiprone. If, for example, the left knee is examined, filming begins with the patient in a right anterior oblique position. A patient restraint is attached to the back edge of the table and wrapped around the distal femur, returning the loose end of the restraint to the attachment. The radiologist applies stress to the knee joint by applying lateral pressure at the ankle to widen the medial aspect of the joint space (Fig. 4–10). An exposure is made of the posterior aspect of the medial meniscus, and the patient is rotated 25 to 30 degrees toward the prone position for a second exposure. The patient is rotated in increments, and spot filming is continued until the meniscus has been demonstrated in profile from the posterior to anterior aspects (Fig. 4–11). Because this process is under fluoroscopic control, the radiologist may choose to rotate the patient in less than 25- to 30-degree increments to further visualize and film the meniscus.

Filming the lateral meniscus (e.g., of the left knee) is similar to filming the medial meniscus, The patient is in a left anterior oblique position with the restraining device attached to the front of the table. The joint is stressed by applying pressure medially at the ankle to open up the lateral aspect of the knee joint (Fig. 4–12), and an exposure of the posterior aspect of the meniscus is made. The patient (and leg) is rotated in increments for a total of 180 degrees during spot filming. When

fluoroscopic filming of the menisci is completed (Fig. 4–13), the Ace bandage is removed and routine AP and lateral views of the knee are taken to demonstrate the bursa and major ligaments (see Fig. 4–9). If warranted, additional filming of these areas may be done with positioning under fluoroscopic control. Tomography may be used, particularly to demonstrate the cruciate ligaments (Fig. 4–14).

## POSTPROCEDURAL CARE

There are no postprocedural orders for knee arthrography other than instructing the patient to notify the physician if pain occurs. An infection may occur postprocedurally, either at the puncture site or in the joint, requiring appropriate treatment. The vast majority of knee arthrographies are uneventful.

## RADIOGRAPHIC FINDINGS

The most common finding of knee arthrography is torn meniscus(i). Torn menisci are classified according to the type of tear that occurs. Vertical and horizontal tears are most common. A vertical tear is visualized when the positive contrast medium passes vertically through the meniscus (Fig. 4–15). The tear may be in-

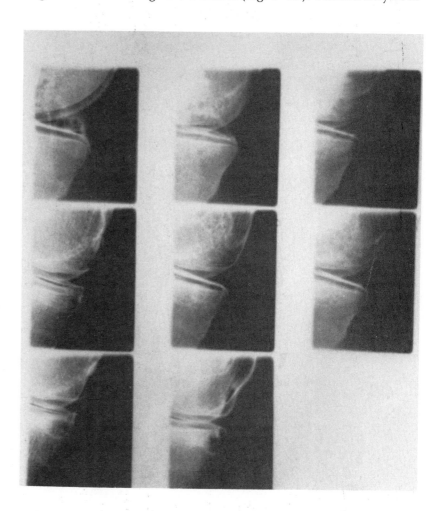

**Figure 4–11.** Medial meniscus, fluoroscopic method.

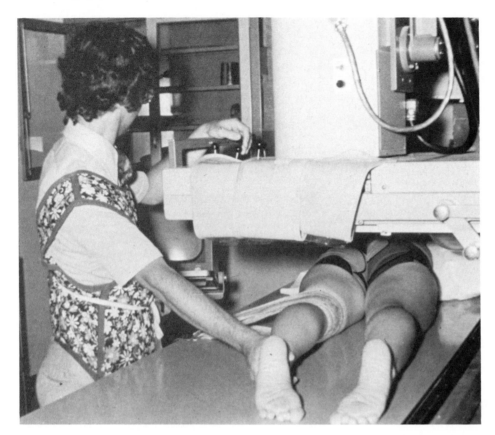

**Figure 4–12.** Lateral meniscus radiography, fluoroscopic method. (Courtesy of Medcom Trainex, Garden Grove, CA.)

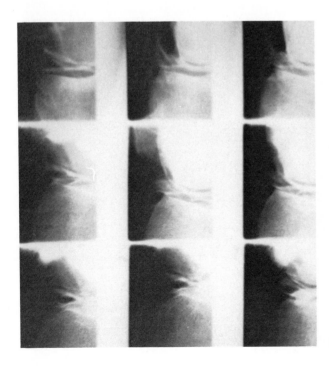

**Figure 4–13.** Lateral meniscus, fluoroscopic method.

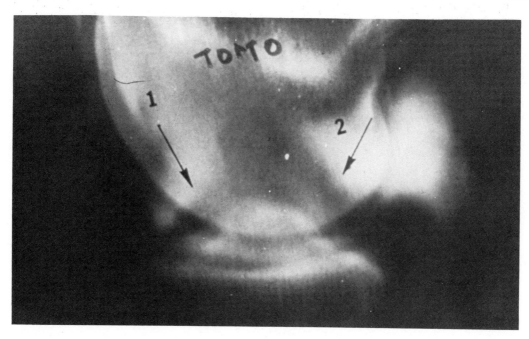

**Figure 4–14.** Tomography of cruciate ligaments: (1) anterior cruciate; (2) posterior cruciate. (Courtesy of Medcom Trainex, Garden Grove, CA.)

complete or may appear in any part of the meniscus. Similarly, horizontal tears are demonstrated by contrast medium visualized as a horizontal line of positive medium through the meniscus (Fig. 4–16). Horizontal tears, like vertical tears, may be in a variety of locations.

Sometimes, the tears are multiple and cannot be classified as either horizontal or vertical but rather are identified as complex (Fig. 4–17). Other, less frequently seen pathologic conditions include capsular tears (Fig. 4–18), ligament tears (Fig. 4–19), popliteal or Baker's

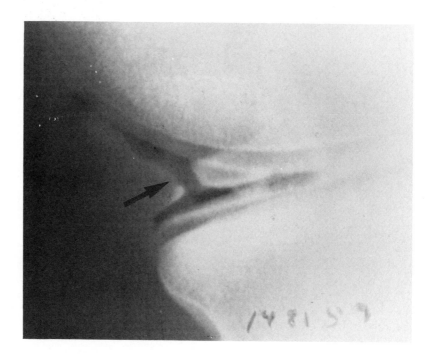

**Figure 4–15.** Vertical tear, meniscus. (Courtesy of Medcom Trainex, Garden Grove, CA.)

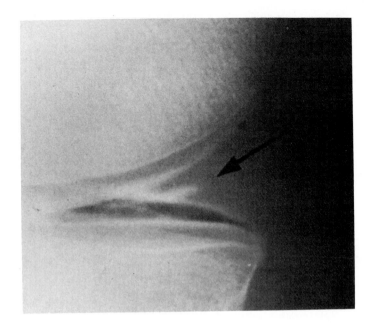

**Figure 4-16.** Horizontal tear, meniscus. (Courtesy of Medcom Trainex, Garden Grove, CA.)

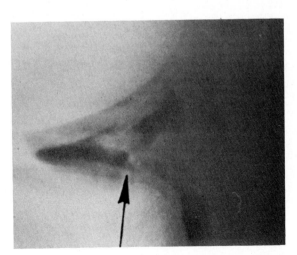

**Figure 4-17.** Complex tear, meniscus. (Courtesy of Medcom Trainex, Garden Grove, CA.)

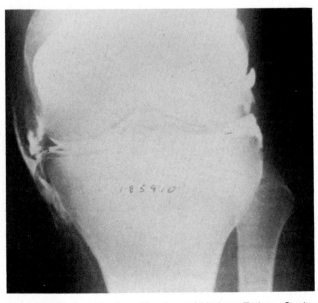

**Figure 4-18.** Capsular tear. (Courtesy of Medcom Trainex, Garden Grove, CA.)

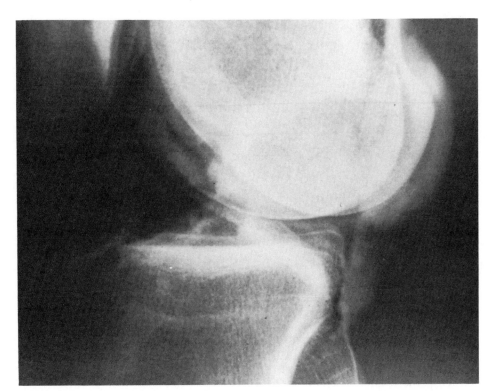

**Figure 4-19.** Anterior cruciate ligament tear with anterior subluxation of tibia. (Courtesy of Medcom Trainex, Garden Grove, CA.)

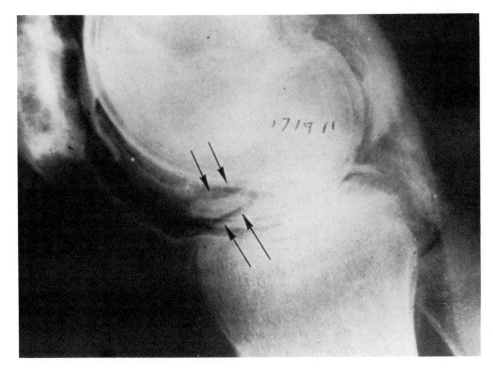

**Figure 4-20.** Loose body. (Courtesy of Medcom Trainex, Garden Grove, CA.)

cyst (Fig. 4–4), discord (seen as an elongated meniscus extending far into the joint space), and loose bodies (Fig. 4–20).

## REVIEW QUESTIONS

1. The knee is a(n) ——— joint.
   A. synarthrodial
   B. amphiarthrodial
   C. synovial
   D. no answer is correct

2. The knee contains ——— meniscus(i).
   A. 1
   B. 2
   C. 3
   D. 4

3. Define "cruciate" as it applies to the knee ligaments.

4. The collateral ligaments of the knee ——— .
   A. prevent anteroposterior hyperflexion of the knee
   B. are attached to the menisci
   C. prevent lateral flexion of the knee
   D. are attached only to the femur

5. Most pathology of the knee joint is the result of ——— .
   A. trauma
   B. joint disease
   C. obesity
   D. standing for long periods of time

6. Filming for arthrography is accomplished by ——— .
   A. vertical beam radiography
   B. horizontal beam radiography
   C. vertical beam fluoroscopy
   D. all answers are correct

7. Stress is applied to the knee joint during arthrography to provide better visualization of the ——— .
   A. ligaments
   B. bursa
   C. menisci
   D. intercondylar eminence

8. Horizontal beam arthrography utilizes ——— cassette(s).
   A. 8″ × 10″
   B. 10″ × 12″
   C. 7″ × 17″
   D. 14″ × 17″

9. The ——— approach for puncture of the knee joint capsule facilitates removal of synovial fluid.
   A. anterior
   B. posterior
   C. medial
   D. lateral

10. Normal synovial fluid is ——— .
    A. opaque
    B. clear
    C. opaque and tinged yellow
    D. clear and tinged yellow

11. If a dual contrast arthrogram is performed on the knee, the suggested amounts of contrast are ——— ml negative and ——— ml positive media.
    A. 100, 50
    B. 100, 100
    C. 80–110, 50
    D. 80–110, 5

12. During an arthrogram, using the horizontal beam method, the leg is rotated ——— degrees between each exposure.
    A. 10
    B. 15
    C. 30
    D. 35

13. During arthrography, using the horizontal beam method, a small table is used when radiographing the ——— .
    A. collateral ligaments
    B. medial aspect of the joint capsule
    C. medial meniscus
    D. lateral meniscus

14. The most common complication to arthrography is ——— .
    A. reaction to contrast media
    B. injury to the joint capsule
    C. infection
    D. injury to the menisci

15. The most common radiographic finding of arthrography is ——— .
    A. torn ligament(s)
    B. torn meniscus(i)
    C. torn joint capsule
    D. loose bodies

16. A Baker's cyst is associated with ——— .
    A. menisci
    B. collateral ligaments
    C. the popliteal area of the bursa
    D. suprapatellar bursa

## BIBLIOGRAPHY

Arthrography of the knee. Squibb X-ray Atlas 2:4, 1976.
Ballinger, P: Merrill's Atlas of Radiographic Positions and Radiologic Procedures, Vol 1, ed 7. Mosby-Year Book, St Louis, 1991.
Bontrager, KL: Textbook of Radiographic Positioning and Related Anatomy, ed 3. Mosby-Year Book, St Louis, 1993.
Gray, H: Gray's Anatomy (The Classic Collector's Edition). Bounty Books, New York, 1977.
Johnson, ME, et al: Human Anatomy. Saunders College Publishing, Philadelphia, 1985.
Kaye, J, et al: Arthrography of the Knee (FTMM). MEDCOM (Trainex), New York (Garden Grove), 1975.
Renografin-60 (Diatrizoate Meglumine and Diatrizoate Sodium Injection USP). ER Squibb & Sons, Princeton, 1985.
Skucas, J: Radiographic Contrast Agents, ed 2. Aspen Publishers, Rockville, MD, 1989.
Westall, DR: Arthrography: A critical study of the technique and possible improvement of knee arthrograms. Radiologic Technology 45(5):311, 1974.

# CHAPTER 5

# Endoscopic Retrograde Cholangiopancreatography

*Patrick J. Apfel, MEd, ARRT(R)*

Endoscopic retrograde cholangiopancreatography (ERCP) can be either a diagnostic or a therapeutic procedure. The procedure may be performed in an endoscopy unit (if fluoroscopy is available) or in an imaging department. For diagnosis, it is used to examine the biliary and pancreatic ducts through a retrograde injection of a contrast medium. This procedure generally follows a nonconclusive study such as cholecystography or an ultrasound examination of the gallbladder or pancreas, or it follows gallbladder surgery. As a therapeutic procedure, it can be used to treat conditions diagnosed by other diagnostic examinations or a diagnostic ERCP. Examples of treatments include, but are not limited to, dilatation of stenosed biliary or pancreatic ducts, removal of biliary or pancreatic duct stones, and cutting of the sphincter muscles (sphincterotomy or sphincterectomy) to increase the size of a narrow orifice or to facilitate stone removal or stent placement.

To perform ERCP, a specialized endoscope known as a duodenoscope is passed through the patient's mouth and guided to the descending duodenum. The papilla of Vater is identified with the endoscope, and a cannula is threaded through the endoscopic tubing and manipulated through the papillary opening into the common bile or main pancreatic duct. Placement of the cannula is verified under fluoroscopy with fractional injections of a contrast medium. Once the cannula is positioned, an appropriate contrast medium is injected until the area of interest (which may be the biliary tree or the pancreatic duct system) is adequately visualized and spot films are taken. This procedure is performed by an endoscopist, generally a gastroenterologist. Nursing personnel assist the physician and attend to the patient. The radiographer is responsible for the imaging equipment and provides general assistance, as needed, during the procedure. A radiologist or the radiographer operates the fluoroscope and exposes spot films as appropriate.

This chapter presents discussions on the diagnostic procedure, equipment, and pathologies identified with ERCP. Although therapeutic applications of ERCP are

**45**

briefly presented where appropriate, a comprehensive discussion of the therapeutic aspects of ERCP is beyond the scope of this text.

## ANATOMY

Endoscopic retrograde cholangiopancreatography examines the biliary tree and the pancreatic duct system. The gallbladder and its ducts (Fig. 5–1) lie in the right upper quadrant of the abdomen and are closely associated with the right major lobe of the liver. The gallbladder collects, stores, and concentrates bile, produced in the liver, for release into the descending duodenum. Contraction of the gallbladder, with injection of bile into the duodenum, occurs by the action of cholecystokinin, a hormone released by the mucosal lining of the duodenum when fats are present. Bile emulsifies, or breaks down, large globules of fat into smaller globules, which can then be digested or broken down chemically. The biliary tree, or duct system, of the gallbladder serves to drain the liver of bile, carry bile to the gallbladder for temporary storage, and deliver bile to the duodenum when the gallbladder contracts. Bile, formed in the functional lobular tissues of the liver, at first drains into very small ducts and then into increasingly larger ducts as they approach the gallbladder (creating a treelike structure). The main ducts composing the biliary tree are the right and left hepatic, common hepatic, cystic (leading to the gallbladder), and common bile (leading to the duodenum) ducts (Fig. 5–1).

The pancreas is an accessory digestive organ that is mostly (tail end) in the left upper quadrant of the abdomen. It lies below the stomach with its head end cradled within the C loop of the duodenum (Fig. 5–1), in the right upper quadrant. It has both endocrine functions (producing the hormones insulin and glucagon) and exocrine functions (producing digestive enzymes). Within the gland, the cells producing digestive enzymes drain into small ducts leading to the main pancreatic duct, which joins the common bile duct to drain into the duodenum (Fig. 5–1). Distal to the junction of the common bile and main pancreatic ducts, the combined duct is expanded into a chamber, the hepatopancreatic ampulla, or ampulla of Vater, which opens into the duodenum. A circular muscle embedded in the wall of the duodenum, the sphincter of Oddi, controls the flow of bile and pancreatic juices into the duodenum. In some individuals, an accessory pancreatic duct drains into the duodenum independently of the main duct. When food is present in the duodenum, the hormones cholecystokinin and secretin are released by the duodenal mucosa and stimulate the pancreas to secrete its digestive enzymes, which aid in the digestion of fats, proteins, and carbohydrates.

## INDICATIONS

Endoscopic retrograde cholangiopancreatography is performed to assess pathologies of either the biliary tree or the pancreatic duct system and to provide therapy to alleviate certain pathologic conditions (e.g., removal of choleliths).

### Diagnostic

Examination of the biliary tree is more common than the examination of the pancreatic ducts. The procedure is indicated when patients exhibit symptoms suggestive of stenosis, dilatation, or obstruction of, or choleliths or small lesions within, the biliary or pancreatic ducts. ERCP can also be performed as a preoperative (for planning) or postoperative (follow-up) procedure. For the biliary tree, generally, ERCP is performed following other gallbladder studies (i.e., cholecystography, cholangiography, and gallbladder ultrasound), which may be inconclusive. It is also useful in examining the biliary ducts following surgical removal of choleliths. During the procedure, the physician also has the opportunity to examine visually the distal esophagus, stomach, and duodenum.

### Therapeutic

Endoscopic retrograde cholangiopancreatography may also be indicated as a therapy to known conditions or conditions diagnosed by the procedure. Sphincterotomy may be performed to repair a stenosis of the sphincter of Oddi or to facilitate stone removal from the bile ducts. A variety of sphincterotomes are used

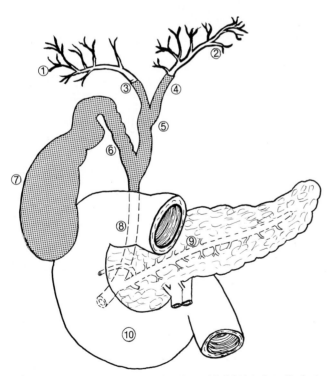

**Figure 5–1.** Gallbladder and related ducts: (1) right intrahepatic duct; (2) left intrahepatic duct; (3) right hepatic duct; (4) left hepatic duct; (5) common hepatic duct; (6) cystic duct; (7) gallbladder; (8) common bile duct. Pancreas and related ducts: (9) pancreatic duct; (10) duodenum.

for the procedure. Stones can be removed either by threading a balloon catheter beyond the stone, inflating the balloon, and then withdrawing the balloon and stone into the duodenum or by using a basket catheter to retrieve the stone. Biliary duct stenoses can be treated by dilatation with a balloon catheter, by stent placement, or by balloon dilatation along with stent placement. Generally, balloon dilatation is successful in dilating a stenosis caused by sclerotic conditions, whereas a stent is required in cases of stenosis caused by nonoperable tumors.

Pancreatic stones can also be removed by using either a balloon catheter or a stone basket for retrieval. Generally, the sphincter of Oddi and the pancreatic orifice sphincter are cut to facilitate the stone removal. Pancreatic duct strictures can be dilated with a balloon catheter, stent placement, or both. Pancreatic pseudocysts may also be drained via placement of a nasopancreatic drain when appropriate.

## CONTRAINDICATIONS

The presence of pancreatic pseudocysts may contraindicate the diagnostic study of the pancreatic duct system. Filling of the pseudocysts with a contrast medium may lead to inflammation and possible rupture and postprocedural infection. Pseudocysts may be detected prior to the procedure with an ultrasound of the pancreas. Acute pancreatitis and septic cholangitis also contraindicate a diagnostic procedure, although these conditions may be relieved by therapeutic procedures (e.g., nasobiliary or nasopancreatic drain placement as appropriate).

Previous contrast media reactions may not contraindicate the study. However, it is recommended that nonionic contrast media be administered and the patient be appropriately premedicated and closely monitored during the procedure for indications of a contrast medium reaction. There is evidence that some contrast medium is absorbed by the pancreatic ductal epithelium into the bloodstream.

Several types of drugs are administered during the procedure (e.g., sedatives, topical anesthetics, etc.). If the patient has a history of allergies to specific drugs, alternates should be substituted.

## PREPROCEDURAL CARE

Because there are certain risks to the procedure (e.g., postprocedural pancreatitis), the procedure and related risks should be thoroughly explained to the patient and an informed consent signed. Because several drugs and a contrast medium are used during the procedure, allergic history is reviewed.

If there has been a previous reaction to an iodinated contrast medium, the procedure may proceed; however, the patient should be premedicated according to protocol. For patients with suspected ductal obstruction or pseudocysts, antibiotics are given about 1 hour before the procedure to preclude cholangitis or pancreatitis. The patient should receive nothing by mouth (NPO) for at least 4 hours before the procedure. An intravenous (IV) fluid line (with a side arm injection site) and normal saline or 5 percent dextrose in water are started and used during the procedure for injection of drugs. Because of patient positioning, the right arm is the preferred site for the IV setup.

## EQUIPMENT AND MEDICATIONS

The major equipment for ERCP may be divided into the imaging equipment and procedural equipment. For imaging, a fluoroscopic unit with a spot radiograph device and tilting table is sufficient.

The equipment for the procedure is extensive and includes patient monitoring devices (Fig. 5–2); the video equipment, duodenoscope, and cannulae (Fig. 5–3); suction equipment; medications, drugs, and contrast medium; and injection materials (syringes and so on). This equipment is generally provided by the endoscopy laboratory.

Because the patient is given a variety of drugs during the procedure, which may affect vital signs, the blood pressure, heart rate, and blood oxygen content are monitored by electronic equipment connected directly to the patient.

The duodenoscope is an endoscope with a wide angle lens and side view capability (as opposed to end view), allowing for easier visualization of the papilla of Vater. The original scopes permitted only one individual to view at a time and are currently being replaced with videoendoscopes. These scopes project the image onto a CRT (TV) screen for better visualization and allow group viewing. The duodenoscope has a channel through its length through which a variety of cannulae or catheters may be advanced for diagnostic or therapeutic purposes. These may have a radiopaque tip to assist in guiding them under fluoroscopy. Diagnostic cannulae are used for the contrast medium injection and specimen collection (e.g., bile or pancreatic juices). Common therapeutic catheters include balloon types to dilate stenotic ducts and remove stones, basket catheters for stone retrieval, and cutting types for sphincterotomy (cutting into the sphincter of Oddi to relieve stenosis).

During the procedure the patient is administered a variety of drugs. Before the insertion of the duodenoscope, the throat is sprayed with a topical anesthetic such as Xylocaine to facilitate passage of the endoscope. A general anesthetic may be used for children and for patients who are unable to cooperate or when the procedure is expected to be lengthy.

Injectable drugs are administered directly into the IV tubing (through a side arm). Sedatives such as meperidine (Demerol), diazepam (Valium), and midazolam (Versed) are administered in small increments and at intervals until the desired effect is achieved. Versed also has a hypnotic effect, causing retrograde amnesia for a period of several hours postinjection. This is a desired effect since endoscopy on a patient who is fully conscious is an uncomfortable experience. Oxygen is

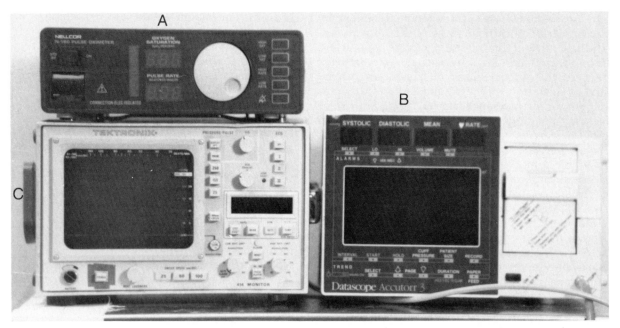

**Figure 5-2.** Monitoring equipment for ERCP: (A) oximeter; (B) blood pressure unit; (C) electrocardiograph.

administered during the procedure, since some of these sedatives are respiratory depressants.

An antispasmodic drug, such as glucagon, is given to relieve spasm of the duodenum and sphincter of Oddi from the presence of the endoscope and cannula.

If it is necessary to reverse the effect of the sedatives, drugs such as naloxone (Narcan) or flumazenil (Mazicon) may be administered. Phentolamine mesylate (Regitine) reverses the effect of glucagon. For more specific information concerning these drugs, their administrations, and recommended doses, see Chapter 19, Catheterization Methodology and Patient Care Management.

A variety of syringes (3 ml to 20 ml) and needles (18 gauge to 25 gauge), sterile water or normal saline (for dilution), and alcohol prep sponges are needed for injection of drugs and contrast medium. Generally, two 50-ml vials of ionic or nonionic, iodinated, water-soluble contrast medium are needed for diagnostic injection.

Nursing notes, including medications and amounts administered, vital signs, and so on, are recorded in the patient's chart.

## INJECTION PROCEDURE

ERCP requires a team made up of an endoscopist (generally a gastroenterologist), two nurses, a radiologist, and a radiographer. Each member of the team has specific duties. The gastroenterologist is the lead physician during the procedure. In addition to performing the endoscopic, diagnostic, and therapeutic aspects of the procedure, this physician directs the administration of the drugs and the contrast medium and the fluoroscopic imaging.

The nursing personnel are responsible for all of the procedural equipment and medications, patient monitoring, preparing and administering the various drugs and contrast medium, and patient charting. Generally, the nursing personnel transport the equipment and patient to the imaging department and the patient to the recovery room following the procedure.

Depending on department protocol, a radiologist or a radiographer may operate the fluoroscope and expose spot films during the procedure. The radiographer is responsible for setting up the imaging equipment and provides general assistance during the examination. When appropriate, the radiographer may operate the fluoroscopic and spot-film equipment.

As the procedure begins, the patient is placed on the table in the reverse of standard placement (i.e., the patient's head is at the "foot" end of the table). This allows the patient to face the physician (when he or she is positioned for the endoscope insertion) and facilitates the arrangement of equipment and personnel in the room. For the insertion of the endoscope, the patient is placed in a left lateral or steep left anterior oblique (LAO) position, with the left arm behind him or her and extended down along the left side. The patient's throat is sprayed with the topical anesthetic, and, under the direction of the gastroenterologist, nursing personnel administer medications. The endoscopic tubing is lubricated and passed through the patient's mouth, esophagus, stomach, and into the duodenum. Once the gastroenterologist maneuvers the endoscope into position within the duodenum, the patient is rolled down into a slight LAO or prone position. The duodenoscope is manipulated until the papilla of Vater is visualized "face on." The cannula is then threaded through the endoscope and inserted through the papilla opening and advanced into the appropriate duct system.

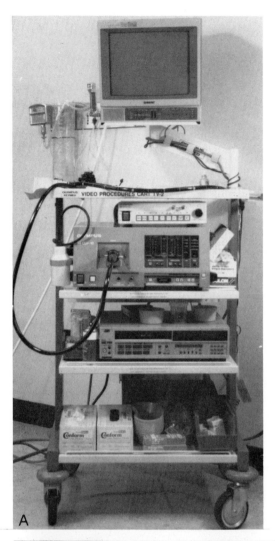

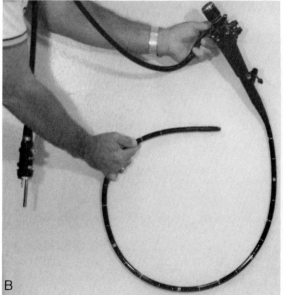

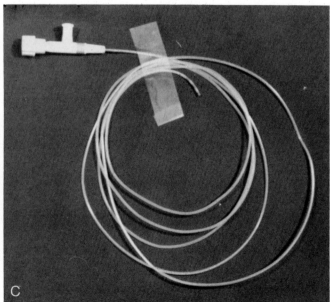

**Figure 5-3.** (*A*) Video equipment; (*B*) duodenoscope; (*C*) injection cannula.

Fractional injections of the contrast medium, under fluoroscopic control, guide and verify proper cannula placement. Once catheter placement is verified, the contrast medium is injected by the endoscopist while the radiologist or radiographer monitors the process with fluoroscopy and obtains appropriate spot films.

## CONTRAST MEDIA

Water-based iodinated contrast agents are used for ERCP. For cholangiography, either highly concentrated contrast medium or diluted medium may be used (30 percent salt concentration, 15 percent iodine concentration), depending on the physician's preference and the suspected pathology. For example, a low concentration medium may be more beneficial in detecting small choleliths. Once cannula placement within the common bile duct is verified by fractional injection under fluoroscopic control, the contrast medium is injected until the biliary tree is adequately visualized.

For pancreatography, a high concentration contrast medium (60 to 76 percent salt concentration, 30 to 38 percent iodine concentration) is recommended. Once the cannula has passed through the orifice of the papilla of Vater, a small amount of contrast medium is injected and cannula placement is verified with fluoroscopy. With the cannula in place, the contrast medium is injected until the pancreatic ducts are sufficiently visualized.

Examples of contrast media used for ERCP include (ionic) Renografin M 60 and (nonionic) Isovue 300. During the fractional injection of the contrast medium for verification of cannula placement, the medium may be diluted to reduce the total amount of contrast medium given to the patient.

## POSITIONING AND FILMING

Filming for ERCP is accomplished by fluoroscopic imaging. Under fluoroscopic control, fractional injections of the contrast medium are administered until there is adequate filling of the appropriate ducts and spot radiographs are taken (Fig. 5–4). The patient is either prone or in a slight LAO position. There is no set routine, and filming continues until sufficient ductal filling is observed or pathology is adequately visualized.

## POSTPROCEDURAL CARE

A patient undergoing ERCP is heavily medicated and must be closely observed and monitored following the procedure. When the examination is completed, nursing personnel transport the ERCP patient to a hospital recovery room. Recommended recovery times are ½ hour for in-hospital patients and 1 hour for outpatients. For patients who have undergone general anesthesia, the length of stay in the recovery room is dictated by their rate of recovery from the anesthetic (i.e., level of alertness and stability of vital signs).

During the recovery room stay, vital signs, including blood pressure, pulse, the heart, and respiration, are monitored. If a topical anesthetic was used to spray the throat, fluids and food are withheld until sensation has returned to the throat to avoid possible aspiration. Once the patient is alert and vital signs are stable, he or she may be discharged from the recovery room.

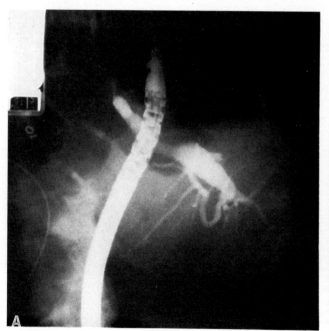 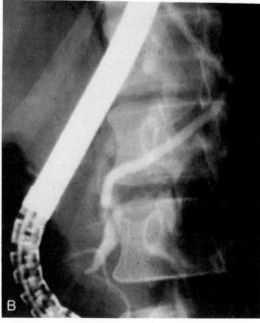

**Figure 5–4.** (*A*) Radiograph demonstrating ERCP of biliary tree; (*B*) radiograph demonstrating ERCP of pancreatic ducts.

# COMPLICATIONS

Possible complications related to ERCP are few. The most common complication to ERCP for the pancreas is pancreatitis, which has a very low incidence (less than 2 percent) and is self-limiting. Postprocedural infection caused by the rupture of pancreatic pseudocysts is also possible. When biliary obstruction is present, postprocedural cholangitis and septicemia may result.

Further complications may occur as a result of reactions to drugs administered during the procedure.

Complications from the endoscopic nature of the procedure include perforation of the upper digestive tract (in cases where a diverticulum or herniations exist) and insertion and injection of contrast medium into the intima of the duodenum (especially when using a cannula with a finely tapered tip).

# RADIOGRAPHIC FINDINGS

Diagnostic findings of ERCP are consistent with indications and include biliary or pancreatic duct stenosis, biliary stones, and lesions within the biliary or pancreatic duct systems. ERCP can also be used as an adjunct to ultrasound or CT in the diagnosis of pancreatitis or cancer of the pancreas. Through ERCP biopsy, disease of the papilla of Vater (e.g., cancer) can be detected.

ERCP is an efficient procedure, since both diagnosis and therapy can occur simultaneously. For example, biliary stones can be detected and removed during a single procedure.

# REVIEW QUESTIONS

1. ERCP examines the ———— .
   A. pancreatic ducts only
   B. biliary tree only
   C. gallbladder only
   D. pancreatic ducts and biliary tree

2. ———— is a therapeutic ERCP procedure.
   A. Stone removal
   B. Duct dilatation with a balloon catheter
   C. Stent placement
   D. All of the above

3. The specific scope used for ERCP is a(n) ———— .
   A. endoscope
   B. cholangioscope
   C. pancreatic endoscope
   D. duodenoscope

4. ERCP is most often used to examine the pancreatic ducts.
   A. True
   B. False

5. A contraindication of ERCP of the biliary duct is ———— .
   A. choleliths
   B. ductal dilation

C. ductal stenosis
D. cholangitis

6. The radiology department is responsible for supplying and maintaining all of the equipment used in ERCP.
   A. True
   B. False

7. A general anesthetic may be used ———— during ERCP.
   A. on children
   B. on patients who are unable to cooperate
   C. when the procedure is expected to be lengthy
   D. all of the above

8. ———— administered during ERCP has a hypnotic effect.
   A. Demerol
   B. Versed
   C. Mazicon
   D. Narcan

9. Oxygen is administered to the patient during ERCP because ———— , given during the procedure, may depress respiration.
   A. Regitine
   B. Mazicon
   C. sedatives
   D. Narcan

10. A drug administered to reduce spasm in the duodenum is ———— .
    A. glucagon
    B. Versed
    C. Narcan
    D. Mazicon

11. An example of an ionic contrast medium used for ERCP is ———— .
    A. Renografin
    B. Gastrografin
    C. Isovue
    D. Cystografin

12. The contrast medium for ERCP is never diluted.
    A. True
    B. False

13. During fluoroscopic spot filming, the ERCP patient is in a ———— position.
    A. supine
    B. left lateral
    C. right lateral
    D. none of the above

14. ERCP is an inpatient procedure only.
    A. True
    B. False

15. Postprocedural care for an ERCP patient requires ———— .
    A. monitoring of blood pressure and pulse only
    B. monitoring of blood pressure and respiration only
    C. administration of Narcan
    D. a recovery room stay

## BIBLIOGRAPHY

Ballinger, P: Merrill's Atlas of Radiographic Positions and Radiologic Procedures, Vol 2, ed 7. Mosby-Year Book, St Louis, 1991.

Bontrager, KL: Textbook of Radiographic Positioning and Related Anatomy, ed 3. Mosby-Year Book, St Louis, 1993.

Cotton, PB. Cited by: Cotton, PB and Williams, CB: Endoscopic Retrograde Cholangio-Pancreatography. Wilson-Cook Medical Inc. Blackwell Scientific Publications, U.K.

Dunn, M (LPN 11): Personal interview, September 1993.

Eisenberg, RL, Dennis, CA, and May, CR: Radiographic Positioning. Little, Brown and Company, Boston, 1989.

Miller, B and Keane, C: Encyclopedia and Dictionary of Medicine, Nursing, and Allied Health, ed 4. WB Saunders, Philadelphia, 1987.

Nemec, FJ (MD): Personal interview, September, 1993.

Scanlon, VC and Sanders, T: Essentials of Anatomy and Physiology. FA Davis, Philadelphia, 1991.

Schapiro, M and Kuritsky, J: The Gastroenterology Assistant: A Laboratory Manual, ed 3. Zephyr Medical Enterprises, Encino, CA, 1989.

Sedin, N (RN): Personal inteview, September 1993.

Sivac, MV: Gastroenterologic Endoscopy. WB Saunders, Philadelphia, 1987.

Skucas, J: Radiographic Contrast Agents, ed 2. Aspen Publishers, Rockville, MD, 1989.

Waye, JD, et al: Techniques in Therapeutic Endoscopy. WB Saunders, Philadelphia, 1987.

# CHAPTER 6

# Hysterosalpingography

*Patrick J. Apfel, MEd, ARRT(R)*

Hysterosalpingography (HSG) is a radiographic examination of the female reproductive system. Specifically, the internal reproductive structures including the uterus, fallopian tubes, and ovaries are examined using a contrast medium. The procedure is diagnostic and, in some cases of infertility, therapeutic in nature. Fallopian tubes that may be obstructed or narrowed may be restored to normal patency during the procedure. Hysterosalpingography is a relatively safe and simple procedure that can be performed on an outpatient basis. Filming can be accomplished using a conventional radiographic room or a radiographic-fluoroscopic room.

## ANATOMY

The female reproductive system includes both the internal organs, which are composed of the paired ovaries and fallopian tubes as well as the singular uterus and vagina, and the external structures, which include the labia major and minora, Bartholin's glands, clitoris (Fig. 6–1), and the breasts. Since hysterosalpingography examines only the internal pelvic female structures, the discussion of anatomy here will center on these areas (Fig. 6–2).

The ovaries are roughly almond-shaped, paired structures approximately 1.5″ long that lie within the pelvic cavity on either side of the uterus. They are supported by a broad ligament suspended from the peritoneum, a suspensory ligament from the pelvic wall, and an ovarian ligament extending from the uterus. The ovaries contain several hundred thousand primary follicles, which can produce mature ova during the woman's childbearing years. When an ovum matures, it ruptures from the follicle (ovulation) into the peritoneal cavity in close proximity to the adjacent fallopian tube. It is swept into, and along the length of, the fallopian tube, where fertilization by a male sperm may take place.

The paired fallopian tubes project, laterally, from the cornu (superior angles) of the uterus. They are approximately 4″ in length and extend toward the ovaries, opening into the peritoneal cavity. The tubes

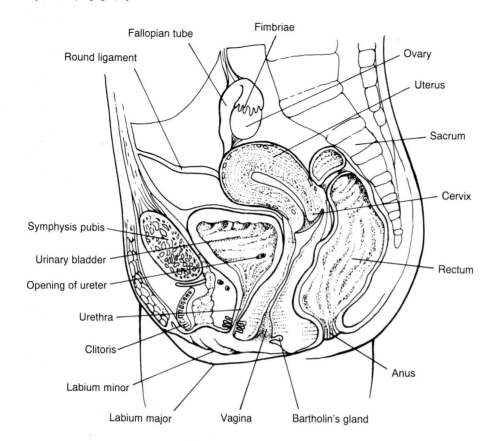

Fallopian tube

Fimbriae

Round ligament

Ovary

Uterus

Sacrum

Cervix

Symphysis pubis

Urinary bladder

Opening of ureter

Rectum

Urethra

Clitoris

Anus

Labium minor

Labium major

Vagina

Bartholin's gland

**Figure 6–1.** Female reproductive system (From Scanlon, VC and Sanders, T: Essentials of Anatomy and Physiology, ed 2. FA Davis, Philadelphia, 1994, with permission.)

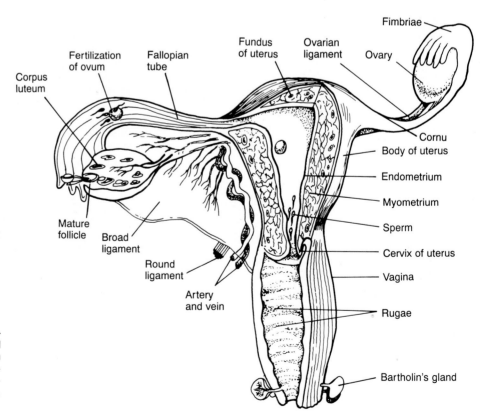

Fertilization of ovum

Corpus luteum

Fallopian tube

Fundus of uterus

Ovarian ligament

Fimbriae

Ovary

Cornu

Body of uterus

Endometrium

Myometrium

Sperm

Mature follicle

Broad ligament

Cervix of uterus

Round ligament

Vagina

Artery and vein

Rugae

Bartholin's gland

**Figure 6–2.** Internal female reproductive organs that are examined by hysterosalpingography. (From Scanlon, VC and Sanders, T: Essentials of Anatomy and Physiology, ed 2. FA Davis, Philadelphia, 1994, with permission.)

terminate in fingerlike projections, fimbriae, one of which is usually attached to or near the ovary. During ovulation, movements of the fimbriae, contractions of the fallopian tubes, and movements of cilia (hairlike projections) within the fallopian tubes create a current in the fluid enclosing the ovary and ovum, sweeping the ovum into the lumen of the fallopian tube. Normally, fertilization of the ovum takes place in the fallopian tube, and the zygote (fertilized egg) is moved into the uterus in 4 to 5 days. Within the uterus, the zygote implants itself into the uterine wall, within 7 or 8 days, where it develops into an embryo, then the fetus. If the zygote does not enter the uterus but continues to develop, an ectopic pregnancy results (e.g., the zygote may remain in the fallopian tube).

In the nongravid woman, the uterus is approximately 2″ long and 3″ wide and shaped somewhat like an upside down pear. In an anterior view, the uterine cavity appears like an inverted triangle. It is divided into three main sections: the fundus or upper portion above the level of the fallopian tubes, the body or midportion, and the lower portion, known as the cervix. The cervical os, or opening, is approximately ¾″ in diameter. The uterus lies between the urinary bladder (anteriorly) and the rectum (posteriorly). Normally, the body of the uterus is folded forward and lies over the roof of the urinary bladder. A uterus that is tilted more forward than normal is anteflexed; a uterus that is tilted more posteriorly than normal is retroflexed. There are eight ligaments, which are actually extensions of the peritoneum, that anchor the uterus within the pelvic cavity. The uterus is a thick-walled structure, made up of three layers of tissue. The outer layer is the epimetrium (actually made up of the peritoneum); the middle layer, made up of smooth muscle, is the myometrium; and the inner layer is the endometrium. During menstruation, the lining of the endometrium is shed and regenerated. In pregnancy, the endometrium makes up a portion of the placenta. During childbirth, the muscular layer of the uterus contracts to expel the fetus from the mother's body.

The vagina is the tube that surrounds, and extends from, the cervix to the vaginal orifice (opening to the outside of the body). It is approximately 4″ in length and serves as a receptacle for sperm during coitus, as an exit for expelling the endometrium during menstruation, and as part of the lower birth canal during delivery. It is not examined during HSG.

## INDICATIONS

Hysterosalpingography is indicated in cases of infertility, habitual abortion, abnormal uterine bleeding, absence of menses, and suspected blockage of the uterine (fallopian) tubes. It is also useful in identifying intrauterine and pelvic masses, fistulae, and congenital abnormalities and for presurgical and postsurgical evaluation. As a therapeutic tool, HSG may restore (fallopian) tubal patency by opening blocked tubes, dilating narrowed tubes, and straightening kinked tubes, which may reverse infertility in some patients.

## CONTRAINDICATIONS

Hysterosalpingography is contraindicated if the patient has pelvic inflammatory disease or active uterine bleeding. Pregnancy generally precludes the procedure, and the examination should not be performed too close to the premenstrual or postmenstrual phase of the menstrual cycle. It may be contraindicated in cases of hypersensitivity to a contrast medium, although the examination may proceed after premedication.

## PREPROCEDURAL CARE

The procedure should be performed within approximately 10 days following the onset of menstruation. This is a relatively "safe" period, because ovulation should not occur at this time. Also, the endometrium is least congested during this period. The bowel should be cleansed with a non–gas-forming cathartic administered the evening before the procedure and with cleansing enemas (until clear) the morning before the examination. Just before the procedure, the vagina should be irrigated, the perineal area cleansed, and the bladder emptied. The procedure should be thoroughly explained to the patient and an informed consent signed.

The patient should be forewarned that she may experience some pain during the procedure. Injectable glucagon may be administered as a premedication to reduce the pain sometimes induced during the contrast medium injection. For the extremely apprehensive patient, a sedative may also be administered at the discretion of the physician.

## EQUIPMENT

Major equipment for HSG may include a conventional radiographic or a radiographic-fluoroscopic room. Ideally, gynecologic stirrups that allow the patient to assume the lithotomy position are desired, but not necessary. Minor imaging equipment consists of 10″ × 12″ cassettes for conventional radiography or fluoroscopic spot filming.

Accessory equipment includes that utilized for cannulation of the uterus and injection of the contrast medium. The cannulation equipment may vary significantly, depending on the type of cannula used by the physician performing the procedure. Sterile trays may be made up and maintained by the imaging department; they are also commercially available. A typical commercially prepared tray will include drapes (one fenestrated), gloves, lubricating jelly, vaginal speculum, gauze sponges, swab sticks, antiseptic solution, uterine sound, two 10-ml syringes, an 18-gauge needle, extension tubing, and a one-way stopcock (Fig. 6–3). A cannula is a tube inserted into the cervical os to inject the contrast medium; it is dilated or blocked to prevent leakage of the contrast medium during injection. There are several types of cannulae that may be used, including a uterine cannula with a rubber "acorn"-type

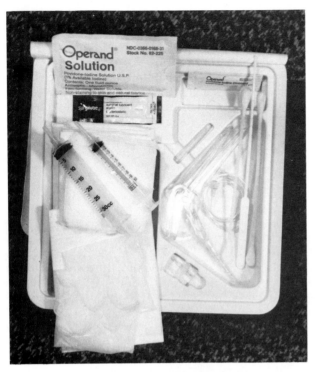

**Figure 6-3.** Hysterosalpingography tray.

plug to seal the cervical os and a tenaculum to maintain counter traction, a vacuum uterine cannula system (Fig. 6-4), a specialized HSG catheter with an inflatable balloon (Fig. 6-5), and a simple Foley catheter. Other equipment needed for the procedure includes the contrast medium, a surgical cap and mask, an adjustable stool, and a floor lamp.

## INJECTION PROCEDURE

Aseptic technique should be maintained during the injection procedure to prevent pathogens from entering the peritoneal cavity. Once the patient is prepped, she is placed supine on the radiographic table. If gynecologic stirrups are available, the patient's legs are positioned appropriately in the leg rests. If no stirrups are available, the patient is positioned with the hips abducted, the plantar surface of the feet together, and the knees flexed approximately 90 degrees. The lower extremities should be supported with positioning sponges if this positioning is used. The table may be lowered into a slight Trendelenburg's position. The physician lubricates the speculum, inserts it into the vaginal orifice, and advances and expands it to visualize the cervix. The vagina and cervix are cleaned using the swab

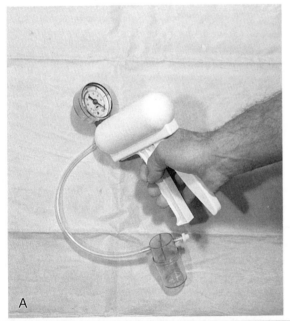

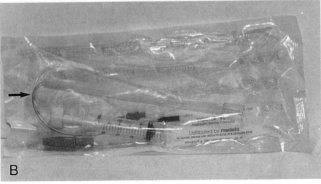

**Figure 6-4.** Vacuum uterine cannula system: (*A*) vacuum pump (used with cannula); (*B*) uterine cannula.

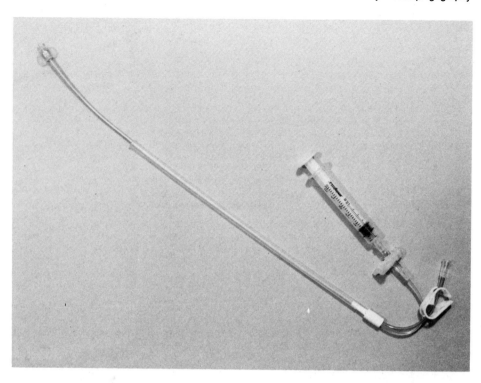

**Figure 6-5.** Hysterosalpingography catheter.

sticks and antiseptic solution. The uterine sound is inserted (through the speculum) to determine the depth and direction of the uterus. Next, the cannula is inserted through the speculum into the cervical canal, and the cannula is anchored in place (according to the type of cannula used) to seal off the cervical os. If a balloon-type cannula is used, one of the 10-ml syringes is used to inflate the balloon. The second 10-ml syringe, extension tubing, and stopcock are used to inject the contrast medium through the cannula into the uterine cavity. The injection is made in increments, and its progress is monitored under fluoroscopy or by conventional filming, until it traverses the fallopian tubes and "spills" into the peritoneal cavity around the ovaries (Fig. 6-6).

## CONTRAST MEDIA

Either a water-soluble iodide (e.g., Sinografin) or iodized oil (e.g., Lipiodol) may be used as a contrast medium for HSG, depending on the physician's preference. Each has advantages and disadvantages. For example, water-soluble media are quickly absorbed (in approximately 1 hour); however, their radiopacity is only moderate. Oily media present good radiopacity but are slowly absorbed, taking up to several months, and may intravasate (enter a blood or lymphatic vessel), causing oily pulmonary emboli. Currently, water-soluble media seem to be the contrast of choice. Their radiopacity can be adjusted by choosing appropriate concentrations. Further, they demonstrate the mucosal pattern better than the oily media and do not present the possibility of emboli formation. Whichever contrast medium is used, approximately 3 or 4 ml is needed to

fill the uterus and a total of 8 to 10 ml is required to fill the fallopian tubes and produce the spill. To reduce pain caused by spasm during injection of the contrast medium, the medium should be warmed to room temperature. To further reduce spasm and subsequent pain, the patient may be premedicated with glucagon.

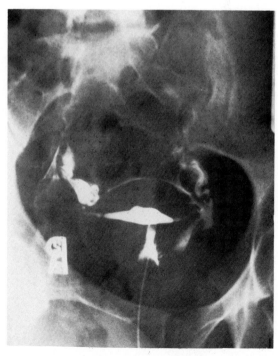

**Figure 6-6.** "Spill" film (normal).

## POSITIONING AND FILMING

A supine scout film of the pelvic cavity is obtained before the injection begins. Postinjection filming for HSG may be accomplished by conventional overhead radiography or fluoroscopic spot filming using 10″ × 12″ cassettes. Filming is coordinated with the injection process and completed when the contrast medium spills into the peritoneal cavity, generally requiring about four films. If overhead radiography is used, two to four fractional injections of contrast medium, each followed by a radiograph, are generally sufficient to complete the study. If fluoroscopy is used, the injection process is monitored with appropriate spot filming as necessary to complete the study. If an oily contrast medium is used and peritoneal spill does not occur, the patient must return for a 24-hour delayed film to confirm possible tubal obstruction. The patient position is supine, and the central ray is directed to approximately 2″ superior to the symphysis pubis. Optional filming includes right and left posterior oblique and lateral positions, as appropriate.

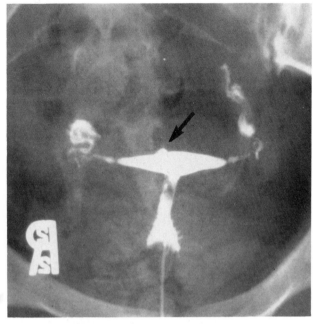

**Figure 6-7.** Diverticulum of the uterus.

## POSTPROCEDURAL CARE

Some patients may experience pain during, and for some time after, the procedure, caused by pressure from the injection or the contrast medium itself. There should be facilities available for outpatients to lie down until the pain subsides. When an oily contrast medium is used, the patient is supplied with a sanitary napkin to absorb any draining contrast medium. This is also true if there is any bleeding caused by the procedure. If pain or bleeding continue for an undue period of time fol-lowing the procedure, the patient should contact her physician.

## COMPLICATIONS

Possible complications of HSG include hemorrhage, spread of a pre-existing infection, and generalized peritonitis. When an oily contrast medium is used, intrava-

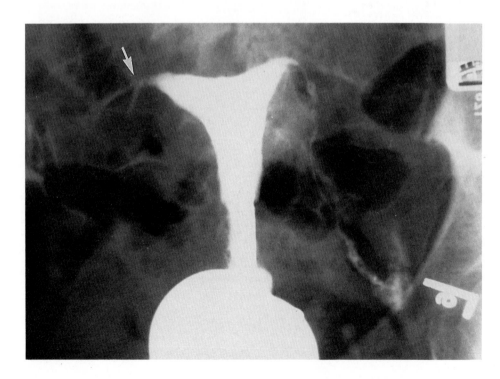

**Figure 6-8.** Tubal obstruction, right fallopian tube.

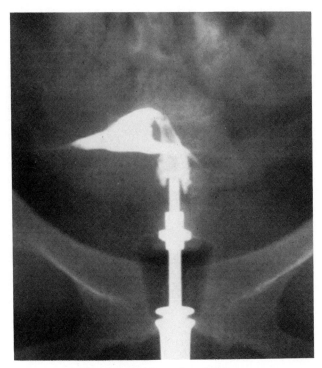

**Figure 6-9.** Anteversion of uterus.

sation may occur (within the uterus) with possible pulmonary emboli formation.

## RADIOGRAPHIC FINDINGS

HSG can detect such congenital abnormalities as a unicornuate uterus (single fallopian tube). Other findings include diverticula (Fig. 6-7) of the fallopian tubes, hydrosalpinx (dilation of the fallopian tube[s] because of partial obstruction), other tubal obstructions (Fig. 6-8), cornual spasm (spasm of the cornu or proximal segment of the fallopian tube), peritubal adhesions, intrauterine tumors (e.g., fibroid tumors or polyps) and retroversion or anteversion (Fig. 6-9).

## REVIEW QUESTIONS

1. Hysterosalpingography examines the _____.
   A. uterus
   B. uterus and fallopian tubes
   C. vagina, uterus, fallopian tubes, and ovaries
   D. uterus, fallopian tubes, and ovaries

2. Ovulation is when an ovum _____.
   A. ruptures from a follicle
   B. is formed
   C. travels to the uterus
   D. is fertilized

3. The inner lining of the uterus is the _____.
   A. epimetrium
   B. epitometrium
   C. endometrium
   D. myometrium

4. The cervix is part of the _____.
   A. female external genitalia
   B. vagina
   C. uterus
   D. fallopian tube

5. Hysterosalpingography is indicated in _____.
   A. habitual abortion
   B. infertility
   C. abnormal uterine bleeding
   D. all of the above are correct

6. Hysterosalpingography is contraindicated _____.
   A. in suspected blockage of a fallopian tube
   B. during pelvic inflammatory disease
   C. in absence of menses
   D. if a fistula is suspected

7. A "safe" time to schedule HSG is approximately _____ following the onset of menstruation.
   A. 2 days
   B. 10 days
   C. 2 weeks
   D. 3 weeks

8. Glucagon may be administered as a premedication for HSG to _____.
   A. reduce patient anxiety
   B. reduce spasm of the uterus or fallopian tubes
   C. reduce hemorrhage
   D. promote drainage of the contrast medium

9. A cannula is used during HSG to _____.
   A. dilate the cervix
   B. drain the uterus
   C. inject contrast medium
   D. dilate the fallopian tubes

10. Aseptic technique is not necessary during HSG.
    A. True
    B. False

11. In HSG, the contrast medium injection continues until _____.
    A. the patient experiences pain
    B. the uterus is visualized
    C. contrast medium spills into the peritoneal cavity
    D. a maximum of 12 ml is injected

12. A disadvantage of an oil-based contrast medium for HSG is _____.
    A. its low radiopacity
    B. it is quickly absorbed
    C. it requires a larger dose than a water-based contrast medium
    D. it may cause pulmonary emboli

13. Routine filming for HSG requires _____ positioning.
    A. supine
    B. prone
    C. lateral
    D. oblique

14. HSG may have a therapeutic effect in cases of
_____.

    A. abnormal uterine bleeding
    B. infertility
    C. absence of menses
    D. habitual abortions

## BIBLIOGRAPHY

Ballinger, PW: Merrill's Atlas of Radiographic Positions and Radiologic Procedures, Vol 2, ed 7. CV Mosby, St Louis, 1991.

Horwitz, RC, Morton, PCG, and Shaff, MI: A radiological approach to infertility—hysterosalpingography. Br J Radiol 52(616):255, 1979.

Johnson, E, et al: Human Anatomy. Saunders College Publishing, Philadelphia, 1985.

Juhl, JH: Paul and Juhl's Essentials of Roentgen Interpretation, ed 4. Harper and Row Publishers, Hagerstown, MD, 1981.

McInnes, J: Clark's Positioning in Radiography, Vol 2, ed 9. Year Book Medical Publishers, Chicago, 1974.

Scanlon, VC and Sanders, T: Essentials of Anatomy and Physiology. FA Davis, Philadelphia, 1991.

Skucas, J: Radiographic Contrast Agents, ed 2. Aspen Publishers, Rockville, MD, 1989.

Snopek, AM: Fundamentals of Special Radiographic Procedures, ed 3. WB Saunders, Philadelphia, 1992.

Spring, DB, Wilson, RE, and Arronet, GH: Foley catheter hysterosalpingography: A simplified technique for investigating infertility. Radiology 131(2):543, 1979.

# CHAPTER 7

# Pedal Lymphography

*Patrick J. Apfel, MEd, ARRT(R)*

The lymphatic component of the circulatory system or the lymphatic system (see Anatomy section of this chapter) represents the major portion of the adult immune system. Lymphography is a radiographic study of the ducts and glands of the lymphatic system. It is a relatively simple but time-consuming procedure, requiring delayed filming. An oily contrast medium is employed to visualize the lymphatic vessels and glands. Locating a lymph vessel for injection is often difficult. Identification of a vessel for injection is enhanced by the use of a "vital dye" selectively absorbed by the lymphatic system. Although this procedure is not often performed, it is useful in demonstrating the internal structure of the nodes, both benign and malignant neoplasms of lymph tissues, and obstruction of lymphatic vessels or nodes. Lymphography can be performed for the cervical area, upper and lower extremities, abdomen, pelvis, and gonads. Clinical evaluation is most difficult in the abdominal and pelvic areas; therefore, most lymphography is performed for these areas. This chapter is devoted to the pedal approach for lymphography of the pelvic, abdominal, and thoracic area (optional). It should be noted that the basic technique for lymphography is similar for all areas examined by this procedure.

## ANATOMY

Some anatomists consider the lymphatics to be components of the circulatory system because they are involved with the circulation of body fluids and the return of these fluids to the blood-vascular component. Other anatomists consider the lymphatics to be their own system, because their functions are considerably different from the blood-vascular system, although the two systems are certainly interdependent. This text will refer to the lymphatic portion of the circulatory system as the lymphatic system. The lymphatic system has several functions including the production of lymphocytes and antibodies. It is responsible for returning vital proteins, interstitial fluids, and blood cells to the circulatory system and for removing and destroying bacterial toxins, pathogens, and pathogenic cells (including cancerous forms) from interstitial fluid by phagocytosis (engulfing and destroying). In normal circulation, blood plasma, blood cells, proteins, and nutrients pass from arterial capillaries into surrounding tissues. About one half of the body's vital proteins leak from blood capillaries into surrounding tissues in one day. The lymph system is the essential system for returning these proteins to circulation (along with fluids, blood cells, etc.).

The lymphatic system is made up of lymph fluid, vessels, and nodes (Fig. 7–1). Lymphatic vessels begin as closed-end capillaries within interstitial spaces (Fig. 7–2), continue as collecting lymphatics, and extend into larger vessels or lymphatics. Lymphatic capillaries con-

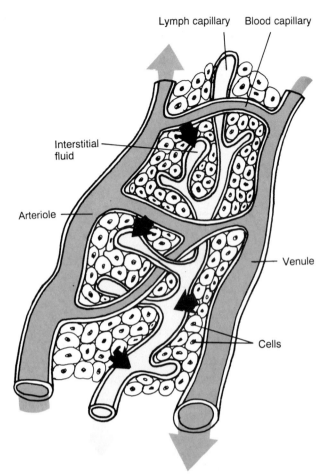

**Figure 7–2.** Lymphatic capillary bed. (Adapted from Scanlon, C and Sanders, T: Essentials of Anatomy and Physiology, ed. 2. FA Davis, Philadelphia, 1994, p 316.)

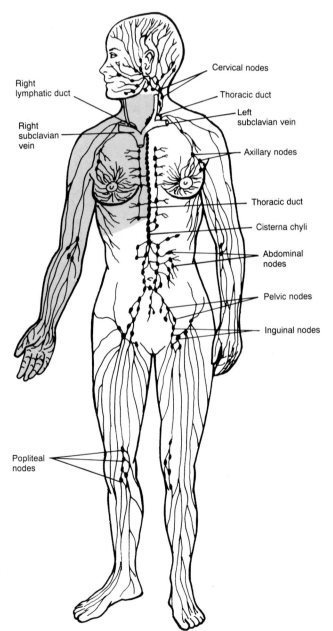

**Figure 7–1.** Lymph system. (Adapted from Scanlon, C and Sanders, T: Essentials of Anatomy and Physiology, ed. 2. FA Davis, Philadelphia, 1994, p 317.)

tain very large pores or openings formed between the endothelial cells making up their wall, thus allowing easy entry of fluids and particulates into the vessels. The lymph is moved along the vessels by several actions including contraction of the lymph vessels themselves, extrinsic compression of the vessels by surrounding muscle or other tissues, and interstitial pressure. All along the length of the vessel system are one-way valves, similar to those found in veins, which keep the circulation of lymph moving in one direction, that is, returning it to the blood circulation. Lymph fluid is returned to the venous blood circulation through two major routes. Most of the lymph from the lower extremities, the abdomen, portions of the chest, the left arm, neck, and head returns through the thoracic duct, which empties into the venous system at the junction of the left internal jugular and subclavian veins (Fig. 7–1). Lymph from the right arm, head and neck mediastinal areas, and lungs returns through the right lymphatic duct, emptying into the junction of the right internal jugular and subclavian veins (Fig. 7–1, *shaded area*).

Lymph is the fluid component of the lymphatic system. It is roughly comparable with blood plasma, from which it is derived. It is clear, tinged slightly yellow, and composed of mostly water (95 percent). As plasma leaks from arterial capillaries, it becomes interstitial fluid. Lymph is that interstitial fluid that has entered the lymph vessels. As lymph flows through lymphatic vessels, it carries essential proteins, blood cells, bacteria and bacterial toxins, and other substances. When it is returned to the blood circulatory system, after filtration, it again becomes plasma. On the average, the total lymph flow in all vessels is about 100 ml/h.

At intervals, along the length of the lymph vessels, are collections of lymphatic tissues termed "nodes" or (incorrectly) "glands." Lymph enters the nodes through afferent lymphatic vessels and leaves through efferent lymphatic vessels. Nodes vary in shape, size, and configuration (occurring either singularly or in clusters). They have an outer cortical layer surrounding an inner medullary area composed of fibrous and

endothelial cells, which make up the reticulum. As lymph fluid passes through the nodes, the reticulum acts as a filter entrapping particulates. Embedded in the reticulum are lymphocytes and macrophages (Fig. 7–3). Both of these types of white blood cells destroy bacterial toxins, bacteria, cancerous cells, and other foreign particles. Additionally, lymph nodes continue to produce new lymphocytes.

The major vessels and nodes examined by pedal injection include those of the inguinal, pelvic, and abdominal areas. The lower extremity and the thoracic area may also be included in the filming procedure if they are of interest.

In the lower extremities, the lymphatic system is divided into deep and superficial components. The deep lymphatics closely follow the deep veins of the leg, passing through the popliteal nodes and eventually the

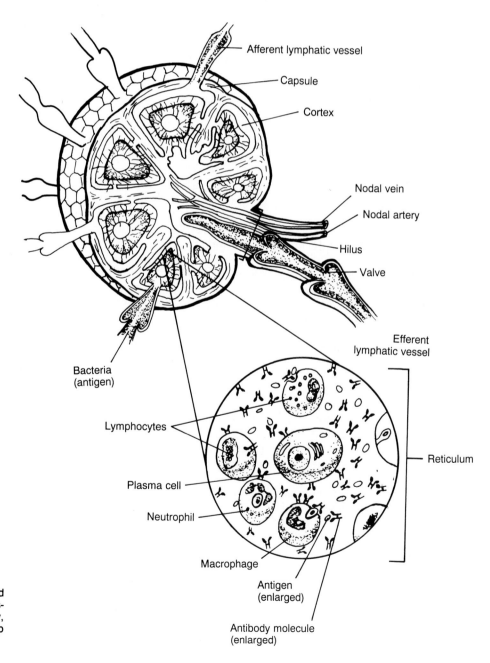

**Figure 7–3.** Lymph node. (Adapted from Scanlon, C and Sanders, T: Essentials of Anatomy and Physiology, ed. 2. FA Davis, Philadelphia, 1994, p 319.)

Afferent lymphatic vessel

Capsule

Cortex

Nodal vein

Nodal artery

Hilus

Valve

Efferent lymphatic vessel

Bacteria (antigen)

Lymphocytes

Plasma cell

Neutrophil

Macrophage

Antigen (enlarged)

Antibody molecule (enlarged)

Reticulum

inguinal nodes. The superficial lymphatics are divided into anterior and posterior segments. The anterior group is subdivided into medial and lateral components. The anterior medial lymphatics closely follow the great saphenous vein and can be visualized after injection of a lymph vessel on the medial aspect of the foot. The anterior lateral lymphatics are visualized after injection of a lymph vessel on the lateral aspect of the foot. The posterior lymphatics pass through the popliteal nodes and continue up the thigh to the inguinal nodes. They can be visualized after injection of a lymph vessel posterior to the lateral malleolus of the ankle.

The inguinal nodes are found below the inguinal ligament and are divided into superficial and deep segments. The superficial nodes have superior and inferior groups with the latter visible during pedal lymphography. The deep and superior superficial groups often are not visualized.

In the pelvic region, the lymphatics and nodes follow the major blood vessels in this area and are named accordingly as the external, internal, and common iliac chains. The external iliac lymphatic is divided into the lateral, intermediate, and medial chains (Fig. 7–4). The medial and lateral chains are best opacified during lymphography. The internal iliac lymphatics and nodes lie along internal iliac blood vessel tributaries and are seldom opacified during lymphography (Fig. 7–4). The external iliac lymphatics extend into the common iliac chains, which follow the common iliac artery. The common iliac lymphatic divides into lateral, intermediate, and medial chains (Fig. 7–4), all of which interconnect.

The common iliac lymphatics extend into the abdomen along the aorta and inferior vena cava and are divided into the right and left para-aortic trunks and midaortic chain. These lie very close to the vertebral column, approximately 3 cm anterior to it, with the para-aortic trunks extending along, but seldom lateral to, the vertebral transverse processes. Cross filling of these trunks often occurs at the lower lumbar area. The nodes are named by their spatial relationship to the aorta. The right trunk lies to the right of the aorta and surrounds the IVC as precaval, interaorticocaval, laterocaval, and retrocaval nodes (Fig. 7–5). The midaortic nodes are divided into preaortic (anterior) and retroaortic (posterior) segments (Fig. 7–5). The left aortic trunk lies on the left of the aorta (Fig. 7–5). The abdominal lymphatics receive tributaries from the lumbar area, kidneys, adrenal glands, gonads, and intestines.

The para-aortic trunks extend to the level of the first and second lumbar vertebrae and terminate at the cisterna chyli. The cisterna chyli is a dilated, saccular lymphatic (Fig. 7–1). It narrows at about the level of the 12th thoracic vertebra to become the thoracic duct, which continues into the area of the neck (Fig. 7–1). The thoracic duct lies to the right of the aorta. At about the level of the fifth thoracic vertebra, it crosses to the left and empties into the junction of the left subclavian and internal jugular veins. The duct varies from 1 to 7 mm in diameter and contains one-way valves near its terminal end. The cisterna chyli and the terminal portion of the thoracic duct may be opacified and visualized on the initial postinjection radiographs.

## INDICATIONS

Lymphography is indicated in cases of suspected malignancies, including lymphoma (e.g., Hodgkin's disease), metastatic disease, and obstruction of lymph vessels or nodes resulting in lymphedema. Note is made that although lymph nodes filter and destroy circulating cancer cells, some of these cells may become entrapped, but not destroyed, and then multiply and cause a new cancer within the node itself. Lymphography is also useful in locating nodes for biopsy or surgical removal.

## CONTRAINDICATIONS

Contraindications to lymphography include known sensitivity to the vital dye, contrast medium, or local anesthetic; respiratory insufficiency; concurrent radiation therapy to the lungs; and conditions resulting in direct, open communication between the lymphatic and blood circulatory systems (e.g., this may occur in cases of severe obstruction of the lymphatic system).

## PREPROCEDURAL CARE

Preprocedural care for lymphography includes an explanation of the procedure and possible complications to the patient. An informed consent should be signed. Solid food should be withheld for 8 hours before the procedure; clear liquids are permitted. A chest radiograph is recommended prior to the procedure to assess the lungs. The patient should be forewarned that the injection process is lengthy (in excess of 1 hour), with initial and delayed filming to follow. Further, patients should be advised that because of the injection of the vital dye, they may void blue-tinted urine and also may see some blue discoloration of the skin on the foot and along the course of lymphatic vessels. These aftereffects of the dye are transient, as the dye is eliminated by the kidneys. If the patient is apprehensive about the procedure, the physician may opt to administer a sedative.

## EQUIPMENT

The major equipment required for lymphography is a conventional radiographic room for imaging (a radiographic-fluoroscopic room may be used). Minor imaging equipment includes an appropriate number and size of standard cassettes. Accessory equipment includes those items needed for pharmaceutic injection (Fig. 7–6). This involves injection of a vital dye, a cutdown procedure to locate and cannulate a lymphatic vessel, and injection of the contrast medium employ-

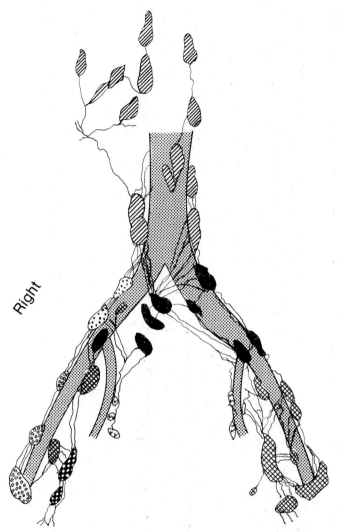

ANTERIOR-POSTERIOR VIEW

**Figure 7–4.** Pelvic lymph nodes.

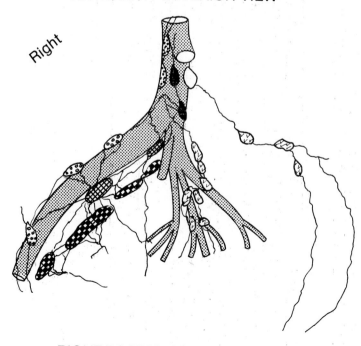

RIGHT POSTERIOR OBLIQUE VIEW

EXTERNAL ILIAC GROUP

Lateral chain

Intermediate chain

Medial chain

COMMON ILIAC GROUP

Lateral chain

Intermediate chain

Medial chain

INTERNAL (HYPOGASTRIC) GROUP

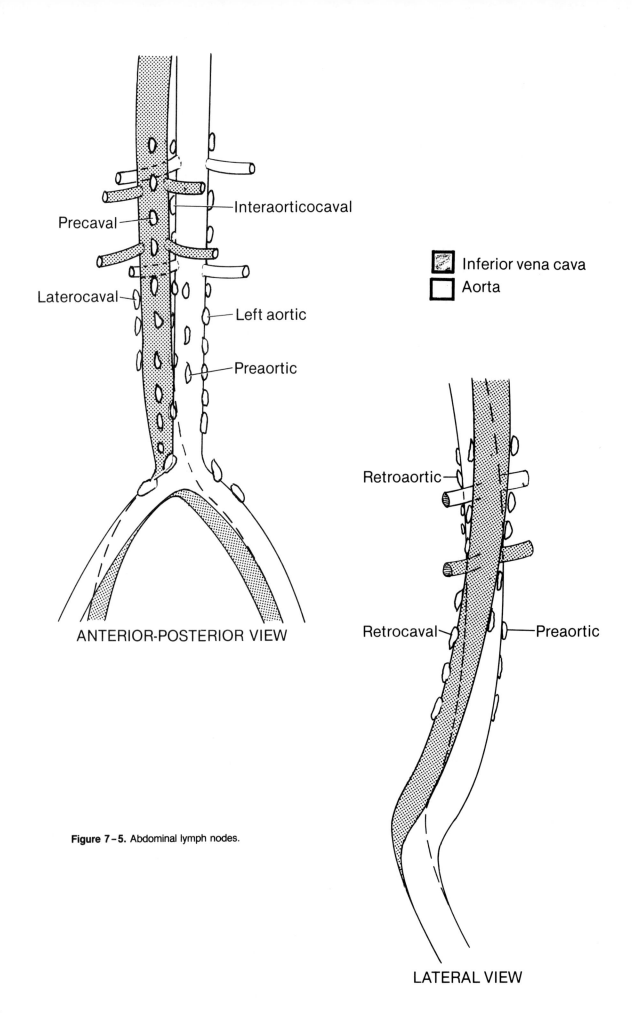

Precaval

Interaorticocaval

Laterocaval

Left aortic

Preaortic

Inferior vena cava

Aorta

ANTERIOR-POSTERIOR VIEW

Retroaortic

Retrocaval

Preaortic

LATERAL VIEW

**Figure 7-5.** Abdominal lymph nodes.

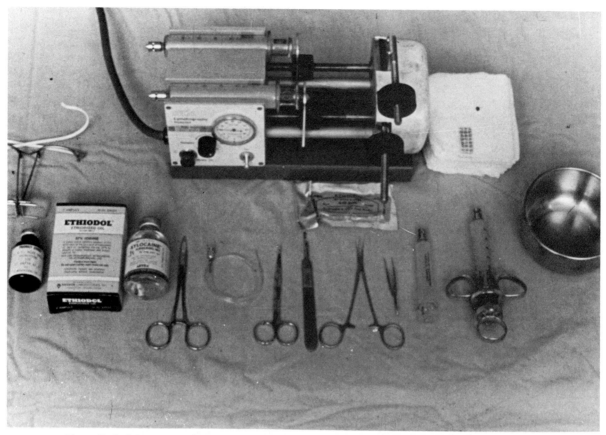

**Figure 7–6.** Accessory equipment for lymphography. (Courtesy of Medcom Trainex, Garden Grove, CA.)

ing an injector pump. There are several vital dyes commercially available, including patent blue V, Evans blue, brilliant blue GFF, and direct sky blue. A tuberculin syringe is used for injection of the dye. The oily contrast medium used for lymphography is Ethiodol, which should be warmed before injection to decrease viscosity. Two 10-ml vials are needed. A razor and an antiseptic solution (e.g., Betadine) are used to prepare the incision-injection site. The equipment for the cutdown and cannulation may vary. The typical sterile cutdown equipment recommended for this procedure includes a local anesthetic (without epinephrine), 27- or 30-gauge lymphography needles, mosquito forceps, scalpel, suture material, 5- and 10-ml syringes, 25-gauge needles, gauze sponges, stocking, and saline solution. Additionally, sterile gloves, gown, and mask are required. A stool, floor lamp, and magnifying glass are also helpful during the cutdown and injection process.

## INJECTION PROCEDURE

Isolation of a lymph vessel for cannulation and injection requires a cutdown procedure. The reader should note that the technique, and the equipment, for the cutdown may vary per the physician performing the lymphogram. The following depicts a representative

scenario of the technique (also see Chap. 19, Catheterization Methods and Patient Management).

Before attempting to locate a lymph vessel, the webbing between the toes is injected with 0.25 to 0.50 ml of the blue dye. To facilitate uptake of the dye by the lymph vessels, the patient is directed to wiggle the toes for several minutes. The dye should visualize the lymphatic vessels within 20 minutes. Because a cutdown is a minor surgical procedure, the dorsum of the foot should be shaved, prepared, and draped appropriately (see Chap. 18, Sterile Technique). A sterile stocking with a "window" cut out over the injection site is the most efficient way to drape the area. The largest lymph vessel on the dorsum of the foot is located and the area around it anesthetized. Either a longitudinal or a transverse superficial incision is made over it. The vessel is isolated by dissecting away surrounding tissue with mosquito forceps (care should be taken to avoid tearing away any tributary vessels). The forceps are placed under the vessel, and it is elevated by carefully opening the jaws of the forceps. Two sutures are placed around the vessel and the forceps removed. A sterile, white bandage or a small piece of white Teflon or other sterile material may be slipped under the vessel to enhance its visualization for the vessel puncture. Tension is applied to the loose suture (toward the ankle) to constrict and dilate the vessel. This suture is taped to the skin with sterile tape. Tension is then applied to the second suture (toward the toes) and the lymphography needle (27 to 30 gauge with attached tubing) is advanced, bevel side up, into the lumen. The needle should be parallel to the vessel and should be advanced only until the bevel is within the lumen to avoid puncturing the opposite side of the vessel. Normal saline is injected slowly at this time, which dilates the vessel, and the needle advanced an additional 2 to 3 mm. The needle is then secured in place by knotting the second suture around the vessel and needle and taping the needle to the foot with sterile tape. To avoid needle recoil, the tubing of the needle may be taped to the patient's toes, or, during the puncture, the skin may be punctured first (to hold the needle in place) and then the vessel. The needle tubing is then attached to an injector pump and the injection initiated. Some local anesthetic may be injected before the contrast medium to prevent the cramping of the calf muscle experienced by some patients.

It is recommended that a radiograph of the foot-ankle area be taken after about 1 minute of injection time to ensure that the contrast medium is within a lymphatic vessel (i.e., as opposed to a vein).

## CONTRAST MEDIA

The medium of choice for lymphography is the iodized oil, Ethiodol. Past use of water-soluble iodides revealed that they quickly diffused from lymphatic vessels and nodes. After injection, Ethiodol remains in the lymph vessels for up to 3 to 4 hours (varies per individual) and in the nodes for periods of weeks to months (in some patients, for over a year). The lymph nodes are best demonstrated approximately 24 hours postinjection. The recommended dose, per lower extremity, is 6 to 8 ml for an adult man with appropriately lower dosages for women and children. Some physicians recommend lesser doses for the elderly or those with a compromised respiratory system. This may be indicated because the contrast medium may reach the lungs through the circulatory system via the thoracic duct drainage into the left subclavian vein, possibly causing oil emboli. Because the contrast medium is viscous and injected at a slow rate, an injector pump is used for the injection. The recommended setting is at a rate of 0.1 to 0.2 ml/min. The total injection time is approximately 1 hour.

## FILMING AND POSITIONING

Filming routines may vary for lower extremity lymphography; however, two sets of routine films are taken. The first set is taken within 1 hour postinjection to demonstrate the lymphatic vessels. A second set is taken 24 hours postinjection to demonstrate the lymph nodes. A suggested routine includes an anteroposterior

(AP) projection of the pelvis and abdomen and right and left posterior oblique (RPO and LPO) positions of the abdomen (Fig. 7–7). Centering for all views is similar to noncontrast views of those areas using 14″ × 17″ cassettes. Additional, or optional, radiography may include a lateral view of the abdomen, an AP of the chest (to demonstrate the thoracic duct), and magnification technique or tomography of selected areas.

## POSTPROCEDURAL CARE

Once the contrast medium injection is completed, the needle is removed, the cutdown incision is sutured, and an antibiotic ointment is applied. The patient is instructed to care for the incision as for any other surgical incision. Sutures are removed in 5 to 7 days. The patient is directed to contact the physician if any infection occurs at the incision site.

## COMPLICATIONS

Complications to lymphography may relate to the (oily) contrast medium used. Pain, and possible vessel rupture, can occur if the medium is injected under too much pressure. Complications of a more serious nature can include pulmonary, cerebral, or hepatic emboli caused by the oily contrast medium reaching these areas through the blood circulation. These can be minimized by using 7 ml (or less) of contrast material per (lower) extremity. Active treatment may be necessary based on patient symptoms.

Infection of the injection site may occur if sterile technique is not maintained.

## FINDINGS

Lymphography is most helpful in confirming previous diagnoses. Pathology in the lymphatic system may be divided into obstructions of the vascular components and those affecting the individual nodes.

Vascular obstructions are best visualized on the initial set of films, while nodal involvements show on the 24-hour series. As in any vessel obstruction, the vessels appear dilated, and collateral circulation may develop (Fig. 7–8). Fistulae may occur and communicate with other areas, for example, the venous system or other hollow organ system (Fig. 7–9). Pathology of the lymph nodes may appear as changes in the size, shape, number, and structure of the nodes. Benign conditions include changes caused by infectious processes, pseudocysts, and replacement of lymph tissues with fat (fibrolipomatosis). Malignant conditions demonstrated include lymphomas (Fig. 7–10), including Hodgkin's disease (Fig. 7–11) and metastases.

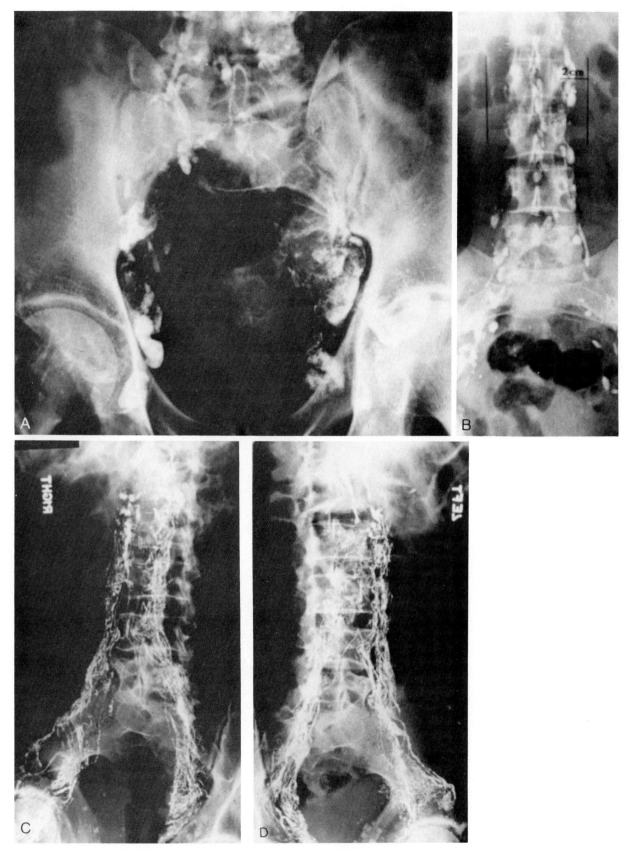

**Figure 7-7.** (*A*) AP projection pelvis; (*B*) AP projection abdomen; (*C*) RPO position abdomen; (*D*) LPO position abdomen. (Courtesy of Medcom Trainex, Garden Grove, CA.)

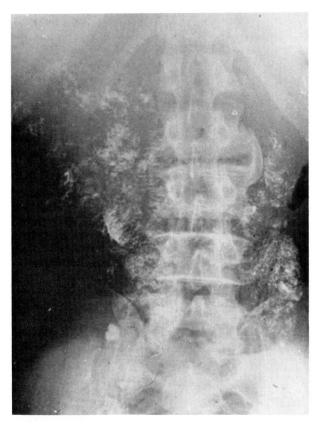

**Figure 7–8.** Obstructed lymph vessel, resulting in reflux into the mesenteric lymph vessels. (Courtesy of Medcom Trainex, Garden Grove, CA.)

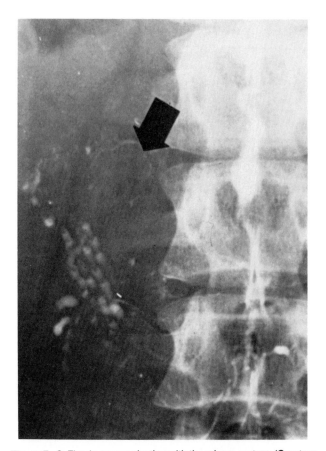

**Figure 7–9.** Fistula communicating with the urinary system. (Courtesy of Medcom Trainex, Garden Grove, CA.)

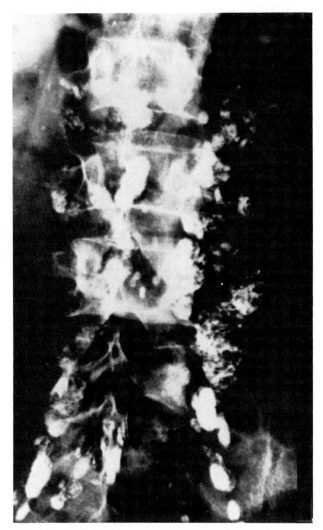

**Figure 7–10.** Non-Hodgkin's type lymphoma. (Courtesy of Medcom Trainex, Garden Grove, CA.)

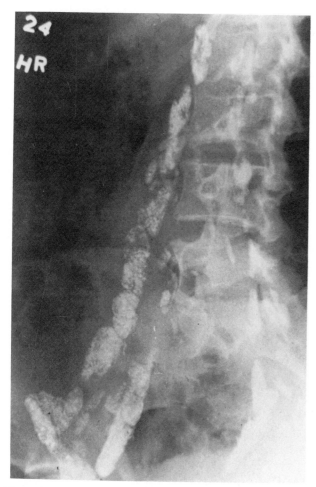

**Figure 7–11.** Hodgkin's disease. (Courtesy of Medcom Trainex, Garden Grove, CA.)

## REVIEW QUESTIONS

1. The lymphatic system is responsible for _____.
   A. removal of pathogenic cells from the body
   B. producing lymphocytes
   C. returning interstitial fluids to the circulation
   D. all of the above

2. Lymph travels in lymphatic vessels by the action of _____.
   A. vessel contractions
   B. extrinsic compressions
   C. interstitial pressure
   D. all of the above

3. Lymph from the lower portions of the body returns to the blood circulation _____.
   A. through the IVC
   B. through the right atrium
   C. at the junction of the right internal jugular and subclavian veins
   D. at the junction of the left internal jugular and subclavian veins

4. Macrophages in the lymphatic system are found _____.
   A. in the cortical layer of a lymph node
   B. in the cisterna chyli
   C. in the reticulum of a lymph node
   D. circulating in lymph

5. A vital dye is used to _____.
   A. opacify the lymphatic system for radiography
   B. mark lymph nodes for surgical removal
   C. aid in visualizing a lymph vessel for contrast injection
   D. outline the area to be radiographed during lymphography

6. Cannulation of a lymph vessel requires _____.
   A. a cutdown procedure
   B. catheterization via a vein
   C. Seldinger technique
   D. a simple puncture

7. The type of contrast medium recommended for lymphography is a (an) _____.
   A. water-soluble iodide
   B. iodized oil
   C. radiolucent medium
   D. barium compound

8. Injection of the contrast medium for pedal lymphography is into a vessel located on (in) the _____.
   A. dorsum of the foot
   B. plantar surface of the foot
   C. webbing between the toes
   D. lateral aspect of the ankle

9. The total contrast medium injection time for lymphography is approximately _____.
   A. 5 minutes
   B. 30 minutes
   C. 1 hour
   D. 4 hours

10. Routine filming for lymphography includes _____ hour(s) postinjection films.
    A. 1
    B. 10
    C. 12
    D. 1 and 24

11. Pulmonary, cerebral, or hepatic emboli are a serious complication of lymphography caused by _____.
    A. the oily nature of the contrast medium
    B. the communication between the lymphatic and circulatory systems
    C. both A and B are correct
    D. thrombus formation in lymphatic vessels

## BIBLIOGRAPHY

Guyton, AC: Anatomy and Physiology. Saunders College Publishing, Philadelphia, 1985.
Johnson, E, et al: Human Anatomy. Saunders College Publishing, Philadelphia, 1985.

Johnsrude, I and Jackson, D: Lymphography (FTMM). MEDCOM (Trainex), New York (Garden Grove), 1975.

Johnsrude, I, Jackson, D, and Dunnick, N: A Practical Approach to Angiography, ed 2. Little Brown & Co, Boston, 1987.

Kadir, S: Diagnostic Angiography. WB Saunders, Philadelphia, 1986.

Miller, B and Keane, C: Encyclopedia and Dictionary of Medicine, Nursing, and Allied Health, ed 4. WB Saunders, Philadelphia, 1987.

Skucas, J: Radiographic Contrast Agents, ed 2. Aspen Publishers, Rockville, MD, 1989.

Tortorici, M: Fundamentals of Angiography. CV Mosby, St Louis, 1982.

# CHAPTER 8

# Myelography

*Patrick J. Apfel, MEd, ARRT(R)*

Myelography is performed to study the spinal canal, spinal cord, and nerve roots through the introduction of a contrast medium. The medium is injected into the subarachnoid space, which surrounds the spinal cord, and allows visualization of the contours of the canal and cord to distinguish possible pathology. By defining the level and extent of abnormalities, myelography is an important method of diagnosis for physicians, particularly for neurosurgeons who need to locate pathologies for surgical treatment. This chapter presents a discussion of myelography of the cervical (C), thoracic (T), and lumbar (L) levels of the spine.

## ANATOMY

The spinal cord is that portion of the central nervous system (CNS) that extends from the base of the brain (medulla oblongata), through the foramen magnum (of the skull) and spinal canal, to the level of the interspace between the first and second lumbar vertebrae, L-1 and L-2 (Fig. 8 – 1). At this level, the cord is constricted to a cone-shaped tip termed the conus medullaris. Below this level, a collection of nerve roots, termed cauda equina, extend from the cord and fill the spinal canal to the level of the second sacral segment. The individual vertebrae of the spinal column and meninges (membranes) enclose and provide protection for the delicate nervous tissues of the spinal cord and cauda equina. A typical vertebra is composed of a vertebral body and a neural arch. Portions of the arch itself can be identified as the pedicle, lamina, transverse and spinous processes, and superior and inferior articular processes (Fig. 8 – 2A). Together the vertebral body and neural arch form an opening, the vertebral foramen. The spinal canal is then shaped by all of the individual vertebrae of the spinal column as they are stacked upon each other with the vertebral foramina aligned to form the canal. The bony canal provides protection for the spinal cord, which passes through it. Along the length of the vertebral column, vertebrae differ in size, shape, and, in some instances, even structure (e.g., in the adult, the first cervical vertebra has no body) from one

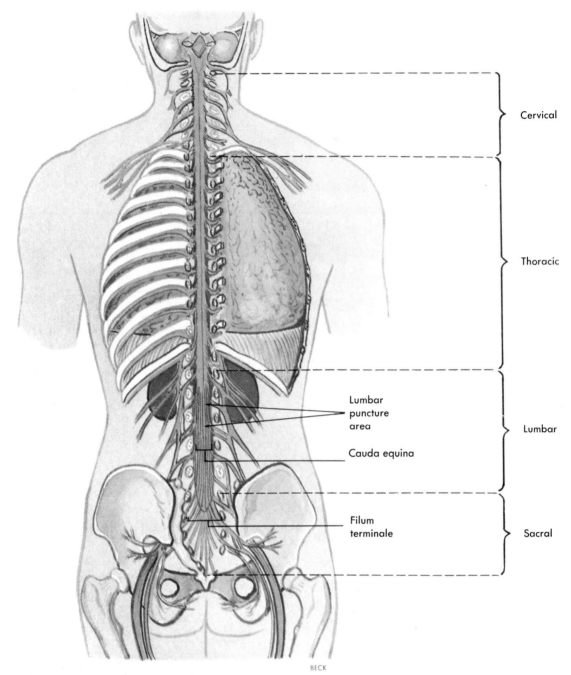

Cervical

Thoracic

Lumbar
puncture
area

Cauda equina

Lumbar

Filum
terminale

Sacral

BECK

**Figure 8–1.** Posterior view of spinal cord. (Adapted from Anthony, CP and Thibodeau, GA: Textbook of Anatomy and Physiology, ed 10. Mosby-Year Book, St Louis, 1979, p 226, with permission.)

level of the spine to the next (Fig. 8–2B). This affects the diameter and shape of the spinal canal and cord. The cord itself varies in width and has two major enlargements. The first is the cervical enlargement, which extends from C-3 to T-2, with the maximum width of approximately 38 mm at the level of C-5, C-6. The second enlargement, termed the lumbar enlargement, extends from T-9 to L-2 with a maximum width of approximately 33 mm at the level of T-12.

The anterior surface of the canal is lined with a strong longitudinal ligament, while the posterior aspect

is lined with the ligamenta flava. Both ligaments run the length of the canal. The cord is surrounded by the same three meninges, or membranes, that cover the brain. The outermost membrane is the dura mater, the middle is the arachnoid, and the innermost is the pia mater. Cerebrospinal fluid (CSF), which is produced in the ventricles of the brain, circulates within the subarachnoid space, below the arachnoid membrane (Fig. 8–3). This fluid acts as a shock absorber to protect the brain and spinal cord from injury and as a barrier to certain harmful substances such as metallic poisons and patho-

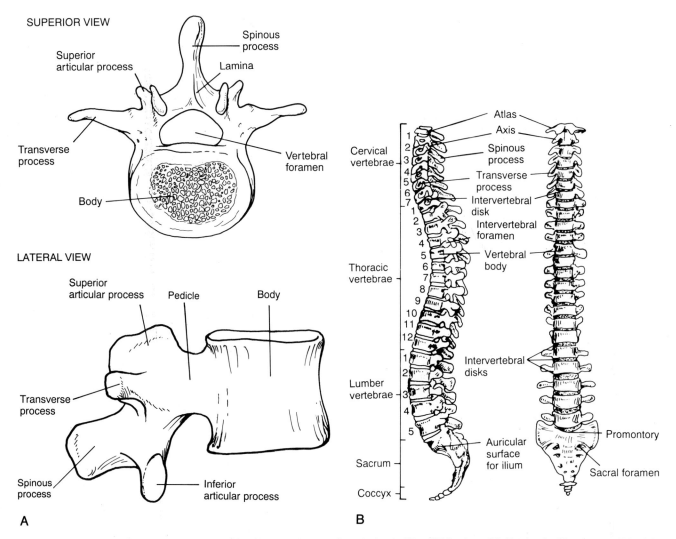

**Figure 8-2.** (*A*) Vertebral structure: superior and lateral views. (Adapted from Anthony, CP and Thibodeau, GA: Textbook of Anatomy and Physiology, ed 10. Mosby-Year Book, St Louis, 1979, p 101, with permission.) (*B*) AP and lateral view of bony spine. (Adapted from Scanlon, VC and Sanders, T: Essentials of Anatomy and Physiology, ed 2. FA Davis, Philadelphia, 1994, with permission.)

gens. CSF is also thought to play a role in metabolism. Thus, the spinal cord itself is protected by bone, ligaments, meninges, and spinal fluid.

Between the vertebral bodies are intervertebral disks, which are responsible for absorbing shock to the spinal column itself. The disks are composed of an outer layer of tough fibrous and fibrocartilage tissues termed the annulus fibrosus. The annulus fibrosus surrounds the inner disk portion composed of a semigelatinous, elastic material termed the nucleus pulposus (Fig. 8-4).

In the adult, the spinal cord is between 18″ and 20″ long. Along the length of the cord itself, 31 pairs of spinal nerves or nerve roots arise from the cord and extend out between the vertebrae to innervate various parts of the body. Openings between vertebrae, which transmit spinal nerves along with blood vessels, are termed intervertebral foramina. The paired spinal nerves are divided into 8 cervical, 12 thoracic, 5 lumbar, 5 sacral, and 1 coccygeal. Because the cord termi-

nates at the level of the interspace between L-1 and L-2, spinal nerves extend from this level through the canal to the level of the second sacral segment. This collection of nerves is termed the cauda equina because it resembles a horse's tail.

The spinal cord and nerves function as a sensory, motor, and reflex system. Messages received by nerves from various areas of the body are transmitted to the brain through the spinal cord. Once the messages are received by the brain, it interprets them and then decides a response, which may be either voluntary or involuntary. This response is then transmitted through the spinal cord and nerves back to the appropriate area. Involuntary responses resulting in actions transmitted from the brain through the spinal cord include those affecting the heartbeat, respiration, digestion, and so on. Examples of voluntary actions are speech, purposeful muscle contractions resulting in voluntary movement, and problem-solving mental processes.

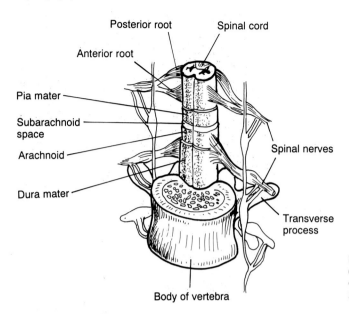

**Figure 8-3.** Transverse section of spinal cord and meninges. (Adapted from Anthony, CP and Thibodeau, GA: Textbook of Anatomy and Physiology, ed 10. Mosby-Year Book, St Louis, 1979, p 233, with permission.)

## INDICATIONS

Myelography is performed when patient symptoms, such as pain or numbness, indicate that a lesion may be present within the spinal canal or is protruding into it. These lesions include both benign and malignant tumors, cysts, herniated nucleus pulposus (HNP), and extradural masses or bone fragments caused by trauma. Most pathology and trauma occur in the cervical and lumbar areas; hence, most myelographic procedures are performed at these levels. Because HNP is the most common pathologic finding of myelography, a discussion of this syndrome is presented.

Herniated nucleus pulposus is a herniation of the pulpy inner portion of the vertebral disk, the nucleus pulposus, into the spinal canal. Each vertebral disk has a tough fibrous outer covering known as the annulus fibrosus. The wall of the annulus fibrosus varies in thickness and is thicker anteriorly than posteriorly. Undue pressure to the disk, caused by improper lifting or bending, or trauma to the disk can result in a fracture to the annulus fibrosus with a herniation or escape of the inner nucleus pulposus. Because the posterior wall of

the annulus fibrosus is thinner than its anterior wall, the tendency is for a disk to rupture posteriorly, that is, toward the spinal cord. Because the strong posterior longitudinal ligament lies along the posterior aspect of the vertebral bodies and disks, the contents of a ruptured disk are somewhat restrained by the ligament and directed laterally. Therefore, most ruptures of the nucleus pulposus occur in a posterolateral direction, exerting abnormal pressures against the spinal nerves or the cord itself (Fig. 8-4).

Symptoms of HNP include numbness, pain, or a burning sensation in a particular area of the body, especially the extremities. These symptoms may be chronic, temporary, or intermittent. Chronic symptoms may be caused by a partial or total disk rupture. Temporary or intermittent symptoms can occur when either the disk does not actually rupture but instead bulges or protrudes during times of stress or the disk actually ruptures but is restrained by the posterior longitudinal ligament. Both conditions exert temporary pressure against the cord itself or the spinal nerves, causing temporary or intermittent symptoms. Most herniations occur at the level of L-5, S-1 interspace or L-4, L-5 in-

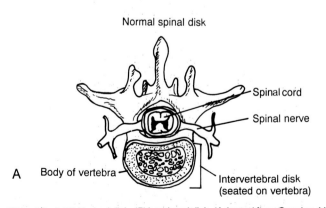

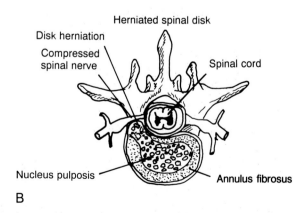

**Figure 8-4.** (A) Normal disk; (B) herniated disk. (Adapted from Scanlon, VC and Sanders, T: Essentials of Anatomy and Physiology, ed 2. FA Davis, Philadelphia, 1994, with permission.)

terspace. Treatment for HNP varies from conservative (i.e., bed rest and reduced physical activity) in less severe cases to surgical removal of the disk, or portions of it, in more severe cases.

## CONTRAINDICATIONS

The contraindications to myelography include sensitivity to iodine or contrast media, arachnoiditis, the presence of blood in the CSF, abnormal intracranial pressure, and a spinal puncture performed within 2 weeks of the present study. Known patient sensitivity to iodine or contrast media can indicate a possible patient reaction to the injection of the contrast medium during the procedure. In a patient with a local infection, injection of contrast material can increase the severity of the condition, or spread the inflammation further. The presence of blood in the CSF indicates bleeding within the canal or an irritation within the canal, which can be further increased by the contrast medium. When increased intracranial pressure exists, a spinal puncture can cause a sudden change in that pressure. This can result in severe complications to the patient as the system attempts to equalize the pressure between the area of the brain and spinal canal. If a previous puncture has been performed recently, there is a chance that contrast medium will extravasate through the old puncture site during the current myelography.

## PREPROCEDURAL CARE

Most patients scheduled for myelography exhibit apprehension of the examination. To reduce their anxiety and fear, a sedative or muscle relaxant may be prescribed for injection 1 hour prior to the procedure.

The exact premedication is determined by the attending physician and is often selected in accordance with the patient's condition and individual needs. A common drug and dosage used is 10 mg of diazepam (Valium) given intramuscularly.

Because there is a chance of reaction to the contrast medium, the procedure should be thoroughly explained to the patient by the physician performing the procedure before the examination proceeds. Explanation of the procedure also helps to alleviate patient anxiety. Once the patient is advised and understands the procedure and possible complications, an informed consent is signed by the patient.

For patients being examined with water-soluble contrast media, all neuroleptic drugs (agents that modify psychotic symptoms) should be withheld for 48 hours before the procedure. To ensure hydration, fluids are encouraged up to the procedure. No food intake is recommended for 2 hours before the examination.

Once the preprocedural care is completed, the patient is brought to the radiographic room and placed on the x-ray table, where the injection site is prepared (see Injection Procedure section of this chapter).

## EQUIPMENT

### Major Equipment

The major equipment for myelography includes a radiographic-fluoroscopic room with a 90-degree two-way tilt table with footrest, ankle boots, and shoulder supports (Fig. 8–5). Filming for myelography includes both radiographic exposures and fluoroscopic spot films. During the procedure the table and patient are tilted into upright and Trendelenburg's positions. This technique uses the force of gravity to move the contrast

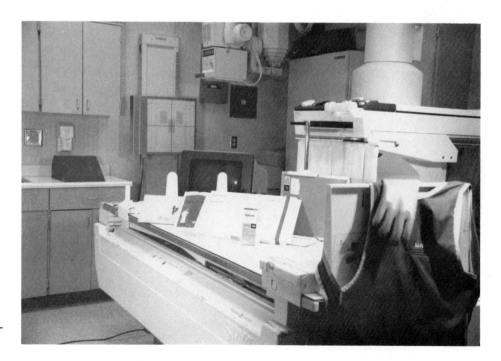

**Figure 8–5.** Fluoroscopic room setup for myelography.

medium along the length of the subarachnoid space and allows visualization of the different levels of the spinal canal and cord. The footboard supports the patient when upright, while the shoulder braces and ankle boots brace the patient when the table is in Trendelenburg's position.

## Accessory Equipment

Accessory equipment for myelography includes a myelography tray, prep razor, contrast medium, antiseptic solution, sterile gloves (worn whenever touching sterile items in the tray), laboratory requisitions for CSF analysis, a firm pillow or large positioning sponge, cassettes and grids or grid cassettes (appropriate number and size for the area under examination), and a cassette holder for cross-table exposures (Fig. 8–5).

Sterile, disposable myelographic trays are commercially available. Reusable trays may be prepared and maintained by the radiology department and sterilized by central supply. To optimize sterile technique and reduce cross-contamination associated with reusable items, it is recommended that disposable units be employed. In either case, the tray must be sterile. Although tray contents may vary somewhat, a typical commercial tray contains the following items: a compartment for antiseptic solution; three prep sponges; a Band-Aid; towel(s); gauze sponges; a fenestrated drape; one 5- and one 20-ml syringe; 18-, 22-, and 25-gauge needles; an 18-gauge spinal needle with stylet; extension tubing; a 5-ml vial of local anesthetic, such as 1 percent lidocaine (Xylocaine); and test tubes (Fig. 8–6).

## INJECTION PROCEDURE

There are two common puncture sites of the spinal canal for myelography, the lumbar and basal cistern regions. Typically, the lumbar area is chosen because it is safer and easier on the patient. The cisternal area is chosen when the lumbar area is contraindicated. This may be because of local infection or because there is a suspected blockage of the spinal canal, which could stop the flow of contrast medium to the upper spinal area, precluding examination of that region. Once the site is chosen, the puncture site is prepared and the patient is positioned for the puncture.

Some of the accessory items and the items on the myelography tray are used to prepare the injection site and perform the puncture. The puncture site is shaved to remove any body hair that may harbor organisms which may be pathogenic if introduced into the body during the injection process. The skin is then cleaned with an antiseptic solution (e.g., Betadine) to further remove any organisms that may be present. The solution is applied with a prep sponge using a circular motion from the center of the injection site outward. This process is repeated three times, using a new prep sponge each time. When finished, the cleaned area should be approximately 4″ to 6″ in diameter. The area is then draped, with the opening of a fenestrated drape centered on the puncture site, and anesthetized using the 5-ml syringe with either the 22- or 25-gauge needle. The skin and underlying tissues are injected with the local anesthetic.

For the lumbar puncture, the patient is prone on the radiographic table with a firm pillow or positioning

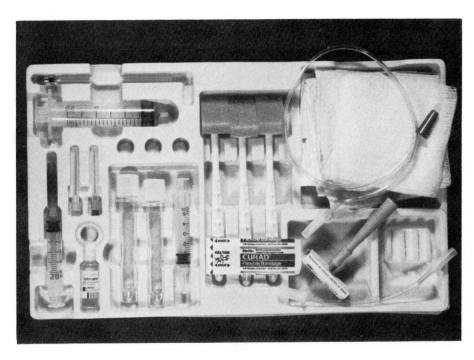

**Figure 8–6.** Accessory equipment for myelography.

sponge under the abdomen. This aids in straightening, or reversing, the normal lordotic curvature of the lumbar spine, which expands the space between adjacent neural arches and allows the spinal needle to pass more easily between them. The common site of injection is at the level of the L-3, L-4 interspace. This level is chosen to avoid damage to the spinal cord by the needle itself, because the cord ends at the interspace between L-1 and L-2. Also, placement of the needle at this level, rather than at the L-4, L-5 or the L-5, S-1 interspace, avoids needle artifacts, which can be confused as disk pathology that commonly occurs at these lower levels. If disk pathology is known to exist at the L-3, L-4 level (from patient history or symptoms or previous studies) or this level is otherwise undesirable, an alternate level may be chosen. During needle placement, the radiologist may use fluoroscopy to guide the needle into the appropriate location. The needle is inserted through the skin and underlying tissues between the neural arches of L-3 and L-4 and into the subarachnoid space. An indication that the needle is within the space is a backflow of spinal fluid through the needle.

For a cisternal puncture the patient is positioned upright or prone with the chin flexed. Preparation for the needle placement procedure is similar to that for the lumbar area, with the radiologist using fluoroscopy to monitor the process. The needle is inserted between the occipital bone and C-1 into the cisterna cerebellomedullaris (cisterna magna). A slight pop can be felt by the physician as the needle punctures the dura mater. Unobstructed flow of CSF back through the spinal needle indicates entrance into the area of the subarachnoid space.

For either puncture, CSF is collected in the test tube(s) by allowing it to drip from the spinal needle. As the spinal fluid is collected, the tubes are numbered in the order they were filled and labeled with the patient's identification (i.e., name, number, and so on). Appropriate laboratory requests are completed, and the CSF is sent to the laboratory for analysis. Specific tests to be performed on the fluid will be a protocol of the individual physician or department. Although CSF laboratory testing will vary, typical analyses include blood cell counts (both red [RBC] and white [WBC]), protein level, sugar level, and a Venereal Disease Research Laboratories (VDRL) test. An elevated RBC, WBC, or protein level can indicate a hemorrhage, an infectious process, or brain tumors, respectively. A low sugar level can indicate meningitis. A positive VDRL can signify syphilis.

Once the CSF has been collected through the spinal needle, the contrast medium is injected, through the same needle, into the subarachnoid space for visualization and filming.

## CONTRAST MEDIA

An ideal contrast medium for myelography would be one that mixes well with CSF, is readily absorbed by the body, is nonreactive with body substances or to the patient, and provides good radiopacity. Although no con-

trast medium currently produced meets all of the requirements mentioned, air or gas, oil-based, and water-soluble agents have been most commonly used for myelography. The type of medium employed is determined by the radiologist to provide the best diagnostic information in consideration of the patient's condition.

## Radiolucent Contrast Media

Procedures using radiolucent media, such as air or gas, are rare. However, radiolucent or negative media can be employed in specific instances, such as when the patient has a sensitivity to iodine, for the detection of a total blockage of the spinal canal above L-4, to visualize a cervical disk herniation, or for certain trauma cases. A radiolucent medium is totally absorbed and is not known to cause patient reaction. Although they are relatively safe, radiolucent media, in general, do not provide good radiopacity, under fluoroscopy, with surrounding tissues in the spinal areas and are difficult to move in the spinal canal. The amount of gas or air used for myelography is 40 to 100 ml, depending on the spinal level under examination.

## Oil-Based Contrast Media

Although oil-based media were used extensively for myelography into the mid-1970s, they have been virtually replaced by water-soluble media. Oil-based media provided good radiopacity but poor visualization of the nerve roots. A definite drawback to this agent was that it had to be removed from the spinal canal when the examination was completed because it was not readily absorbed (the absorption rate is roughly 1 ml/y) or excreted by the body. To facilitate removal of the contrast medium, the spinal needle was left in place during the procedure, which required obvious caution in moving the patient and precluded supine positioning. The oil-based medium of choice for myelography was bottled under the trademark name of Pantopaque.

## Water-Soluble Contrast Media

Water-soluble contrast media have been in use in the United States since the late 1970s (longer in the European countries). The popularity of this medium can be attributed to its low viscosity, its ability to provide excellent visualization of nerve roots, and the fact that it is rapidly absorbed and excreted by the body. Aqueous media are totally absorbed and excreted within 48 hours; therefore, there is no need to remove the water-soluble medium when the procedure is finished. This allows more flexibility in patient positioning because the spinal needle can be removed once the contrast medium is injected and the patient can be easily moved into any position. A drawback to aqueous media is that because they are absorbed rather quickly, the filming procedure must be expedited. Absorption begins approximately 30 minutes after injection. Refilming for additional information may require the injection of more medium. There is good radiopacity for about 1 hour, with a hazy radiographic appearance after 4 to 5 hours. There is no radiographic visualization of the medium after 24 hours. The recommended dose varies from 7 to 17 ml, depending on the concentration used and the area of the canal to be examined. The injection process is slow, taking about 1 to 2 minutes. This is done to avoid excessive mixing of the medium with CSF, which results in a loss of optimal radiographic contrast.

For injection, the contrast medium is drawn up in the 20-ml syringe. The vial containing the medium is kept until the procedure is completed. The lot number of the contrast medium is recorded, if this is required by department protocol.

## FILMING AND POSITIONING

Filming routines, both fluoroscopic and radiographic, vary according to the physician's preference, the area examined, the type of contrast medium employed, and the patient's condition. If employing air or gas as a contrast medium, tomography of the area of interest provides optimal visualization. Lateral positions are primarily used, and the whole procedure, including the injection process, can be performed in a tomographic room.

Following injection of water-soluble medium, the spinal needle is removed, and the patient may be positioned either prone, supine, or lateral and in either anterior and posterior oblique positions. During fluoroscopy, the table and patient can be tilted from upright to Trendelenburg's position to facilitate flow of contrast to the area of interest. Whenever the table is in Trendelenburg's position, the patient's chin *must remain hyperextended* to prevent the contrast medium from entering the area of the head. Once fluoroscopic spot filming is completed, routine radiographs are taken by the radiographer. Radiographic positioning is dictated by the area of interest. Under fluoroscopic control, the radiologist tilts the table at the appropriate angle to pool the contrast medium at the level of interest for routine radiography.

Recommended radiography for the cervical region includes two lateral views with the patient's chin hyperextended. The views are a transcervical (cross-table) lateral and a swimmer's lateral, with the central ray directed to the level of C-4 for the transcervical and to the level of C-7 for the swimmer's lateral (Fig. 8–7A).

A general routine for the thoracic region includes a right lateral decubitus (RLD), left lateral decubitus (LLD), either AP or PA projection, and a right or left lateral with the central ray to T-7 (Fig. 8–7B). Decubitus positioning is recommended rather than supine or prone positioning for an AP or PA projection because contrast medium at the thoracic level would tend to pool in certain areas because of the normal kyphotic curvature of the thoracic spine. In a decubitus position

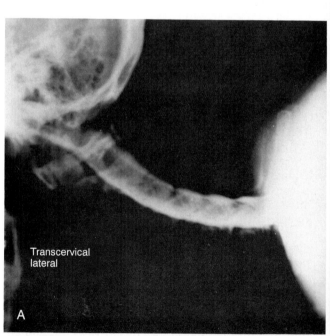
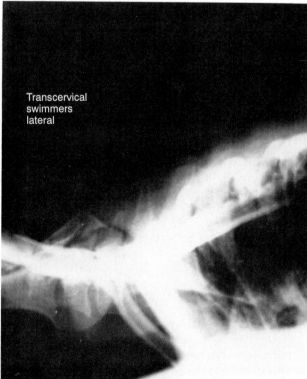

**Figure 8–7.** Radiography of cervical area (*A*); thoracic area (*B*); and lumbar area (*C*).

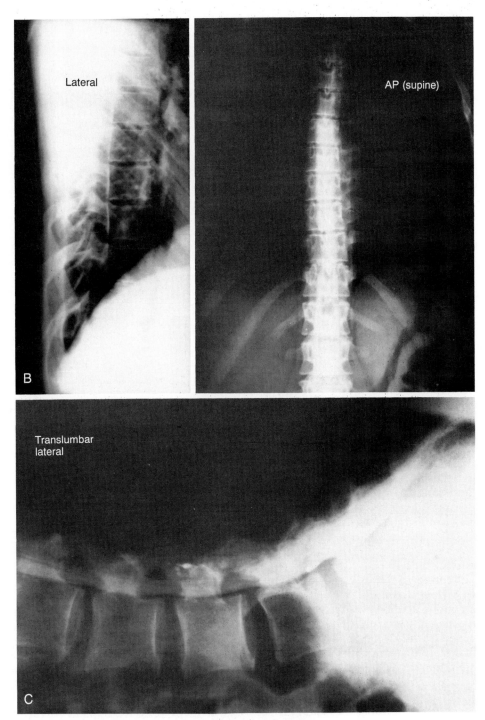

**Figure 8–7** *Continued.*

(with the spine parallel to the table top), the contrast medium fills only the dependent half (or down side) of the thoracic area. Because the RLD position demonstrates only the right half of the spinal canal, an LLD is required for complete visualization of the entire thoracic area (in an AP or a PA projection). The decubiti positions also allow for good visualization of the bases of the nerve roots on the dependent side of the spinal cord. The lateral view can be taken as either a right or left lateral with positioning similar to a lateral of the thoracic spine.

The lumbar area generally requires only a semierect translumbar, or cross-table, lateral view with the central ray directed to L-3 (Fig. 8–7C). Additional or optional radiography may include PA or AP projections and oblique and decubitus positions.

## POSTPROCEDURAL CARE

When the spinal needle is removed, the puncture site should be covered with a bandage. Care of the patient following an air-gas contrast medium injection for myelography is essentially the same care given to any patient having a spinal puncture. The patient should remain hospitalized for observation and lie flat in bed for 24 hours.

When myelography employing a water-soluble medium is completed, the patient should be maintained in a semierect position of 15 to 30 degrees while being transported by gurney and while in bed. The patient should be restricted to bed for several hours and observed for 12 hours after the procedure. After about 8 hours the patient may lie flat. Fluids and food should be encouraged.

## COMPLICATIONS AND PRECAUTIONS

The passage of air through the subarachnoid space into the ventricles of the brain can cause the patient to experience a severe, temporary headache. Therefore, a severe semierect or totally erect position should be avoided during and after the procedure. Other side effects and complications as a result of myelography vary in extent from minor to severe. Complications can generally be divided into either procedural or reaction effects.

There are several complications that may be a direct result of the procedure. Any spinal puncture may produce headaches and nausea. Injection of the contrast medium into the inappropriate space (i.e., epidural or subdural) presents a problem because the medium can obscure visualization of the structure(s) being examined. Spinal needles may also be inadvertently positioned so as to cause irritation to nerve tissue and consequent patient discomfort. Excessive subarachnoid bleeding because of the puncture process can increase the severity of arachnoiditis when present. Inadequate filling of the subarachnoid space can result in poor visualization of structures or pathology. Pathology of other levels of the spinal canal (i.e., other than that level ordered for examination) can be missed unless the entire canal is surveyed with fluoroscopy during the procedure.

Adverse reactions to the contrast medium can be minor or severe. Caution is advised in pregnant or nursing women because safe use of water-soluble media in these individuals has not been established. The most frequently occurring reactions to water-based media are headaches, nausea, and vomiting. Less frequently, exaggeration of previously existing symptoms (sciatica, leg pain, and so on) occurs on a temporary basis. Reports of chest pains, abnormal heart rates, changes in blood pressure, seizures, aseptic meningitis, allergic symptoms (such as nasal congestion and dyspnea), and central nervous system abnormalities (including hallucinations, depression, and disorientation) have occurred. It is important to note that the occurrence of the latter symptoms is rare. Care should be taken to

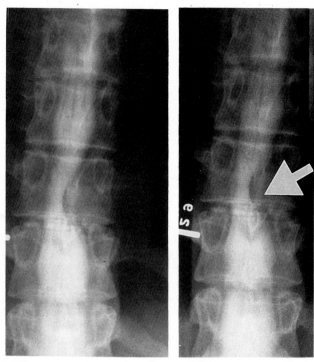

**Figure 8–8.** Herniated nucleus pulposus from T-10 to T-11 interspace.

avoid spilling the medium into the cisternal and ventricular areas (may cause seizures). It is also advised to move the patient slowly (i.e., avoid abrupt position changes) to prevent excessive mixing of the contrast medium with the CSF.

## FINDINGS

Radiographic findings are consistent with indications. Pathologies include benign and malignant tumors, cysts, HNP, and abnormalities caused by trauma. Typical findings include meningocele (herniation of meninges), meningioma (tumor along meningeal vessels), glioma (nerve tissue tumor), and metastatic lesions. A cyst frequently found is one of the nerve root sheath (covering). Trauma, resulting in pressure on the spinal cord, can be represented by fractures of the neural arch with a depressed arch or arch fragments encroaching on the spinal cord or by misalignment of vertebrae (e.g., spondylolisthesis) with subsequent pressure applied to the cord. The most common finding is HNP (Fig. 8–8). Degrees of herniation vary in severity and treatment. Most disk ruptures occur in the lumbar region because of poor lifting or bending movements.

## REVIEW QUESTIONS

1. The spinal cord itself extends _____.
   A. the length of the spinal canal
   B. from the foramen magnum to L-1
   C. from the medulla oblongata to L-1, L-2
   D. from the medulla oblongata to the second sacral segment

2. CSF is produced in the _____.
   A. ventricles of the brain
   B. spinal cord itself
   C. subarachnoid space
   D. subdural space

3. The outer portion of an intervertebral disk is termed the _____.
   A. cauda equina
   B. annulus fibrosus
   C. nucleus pulposus
   D. nucleus fibrosus

4. State the three membranes surrounding the spinal cord, starting with the inner membrane.

5. Most pathology and trauma occur in the _____ and _____ levels of the spinal cord.
   A. cervical, thoracic
   B. cervical, lumbar
   C. thoracic, lumbar
   D. lumbar, sacral

6. Herniation of an intervertebral disk is termed _____.
   A. HPN
   B. HAN
   C. HNP
   D. NPH

7. When an intervertebral disk herniates, it tends to do so in a(n) _____ direction.
   A. posterior
   B. lateral
   C. posterolateral
   D. anterior

8. Most intervertebral disk herniations occur at the level of _____ interspace.
   A. C-1, C-2
   B. C-5, C-5
   C. L-3
   D. L-5, S-1 or L-4, L-5

9. The typical puncture site for myelography is at the level of the _____, _____ interspace.
   A. C-1, base of skull
   B. T-12, L-1
   C. L-3, L-4
   D. L-5, S-1

10. A cisternal puncture for myelography is _____.
    A. never done
    B. done to evaluate only the cervical area
    C. done to evaluate the cervical and thoracic areas
    D. done if there is a suspected blockage of the lower canal

11. Contrast medium, for myelography, is injected into the _____.
    A. epidural space
    B. subdural space
    C. subarachnoid space
    D. no answer is correct

12. A positive VDRL analysis indicates _____.
    A. arachnoiditis
    B. brain tumors
    C. syphilis
    D. meningitis

13. _____ contrast media can be used for myelography.
    A. Radiolucent
    B. Oil-based
    C. Water-soluble
    D. All of the above

14. An advantage of using an aqueous medium for myelography is _____.
    A. nerve roots can be visualized
    B. it is absorbed and excreted
    C. supine and prone positions are possible
    D. all answers are correct

15. Conventional radiographs of the cervical area for myelography include _____.
    A. AP projection and lateral position
    B. AP projection, lateral, and oblique positions
    C. lateral position only
    D. lateral and swimmer's lateral positions

16. Conventional radiographs of the thoracic area for myelography include _____.
    A. AP projection and lateral position
    B. AP projection, lateral, and swimmer's lateral positions
    C. RLD and LLD positions
    D. RLD, LLD, and lateral positions

17. Conventional radiographs of the lumbar area for myelography include _____.
    A. AP projection and lateral position
    B. AP projection, RPO, LPO, and lateral positions
    C. lateral, RLD, and LLD positions
    D. translateral only

18. The most common radiographic finding of myelography is _____.
    A. metastatic cancer
    B. meningocele
    C. herniated disk
    D. glioma

## BIBLIOGRAPHY

Ballinger, P: Merrill's Atlas of Radiographic Positions and Radiologic Procedures, ed 7. Mosby-Year Book, St Louis, 1991.

Bontrager, K and Anthony, B: Radiographic Positioning and Related Anatomy, ed 3. Mosby-Year Book, St Louis, 1993.

Donovan Post, J: Radiographic Evaluation of the Spine: Current Advances with Emphasis on Computed Tomography. Masson Publishing, New York, 1980.

Gray, H: Gray's Anatomy, Classic Collector's Edition. Bounty Books, New York, 1977.

McInnes, J: Clark's Positioning in Radiography, Vol 2, ed 9. Year Book Medical Publishers, Chicago, 1974.

Miller, B and Keane, C: Encyclopedia and Dictionary of Medicine, Nursing and Allied Health, ed 4. WB Saunders, Philadelphia, 1987.

Omnipaque injection (iohexol), Winthrop-Breon, New York, NY, 1985.

Pantopaque Iophendylate injection USP. Lafayette Pharmaceuticals, Lafayette, IN, 1980.

Skucas, J: Radiographic Contrast Agents, ed 2. Aspen Publishers, Rockville, MD, 1989.

# CHAPTER 9

# Sialography

*Patrick J. Apfel, MEd, ARRT(R)*

Sialography is an infrequently performed radiographic study of the salivary glands. The glands and their respective ducts can become inflamed or obstructed by a variety of pathologies. Because the density of the glands and ducts is similar to that of surrounding tissues, a contrast medium is used to visualize these structures. Although sialography is a safe and simple procedure, it is sometimes difficult to perform because the ducts leading to the glands are often hard to locate and catheterize.

## ANATOMY

There are three pairs of salivary glands surrounding the area of the mouth (Fig. 9–1). The largest pair are the parotid glands, which are lateral to the mandible and lie anterior and inferior to the ear. For the most part, they extend over the external surface of the ramus of the mandible. Their shape is somewhat like an inverted triangle with the base of the triangle extending across the superior portion of the mandibular ramus and with the tip of the triangle pointing to the mandibular angle. Each gland is drained by the parotid (also termed Stensen's) duct, which is approximately 7 cm in length. This duct runs from the gland to an opening in the parotid papilla (a nipplelike tissue mound) located on the inner aspect of the cheek adjacent to the second upper molar. Within the gland the duct extends in branches through the glandular tissues.

The second largest pair of glands are the submandibular (also termed submaxillary) glands. These glands are considerably smaller than the parotid glands and lie under the floor of the mouth, internal to and slightly inferior to the body of the mandible. They extend anteriorly from the angle of the mandible toward the mandibular symphysis. The glands are drained by the submandibular (Wharton's) duct, which opens in a slightly mobile papilla lateral to the frenulum, the membrane that attaches the tongue to the floor of the mouth. The duct is approximately 5 cm long and within the gland extends in branches. The orifice of the duct is often difficult to locate.

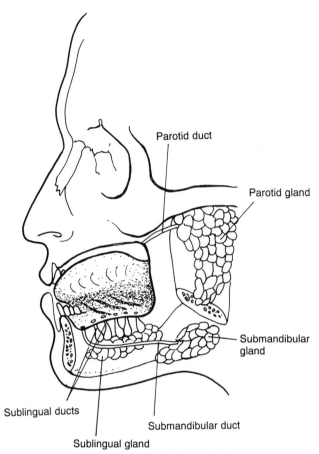

Figure 9-1. Diagram of salivary glands.

The third and smallest pair of glands are the sublingual glands, lying beneath the floor of the mouth under the area of the tongue. They are located on either side of the mandibular symphysis and extend posteriorly from it. These glands are drained by several ducts. The primary duct is Bartholin's, which opens on the floor of the mouth, lateral to Wharton's duct. In addition, there are a series of ducts, termed the ducts of Rivinus, which open along the floor of the mouth, beneath the tongue. Identification of the orifice of Bartholin's duct is difficult.

Although they are not examined by sialography, there are minor salivary glands located in the tongue and lining of the mouth.

## INDICATIONS

There are several indications for sialography. These include inflammatory lesions, either obstructive or nonobstructive, with symptoms of recurrent pain or swelling in the area of the parotid or submandibular glands; a palpable mass in the area of the glands; symptoms indicating calculi (e.g., pain or swelling) or infection; and dryness of the mouth and eyes of unknown origin.

## CONTRAINDICATIONS

Sialography is contraindicated when the patient has parotitis (mumps), which is a viral disease affecting primarily the parotid glands. This condition may also affect the submaxillary glands, gonads, and central nervous system.

## PREPROCEDURAL CARE

Preprocedural care is minimum with no premedication or fasting required. As with any contrast medium examination, the procedure and any possible complications should be explained to the patient and an informed consent signed.

## EQUIPMENT

### Major Equipment

The major equipment required for sialography is a radiographic and fluoroscopic room. Although the procedure can be accomplished in a conventional radiographic room, a specialized head unit or fluoroscopy may also be used. The choice of major equipment to be used is determined by the department's or radiologist's protocol.

### Accessory Equipment

The accessory equipment includes those items necessary for catheterization of the ducts, injection of the contrast medium, and filming of the glands (Fig. 9-2).

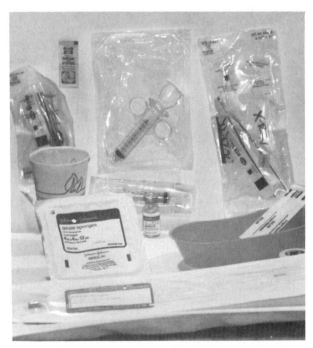

Figure 9-2. Accessory equipment for sialography.

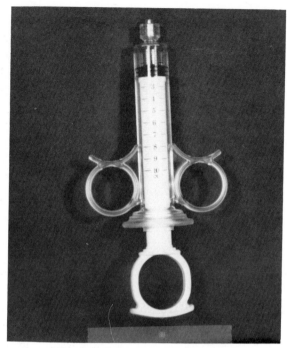

**Figure 9-3.** Pressure control syringe.

Suggested items for catheterization include a sialo-gogue, tincture of benzoin, lacrimal probes, blunt nee-dles, Rabinov sialography catheters, forceps, and a light. For the injection process, a 10-ml syringe, the contrast agent, and gauze or tissue are required. If an oil-based contrast medium is employed, a glass pressure control syringe (Fig. 9-3) is suggested for the injection to maintain a continuous low pressure. In filming the glands, $8'' \times 10''$ cassettes are generally adequate for routine and fluoroscopic imaging. The number of cas-settes required depends on the filming protocol for the gland(s) being examined.

## INJECTION PROCEDURE

Of the three pairs of salivary glands, only the parotid and submandibular glands are examined with a con-trast medium. The parotid gland is the easier gland to examine because its ductal opening is larger and rela-tively easy to locate as compared with that of the sub-mandibular duct.

The sublingual glands are not examined with a con-trast medium because of the difficulty in locating the orifice of Bartholin's duct and in distinguishing it from the opening of Wharton's duct. Limited radiography, without a contrast medium, can be done on the sublin-gual glands to demonstrate obvious pathology such as a radiopaque calculus.

Most of the difficulty during sialography is encoun-tered by the radiologist in locating the ductal openings. A bright light is needed to illuminate the area within the mouth during this process, for example, an adjust-able floor lamp or head lamp. To facilitate locating the opening of a salivary duct, a sialogogue (or secretory stimulant) such as a lemon is used to dilate the open-ing. Prior to catheter insertion, the patient is directed to suck on the lemon wedge. This stimulates secretion of saliva and consequent opening of the duct. If the duct is not sufficiently opened by this stimulus, a lacrimal (tear duct) probe, which has a blunt, tapered tip, or a blunt-tipped needle can be employed to dilate the duct. If the duct is still difficult to locate, tincture of benzoin can be used in the area of the duct to tint the tissues to aid in visualization of the duct opening.

When the duct is located and dilated, the appropriate Rabinov catheter is inserted. These catheters are spe-cially designed for sialography. They are tapered, blunt, metal-tipped catheters with a clear, flexible tub-ing attached to accommodate a syringe for injection. For the parotid gland, the Rabinov no. 32 is used. This catheter's tip has a side hole and is 0.032″ in diameter. When examining the submandibular gland, the no. 16 Rabinov is used. The tip on the no. 16 has an end hole and is 0.016″ in diameter. Once the catheter is in-serted, its tapered conformation aids in keeping it within the duct. For the injection, a 10-ml syringe with the appropriate contrast agent is attached to the cath-eter tubing and the contrast is injected. A glass, pres-sure control syringe is recommended to maintain the low pressure desired when injecting an oily medium. When a water-soluble medium is used, it may be in-jected via a syringe or by a hydrostatic method, which is similar to an IV drip method of injection. If the hydro-static injection is employed, an open syringe (i.e., less the plunger) connected to the Rabinov catheter, by ap-propriate tubing, can be suspended above the level of the patient's head. The flow of contrast medium during the injection can be controlled by a simple in-line valve or clamp.

The contrast medium is injected until the patient ex-periences pressure or pain within the gland. When the duct and gland are filled with contrast medium, via a sy-ringe, the syringe is disconnected from the catheter and small forceps are clamped on the catheter tubing to prevent escape of the medium. The forceps may be taped to an area on the patient's face where it will not superimpose over the gland being examined, or the pa-tient may hold the forceps to prevent accidentally dis-lodging the catheter. The patient may also be directed to hold some positive pressure on the catheter to keep it in place. If the hydrostatic method of injection is used, the drip setup is left in place until the procedure is completed.

Once the contrast medium has been injected, filming proceeds. When the postcontrast injection filming is finished and the examination is satisfactory, the patient is given another lemon wedge. This causes the gland to contract and secrete more saliva, which expedites drainage of contrast medium from the gland and duct system. An appropriate postdrainage film is taken at this time to complete the examination.

## CONTRAST MEDIA

For sialography, an oil-based or a water-soluble me-dium may be used. A common oil-based medium that can be used is Ethiodol. This medium has the advantage of having a high viscosity, which allows it to remain in the ductal system for a time sufficient for radiography. However, if this medium extravasates or spills outside the gland or duct, it can cause a foreign-body-type reaction and granulomatous (tumorlike tissue) formation. Also, with extravasation, the free contrast medium may obscure the area being examined for some time.

A water-soluble medium, such as Sinografin, may also be used. Because it is more soluble, extravasation causes less of a problem than with an oil-based medium. A disadvantage of this medium, also related to its solubility, is that it is rapidly absorbed and may require additional injection of medium. Therefore, when using a water-soluble medium, it may be advisable to use the hydrostatic injection method to replace the contrast medium as it is absorbed.

The amount of contrast medium varies for each gland, with 0.5 to 1.5 ml used for the parotid and 0.2 to 0.5 ml used for the submandibular gland.

## FILMING AND POSITIONING

Radiography of the gland(s) can be accomplished by using a conventional radiographic tube, a specialized head unit, fluoroscopy, or a combination of fluoroscopy and conventional radiography. If fluoroscopy is used, the radiologist can monitor the injection process, ensuring complete filling of the gland and ducts. Under fluoroscopic control, the patient can be positioned to best demonstrate the desired anatomy without superimposition of adjacent structures such as the bony mandible. Generally, even when fluoroscopy is employed, overhead radiography is also used to produce a complete study.

The filming procedure closely resembles that of a routine, underexposed mandible series with appropriate adjustments of the central ray to demonstrate the gland(s) being examined. Additionally, specific views of the gland(s) may be required. Other considerations for visualizing any of the glands without superimposition of bony structures include tomography and subtraction technique. Before the injection of a contrast agent, scout films of the mandible area are taken. Suggested routine views include an AP projection, true lateral and lateral oblique positions of the side of interest. These scout films may demonstrate the presence of calculi in the duct or gland and preclude continuing the examination with a contrast agent. This judgment lies with the radiologist, because the presence of calculi in the general area of the duct or gland may require the injection of contrast medium to verify that the calculi are indeed within these structures.

Because the area of interest is soft tissue accentuated by a contrast medium, a low milliampere-seconds (mAs), medium kilovoltage (approximately 70) technique is used for Bucky radiography. The films may also be taken table top, with an appropriate technique.

The choice of Bucky or table-top exposures is per department protocol.

## Parotid Gland

The following are suggested contrast films of the parotid gland:

A true AP or PA projection with the central ray directed through the ramus of the mandible of the affected side (Fig. 9–4A).

A true lateral (which is a universal view for all three glands) with the central ray directed through the parotid gland (Fig. 9–4B).

A tangential AP projection with the head rotated 10 to 15 degrees toward the affected side so that the body of the mandible is perpendicular to the film and not superimposed over the area of interest and with the central ray directed through the gland. This view may also be taken as a blow-out view with the patient directed to puff out the appropriate cheek with air, thus providing a background of air around the contrast-filled gland and duct for better visualization.

A lateral oblique, or axiolateral (also universal for all three glands), with the patient's head tilted toward the affected side approximately 35 degrees from a true lateral position, to project the body of the opposite side of the mandible away from the area. The head is also rotated 5 to 10 degrees from a true lateral away from the affected side to avoid superimposition of the upper cervical spine over the area. The central ray is directed through the area of the parotid gland of interest.

An optional position for the parotid gland is an AP Towne, with the central ray directed through the appropriate parotid gland.

Once the contrast films are completed, the patient is given a lemon wedge, and following expectoration of saliva and contrast medium, an appropriate postdrainage film is taken to complete the study.

## Submandibular Gland

Recommended views for the submandibular gland are as follows:

A true lateral (of the mandible) with the central ray directed through the area of the gland.

A lateral oblique (Fig. 9–4C) with the central ray through the area of the gland.

Optional views that can be used to demonstrate the gland are a submentovertex projection, a Water's position, and a submentovertex projection using an intraoral or dental film.

For all of these positions and projections, the central ray is directed through the area of the appropriate gland. When the contrast filming sequence is completed, the patient is given another lemon wedge. Following expectoration of saliva and contrast medium, an appropriate postdrainage film is taken to complete the examination.

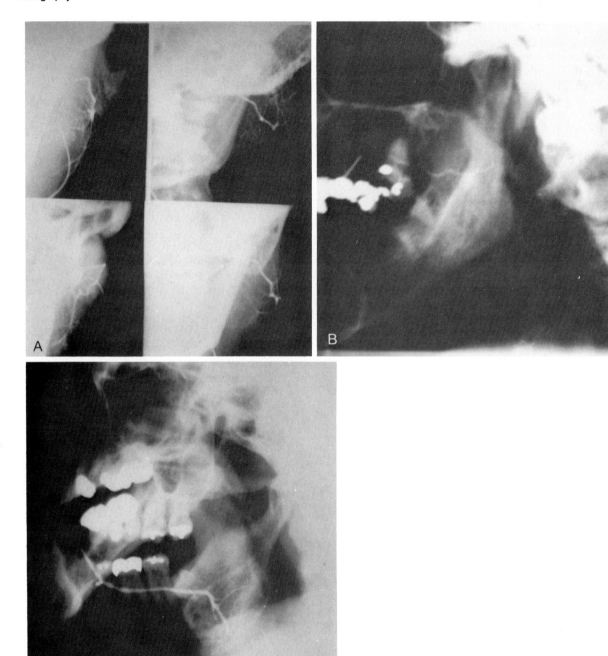

**Figure 9–4.** (*A*) AP view of parotid gland; (*B*) lateral view of parotid gland; (*C*) lateral oblique view of submandibular gland.

## Sublingual Gland

The sublingual gland is not examined with a contrast medium; therefore, if radiography of this gland is desired, the scout film series is generally adequate. An additional projection that may be helpful to demonstrate the gland is the submentovertex projection using an intraoral film. As with the other glands, the central ray is directed through the area of the appropriate gland for all views and projections. A soft tissue, low mAs, medium kilovolt technique is used.

## POSTPROCEDURAL CARE

Once the postdrainage film shows that the gland being examined is emptying sufficiently, there is little postprocedural care for the patient.

## COMPLICATIONS

Complications with this examination are generally procedural. This includes difficulty in locating and

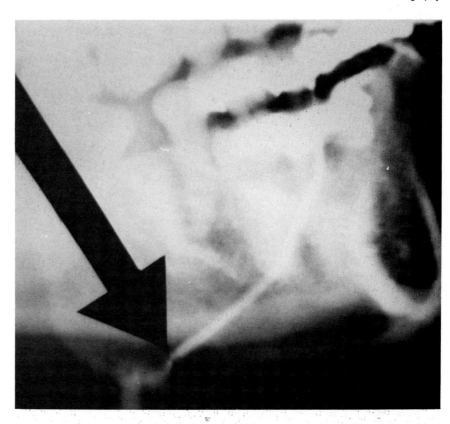

**Figure 9–5.** Inflammatory lesion of submandibular duct with obstruction.

catheterizing a duct or catheterizing the wrong duct and underfilling or overfilling the gland. Extravasation of contrast agent can obscure adequate visualization of the duct and associated gland. In certain pathologic conditions (e.g., Sjögren's disease), when an oily contrast medium is used, the procedure may cause a short-term granulomatous foreign-body-type reaction.

## FINDINGS

Several radiographic findings are demonstrated by sialography. Inflammatory lesions, which can be obstructive or nonobstructive, are the most common finding. Generally, inflammatory changes without calculi are more prevalent. If severe enough, inflammatory lesions can cause a stricture of the duct with subsequent obstruction (Fig. 9–5). Inflammation can be caused by pathologic conditions or even simple mechanical conditions such as poorly fitting dentures. If calculi are present, there is generally concurrent inflammation with partial to complete obstruction, depending on the size of the calculi. Most calculi are radiopaque, but they can be radiolucent.

Mass lesions can also be demonstrated by sialography. These masses may be either cancerous or benign and may be intrinsic or extrinsic to the gland or duct. The incidence of cancerous lesions is inversely related to the size of the gland. That is, if there is a palpable mass present, the larger the gland involved the less chance of malignancy and the smaller the gland involved the greater the chance of malignancy.

Other radiographic findings include hypertrophy of the masseter muscle of the mandible and Sjögren's syndrome. Hypertrophy of the masseter muscle represents an extrinsic pressure to the parotid gland, which can cause pressure and inflammation of the gland or duct. Sjögren's syndrome is characterized by bilateral enlargement of the affected glands, with increased alveolar pressure and slow emptying of the glands (i.e., longer than 10 to 15 minutes).

## REVIEW QUESTIONS

1. Name the three pairs of salivary glands.

2. State the two names for the duct that drains the parotid gland.

3. The alternate name for the submandibular gland is (the) _____.
   A. parotid
   B. submaxillary
   C. sublingual
   D. Wharton's

4. State the two names for the duct that drains the submandibular gland.

5. The primary duct that drains the sublingual gland is (the) _____.
   A. Bartholin's duct
   B. Wharton's duct
   C. duct of Rivinus
   D. duct of Rabinov

6. Name a pathology that contraindicates sialography.

7. The salivary gland that is not examined with a contrast medium is the _____.
   A. parotid
   B. submaxillary
   C. sublingual
   D. submandibular

8. What is a sialogogue?

9. The catheter used for the examination of the salivary glands is _____.
   A. Sjögren's
   B. Rabinov
   C. Rivinus
   D. parotid

10. Give an example of both an oil-based and a water-soluble contrast medium used in sialography.

11. Name two positions that are universal views used for all three salivary glands.

12. Name three pathologies that can be demonstrated with sialography.

## BIBLIOGRAPHY

Ballinger, P: Merrill's Atlas of Radiographic Positions and Radiologic Procedures, Vol 2, ed 7. CV Mosby, St Louis, 1986.

Guyton, A: Anatomy and Physiology. CBS College Publishing, Philadelphia, 1985.

Manashil, G: Sialography: A simple procedure. Eastman Kodak Medical Radiography and Photography 52:34, 1976.

McInnes, J: Clark's Positioning in Radiography, Vol 2, ed 9. Year Book Medical Publishers, Chicago, 1974.

Miller, B and Keane, C: Encyclopedia and Dictionary of Medicine, Nursing and Allied Health, ed 4. WB Saunders, Philadelphia, 1987.

Skucas, J: Radiographic Contrast Agents, ed 2. Aspen Publishers, Rockville, MD, 1989.

Sterling, S: Some radiological considerations in sialography. Radiol Technol 42:57, 1970.

# CHAPTER 10

# Lower Extremity Venography

*Patrick J. Apfel, MEd, ARRT(R)*

Venography is a radiographic study of the venous portion of the circulatory system. Vascular patterns and possible pathologies are outlined through the use of a contrast medium. Venography can be performed in various areas of the body, including both the superior and inferior venae cavae, the portal system of the liver, the kidneys, the thyroid gland, dural membranes, and the extremities. The most common procedure performed in a diagnostic imaging department is venography of the extremities, particularly the lower extremity. In lower extremity venography, the deep venous system from the ankle to, and including, the pelvic area is examined. Optionally, the inferior vena cava (IVC) may be included. This chapter deals with the anatomy and pathologies demonstrated by lower extremity venography.

## ANATOMY

The circulatory system of the body includes the cardiovascular and lymphatic components. The cardiovascular component involves the heart, arteries, veins, and blood. Of the blood vessels, the arteries are generally responsible for transportation of blood from the heart to the various areas and organs of the body. Veins constitute those blood vessels that generally return blood from the various parts of the body and organs to the heart for recirculation. In general, veins transport deoxygenated blood and waste products, and arteries carry oxygenated blood and nutrients, the exception being in the pulmonary circulation (lungs), where veins carry oxygenated blood and arteries carry deoxygenated blood. Veins differ from arteries in their structure. A major difference is that veins contain one-way valves to prevent a backflow of blood (Fig. 10–1), whereas arteries do not. Although both vein and artery walls have three layers (or coats), veins have thinner walls than arteries. The layers comprise an inner layer of endothelial tissue (tunica intima); a middle layer made up of muscle, elastic, and fibrous tissue (tunica media); and an outer layer of fibrous connective tissue (tunica adventitia) (Fig. 10–2). The major difference in the thickness of the vessel walls is that the muscle,

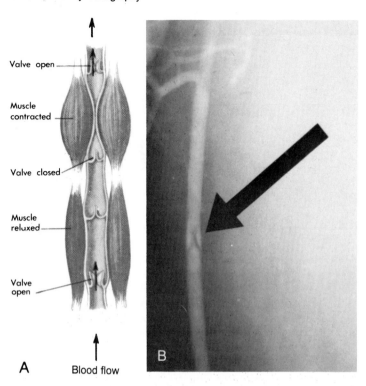

**Figure 10-1.** (*A*) Diagram of venous valves (From Miller, BF and Keane, CB: Encyclopedia and Dictionary of Medicine, Nursing, and Allied Health, ed 4. WB Saunders, Philadelphia, 1987, Plate 7, with permission); (*B*) femoral vein with venous valves.

elastic, and connective tissue components are thicker in arteries than in veins because arteries must withstand a greater blood pressure than veins.

Veins and arteries form a continuous closed system of vessels for transportation of blood to and from the heart. As blood is pumped from the left ventricle of the heart, it travels through arteries that are relatively large. The aorta is the first major artery extending from the heart and is approximately 1 inch in diameter. As blood travels distal to the aorta, it moves through a succession of increasingly smaller arteries and arterioles. The most distal arterial vessels, termed capillaries, are so small (about 10 $\mu$m in diameter) that blood cells must travel through them in a single file. As arterial capillaries end, venous capillaries begin (Fig. 10-3). Blood flowing back to the heart from the lower extremities travels from venous capillaries through a succession of venules and increasingly larger veins, which terminate with the inferior vena cava at the right atrium of the heart.

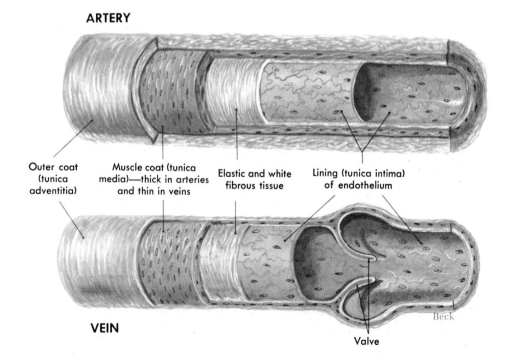

**Figure 10-2.** (*A*) Artery wall structure; (*B*) vein wall structure. (From Anthony, CP and Thibodeau, GA: Textbook of Anatomy and Physiology, ed 10. Mosby-Year Book, St Louis, 1979, p 380, with permission.)

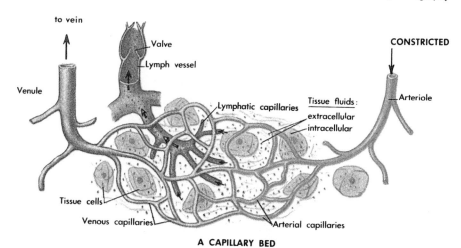

**Figure 10-3.** Diagram of arterial-venous capillary bed. (From Miller, BF and Keane CB: Encyclopedia and Dictionary of Medicine, ed 4. WB Saunders, Philadelphia, 1987, Plate 7, with permission.)

Blood moves through arteries primarily because of the force exerted by the heart as a pump. Pressure in arteries measures approximately 120 millimeters of mercury (mm Hg) in the average, healthy individual, whereas in veins it is as low as 10 mm Hg or less. By the time blood from the lower extremities reaches the right atrium of the heart, the venous pressure is close to zero. Because most of the pressure produced by the heart is lost by the time blood reaches the venous system, additional mechanisms aid in moving the blood through veins. Venous blood circulation in the upper portion of the body is aided by gravity and muscular contractions. In the lower portion of the body, venous blood flow is augmented by contractions of surrounding muscles (Fig. 10-1), by pressures exerted during respiration, and by physical movements of the bowel. In the lower extremity, blood movement back toward the heart is aided by muscular contractions of the leg and thigh muscles.

The veins of the lower extremities are divided into deep and superficial segments. The deep veins are separated from the superficial veins by the crural fascia (a sheet of fibrous tissue similar to that surrounding muscles). The superficial and deep components are interconnected by perforating veins, named so because they perforate the crural fascia. Blood flow between the two segments is from superficial to deep veins and is controlled by one-way valves within the perforating veins. Lower extremity veins may vary in number, size, and configuration from one individual to another. The larger veins (main trunks) are often paired, but sometimes singular. Trunks may vary greatly in diameter and appearance, with some varying in width along their length and others appearing very uniform. Valves vary in number and proximity. The number of interconnecting branches can also vary. Veins are commonly located adjacent to arteries, at times almost in a mirror image, and their names are often similar to the adjacent arteries.

During lower extremity venography, generally only the deep veins are examined. The major deep vessels visualized during lower extremity venography are the anterior and posterior tibial, popliteal, femoral, external, and common iliac, as well as tributaries of these vessels (Fig. 10-4). The inferior vena cava may also be examined as an option. If superficial veins are of interest (e.g., saphenous veins), tourniquets above the ankle may be omitted during the injection of contrast medium (see Injection Procedure section in this chapter).

## INDICATIONS

Venography is indicated when symptoms of obstruction, varicose veins, and congenital abnormalities of the venous system are evident. These symptoms can include pain, swelling, and discoloration of the extremity. Venography is also useful in evaluating the great saphenous vein for possible use in arterial graft surgery.

## CONTRAINDICATIONS

Contraindications to venography are typically related to the contrast medium. These are sensitivity to the agent itself, and advanced hepatic failure, renal failure, or both. Phlebitis may also contraindicate the procedure.

## PREPROCEDURAL CARE

There is no premedication for this procedure. If there is excessive swelling in the foot, it may be wrapped with elastic bandage for up to 24 hours before the procedure. For lesser edema, massage can help reduce the swelling to aid in visualizing small veins on the dorsum of the foot for injection. If swelling is not present and veins are difficult to locate for injection, a tourniquet may be applied above the ankle and warm compresses to the foot to dilate the vessels.

As with any examination involving the injection of contrast medium, prior to the procedure, the exami-

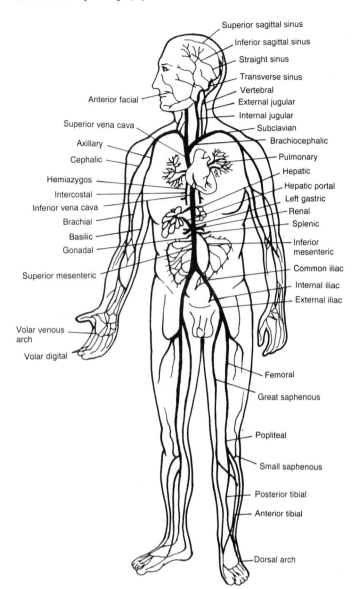

**Figure 10–4.** Diagram of major veins of body. (From Scanlon, VC and Sanders, T: Essentials of Anatomy and Physiology, ed 2. FA Davis Company, Philadelphia, 1995, p 289, with permission.)

nation and any possible complications should be thoroughly explained to the patient and an informed consent signed.

## EQUIPMENT

### Major Equipment

The major equipment needed to perform venography includes a radiographic-fluoroscopic room with a spot film device, or high speed camera, and a 90-degree tilting table with a footrest. Although this procedure can be performed with a conventional radiographic unit (i.e., without fluoroscopy), the use of a fluoroscopic unit is most common and is presented in this chapter.

### Accessory Equipment

Typical accessory equipment required for venography includes high speed camera film or 14″ × 14″ cassettes, a block to support the unaffected leg, and items necessary for the injection of the contrast medium. The injection equipment includes the contrast medium, a 5 percent dextrose solution or normal saline (used as a venous flush), an IV pole, IV tubing, a three-way stopcock, two 50-ml syringes, a 19-gauge needle, an 18- and a 21-gauge butterfly needle, prep sponges, two tourniquets, and tape (Fig. 10–5).

## INJECTION PROCEDURE

Before the start of the examination, the flushing solution with IV tubing and three-way stopcock is sus-

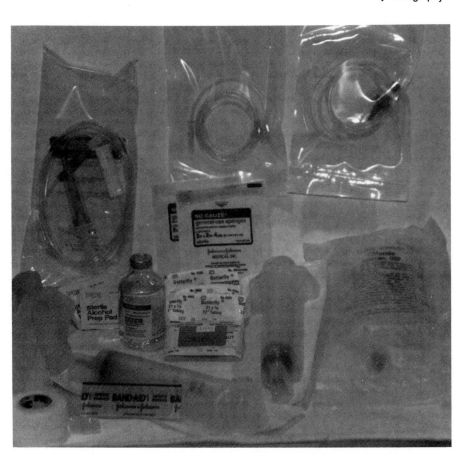

**Figure 10–5.** Injection equipment for venography.

pended from the IV pole placed close to the x-ray table. The table is positioned at 90 degrees (upright) with the patient standing on the footboard and with the full weight of the body supported by the unaffected leg. This is accomplished by having the patient stand on a block, on the footboard, with the body weight supported by the unaffected leg while the affected leg is suspended above the footrest. A tourniquet is placed tightly just above the ankle of the affected extremity. A distal superficial vein on the dorsum of the foot is chosen for injection. Any edema present may be massaged away (if edema cannot be reduced, a cutdown procedure may be necessary to locate and inject a vein [see Chap. 19, Catheterization Methods and Patient Management]). The area is cleaned with an alcohol prep. The physician inserts a butterfly needle into the vein. When a backflow of blood indicates that the needle is within the lumen of the vessel, the butterfly tubing is connected to one of the remaining openings of the three-way stopcock and the needle is taped in place. To further ensure that the needle is within the lumen of the vessel, the flushing solution can be infused through manipulation of the stopcock. A second tourniquet is placed tightly above the ankle. Tourniquets are applied to compress superficial veins, thereby shunting the contrast medium during injection into the deep system through the perforating veins. This results in visualization of the deep venous system without superimposition of contrast medium in the superficial veins.

The contrast medium is injected through the remaining opening of the three-way stopcock after it is manipulated to accommodate the flow of medium. The injection process begins with the patient in a semierect position, at approximately 60 degrees, which allows the effect of gravity to slow the progress of medium up the veins of the extremity (Fig. 10–6A). This first position allows fluoroscopic visualization and filming of the veins in the area of the calf. The table is then lowered to a 45-degree position, and the veins of the knee area are visualized and imaged (Fig. 10–6B). While continuing the injection, the table is again lowered, to approximately 20 degrees, to demonstrate and film the veins of the thigh (Fig. 10–6C). Finally, the table is lowered into the horizontal position and the pelvic and lower abdominal veins are visualized and filmed (Fig. 10–6D). If the inferior vena cava is to be included in the examination, the table can be left horizontal or lowered to a Trendelenburg position. The femoral vein may be compressed and the extremity elevated. When ready for an exposure, the compression is released, allowing contrast medium to flow into the IVC. An exposure is made when the vessel is sufficiently visualized. Incomplete filling of some segments of vessels, which may not be pathologic, may occur during the procedure. Additional contrast medium may be injected as necessary, or compression may be applied by a tourniquet or palpation (applied pressure from hands or fingers) to permit filling of nonopacified areas (e.g., a tourniquet ap-

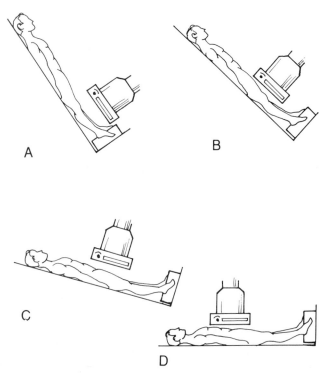

**Figure 10-6.** Table angulations for venography: (*A*) 60 degrees demonstrates area of calf; (*B*) 45 degrees demonstrates area of the knee; (*C*) 20 degrees demonstrates area of the thigh; (*D*) 0 degrees demonstrates area of the pelvis and lower abdomen.

plied above the knee will retain contrast medium in the calf area and aid in filling the veins).

Following filming of the veins, contrast medium is flushed from the veins by infusing approximately 50 ml of 5 percent dextrose or normal saline.

## CONTRAST MEDIA

A low density, water-soluble, iodine-based contrast medium such as Renografin 60 is used for venography. The amount of medium injected varies from 50 to 100 ml per extremity according to the extent of the venous system that is to be examined. A nonionic medium may be used if the patient is subject to a contrast medium reaction. Use of a nonionic medium may also reduce the pain often experienced during injection of an ionic medium, preclude some postvenography complications such as phlebitis, and, in patients with thrombophlebitis, reduce the normal exacerbation of their symptoms experienced with injection of an ionic medium.

## FILMING AND POSITIONING

Filming can be accomplished by overhead radiography, by fluoroscopic spot filming (14″ × 14″ cassettes), or by using a high speed camera with either cut or roll film. Filming occurs during the injection procedure in conjunction with the injection process. A typical film-

ing sequence includes the following projections and positions: an anteroposterior (AP) and lateral of the calf to include the knee; an AP and lateral centered at the knee; an AP and lateral of the thigh; an AP of the pelvis (Fig. 10-7); and an AP of the abdomen (optional to visualize the IVC).

If routine radiographs are taken using the overhead tube and table Bucky diaphragm, 14″ × 17″ cassettes are used. This method of filming is rarely used because coordination and speed are too critical during the injection and filming process to ensure an adequate examination. Further, adequate visualization of the venous system cannot be determined until the films are processed, and if there is inadequate filling of the vessels with contrast medium, additional contrast medium injection and filming are necessary.

Fluoroscopy and filming with a spot filming device or high speed camera is the preferred method for imaging the venous system. Fluoroscopic control is used to correlate vessel filling with imaging. Under fluoroscopic control, filming is coordinated with the table angulations and contrast medium injection to allow optimal demonstration of the veins.

## POSTPROCEDURAL CARE

Unless complications result, postprocedural care for venography is minimal. Generally, the only care taken following venography is to ensure that no hematoma results when the injection needle is removed. Compression at the site for several minutes generally prevents a hematoma from developing. A small bandage or dressing should be applied to the puncture site when the procedure is completed.

## COMPLICATIONS

Complications can result because of a toxic effect of the contrast medium on the venous epithelium. The medium may cause a phlebitis in nonsymptomatic patients and an increase in symptoms in patients with thrombophlebitis. To avoid this, the contrast medium is flushed from the venous system with 5 percent dextrose in water or normal saline. Care should be taken to flush the veins of as much of the contrast medium as possible to lessen the chance of contrast medium–induced complications. Phlebitis itself may occur at the venous puncture site or anywhere along the course of the vessel. On occasion, skin has been known to slough later at the injection site, even when there has been no extravasation of contrast medium.

As in any study using an intravenous contrast medium, possible complications can result from systemic reactions to the contrast medium.

## FINDINGS

Typical pathologies demonstrated by venography include obstructions (Fig. 10-8), phlebitis, vein varicosities, and congenital abnormalities.

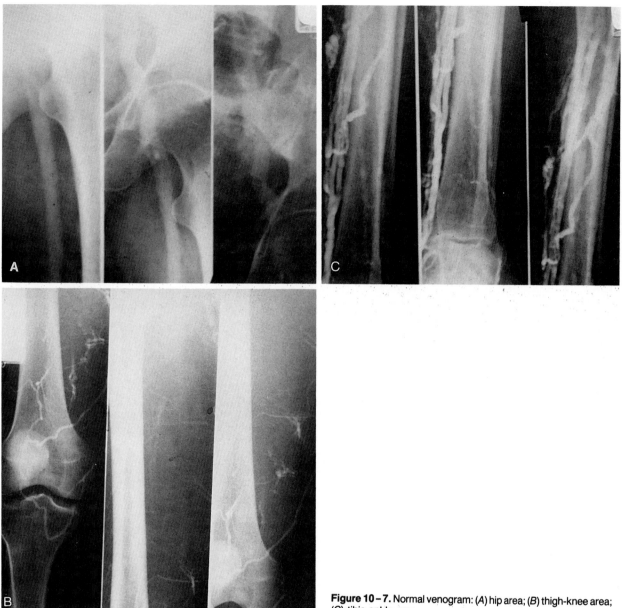

**Figure 10–7.** Normal venogram: (A) hip area; (B) thigh-knee area; (C) tibia-ankle area.

Obstructions can be caused by phlebitis, thrombosis, tumor invasion, or extrinsic compression (by bone, muscle, and so on). Phlebitis is an inflammation of a vein that can cause reduced blood flow and can be further complicated by a thrombus. If phlebitis occurs in a deep vein and affects the inner lining, a thrombus may be formed, resulting in thrombophlebitis. Thrombi formed in the lower extremities can result in partial to complete obstruction of the affected vein. Detection of deep venous system thrombi is important, because these can be responsible for pulmonary emboli if the thrombi break loose and make their way into the pulmonary circulation. Extrinsic compression can be caused by any structure adjacent to the veins, such as bone, muscle, and tumors. Compression of the vein can lead to a thrombus formation and the complications related to a thrombus.

The extent of vein varicosities can also be detected by venography. Varicose veins (Fig. 10–9) are swollen, distended, knotted, and collapsed vessels. They are a result of sluggish blood flow in combination with defective valves and weakened vein walls.

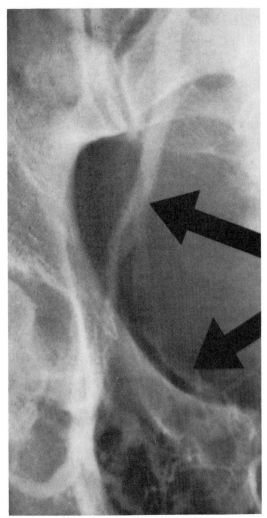

**Figure 10-8.** Thrombus with obstruction.

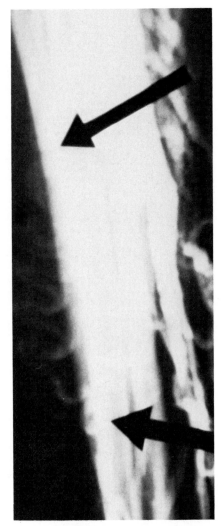

**Figure 10-9.** Varicose vein.

Congenital abnormalities such as malformations and incomplete or underdeveloped vessels can also be demonstrated by venography.

## REVIEW QUESTIONS

1. Veins that transport oxygenated blood are found in the ____.
   A. lower extremity
   B. cardiac circulation
   C. pulmonary circulation
   D. portal circulation

2. The crural fascia is a membrane that ____.
   A. separates veins from arteries
   B. separates superficial from deep veins
   C. forms the outer layer of venous walls
   D. forms the inner layer of venous walls

3. Perforating veins ____.
   A. perforate the crural fascia
   B. connect superficial and deep veins

C. both A and B
D. none of the above

4. Circulation in the lower extremity is from deep to superficial veins.
   A. True
   B. False

5. Identify the major vessels examined by venography.

6. State two structural differences between veins and arteries.

7. Give two indications for venography.

8. Two tourniquets are used in venography to ____
   A. dilate a vein for injection
   B. dilate all lower extremity veins for better visualization
   C. slow the progress of blood up the extremity
   D. force blood into the deep venous system

9. Injection of a contrast medium into the veins can cause ____.

A. obstruction
B. varicose veins
C. phlebitis
D. poor circulation

10. Give two examples of flushing solutions used during venography.

11. A recommended filming sequence for venography includes _____.

12. Give the four fluoroscopic table angulations recommended for venography and the area imaged for each of the angulations.

## BIBLIOGRAPHY

Abrams, H: Abrams Angiography Vascular and Interventional Radiology, ed 3, Vol 3. Little, Brown & Co, Boston, 1983.

Johnson, E, et al: Human Anatomy. WB Saunders, Philadelphia, 1985.

Johnsrude, I, Jackson, D, and Dunnick, N: A Practical Approach to Angiography, ed 2. Little Brown & Co, Boston, 1987.

Kadir, S: Diagnostic Angiography. WB Saunders, Philadelphia, 1986.

Katzen, B: Interventional Diagnostic and Therapeutic Procedures (Comprehensive manuals in radiology). Springer-Verlag, New York, 1980.

Miller, B and Keane, C: Encyclopedia and Dictionary of Medicine, Nursing, and Allied Health, ed 4. WB Saunders, Philadelphia, 1987.

Skucas, J: Radiographic Contrast Agents, ed 2. Aspen Publishers, Rockville, MD, 1989.

White, R: Fundamentals of Vascular Radiology. Lea & Febiger, Philadelphia, 1976.

# PART THREE

# ARTERIOGRAPHY

# EQUIPMENT

## CHAPTER 11

# Physical Facilities

*Marianne R. Tortorici, EdD, ARRT(R)*

The needs of an angiographic room differ significantly from those of a conventional radiographic or fluoroscopic room. The primary differences are in the size of the room and the specialized equipment. Angiographic rooms are much larger than conventional radiographic rooms and contain more sophisticated equipment. As in the case of conventional radiographic rooms, the physical facilities of an angiographic room should be designed from a practical point of view. The selection of equipment is based on the recommendations of engineers, architects, radiologists, technologists, and other experts. Difficulties may arise when individuals who must operate the equipment are not consulted during the planning phase. However, consultation with the personnel who operate the equipment does not guarantee that the facilities will be trouble free. This is especially true if these individuals are unfamiliar with the variety of equipment available and the limitations of each piece of equipment. Generally speaking, by consulting with experts and technologists, the need for renovations or reconstruction at a later time is often avoided.

The objective of this chapter is to identify the major factors that should be considered when designing an angiographic room. The information presented serves as a foundation from which readers can build to meet the specific needs of their particular institutions.

### STRUCTURAL LAYOUT

Unless an angiographic room is built from "scratch," the size and location of the room are determined by the current facilities. Often this results in rooms that are small and poorly located. The ideal angiographic room should have a minimum of 500 square feet, with an adjacent control room of no less than 60 square feet. The angiographic room should be constructed so that it has sufficient counter and cabinet space (average cabinet space covers the length of one wall). The room should be located near the conventional imaging department, a processing area, and surgical room (Fig. 11–1). If prefabricated catheters and reusable accessory equipment are used, a small utility room for storing, steriliz-

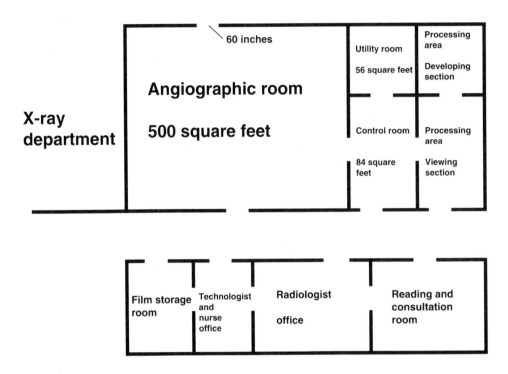

**Figure 11-1.** Angiographic room layout.

ing, and fabricating equipment should also be adjacent to the angiographic room. Other rooms that should be readily accessible are an office(s) for the angiographic team and a viewing room.

The location and number of entrances for these rooms vary. Some angiographic rooms have an entrance for the patient, an entrance to the control room, and a doorway connecting the angiographic room to the surgical room; others have an additional door connecting the processing area to the control room (Fig. 11-2). It is suggested that the angiographic room itself have at least one door dedicated for the patient to enter and exit. In a hospital environment, this door should be large enough to accommodate a hospital bed.

The control area should have a minimum of two doors, one opening into a hallway and the other leading to the angiographic room. Other entrances are optional and depend on the imaging department's needs. For example, if a large number of emergency trauma

patients are treated, it may be advantageous to have a door connecting the angiographic room to surgery, providing ready access for patients requiring immediate surgery after the angiography. An entrance from the control room to the processing area is convenient but is not essential. However, it is strongly recommended that a processing area be located close to the angiographic room and that it be used primarily for angiographic processing.

Maintaining a clean angiographic room is extremely important because the room is used for procedures that require aseptic technique. It is not unusual for the floors, walls, or doors to have blood or contrast medium on them during a procedure. Therefore, the doors, walls, and floors should be of a material that is easily cleaned.

Some angiographic rooms are designed for outpatient procedures. In these departments, it is common to have a place where patients are kept for preprocedural

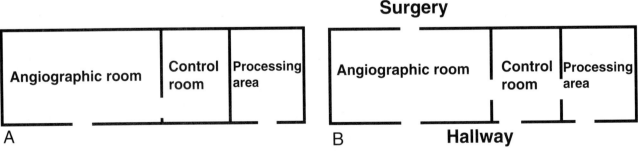

**Figure 11-2.** Two types of room entrances.

preparation and postprocedural monitoring. The patient monitoring room may be a separate room within the imaging department or may be located outside the department. It should contain enough space to accommodate at least two gurneys, a desk for record keeping, an oxygen supply, an emergency drug cart, a suction machine, and equipment to monitor the patient (e.g., blood pressure cuff). Many facilities use the surgical recovery room for postprocedural monitoring. It is common to have a registered nurse perform the monitoring procedures.

Angiographic room accessories should include an oxygen supply, air-conditioning system, sink, contrast medium warmer, and floor troughs. An oxygen supply, preferably piped in from a central location, suction equipment, and an emergency cart are necessary in the event a patient has a severe reaction to the injection of a contrast medium. Air-conditioning is needed to maintain room temperature and cool the equipment, which generates a great deal of heat. Central air-conditioning is recommended because it is more effective than a window-type cooling unit. A sink with both hot and cold water is useful for cleaning equipment and washing hands. A contrast medium warmer helps maintain the contrast medium at the proper temperature prior to injection. Covered floor troughs are used to store the electric wiring components to prevent individuals from tripping over exposed cables, to decrease the possibility of electric shock, and to allow for easy access to the wires should repairs or additional wiring be needed.

## CONTENTS OF THE ROOM

The primary components of major equipment in an angiographic room are x-ray tubes, generators, transformers, an x-ray table, an image intensifier, television monitors, a serial film changer, and an electromechanical injector (see Chaps. 12 and 13, respectively, for information regarding serial film changers and electromechanical injectors). Optional major additions include cineangiography equipment, a video recorder, computer equipment used for DSA, and cardiac catheterization equipment. Disposable or reusable supplies include guidewires, catheters, needles, adaptors, and other supplementary equipment. The exact contents of the room depend on the procedures performed there, the size of the room, and the personal preferences of the angiographer. The intent of this section is to provide the reader with a general understanding of the equipment needed for an angiographic room. No attempt is made to present an in-depth discussion of the equipment. For more specific information about the equipment, the reader is advised to consult the references listed at the end of this chapter.

## X-Ray Tubes

Many angiographic rooms have a minimum of two overhead x-ray tubes and one fluoroscopic tube. Recent developments have introduced C-arm x-ray units

that have an x-ray tube connected by a curved (C-shaped) metal bar or arm to an image intensifier and a serial film changer (Fig. 11–3). This type of setup has the advantage of allowing patients to maintain a comfortable position while the x-ray tube can be moved around them for quality filming. If a patient is comfortable, the examination can be performed with speed and ease. The tube and intensifier are mounted on a movable bar. This allows the tube or intensifier to be moved so that the source-to-image receptor distance can be changed to improve image quality. One disadvantage of the C arm is that the radiologist usually receives more radiation than with the usual conventional overhead fluoroscopic unit.

The x-ray tubes used for image intensification in either the C-arm or the under-the-table mount should have the capability to magnify the image. The x-ray tubes employed for serial film exposures differ from the normal radiographic tube in the angle of the anode. Angiographic x-ray tubes have a smaller anode angle, usually 10 degrees (see the following section on Magnification Tubes).

X-ray tubes employed for serial filming should have the capacity to expose as many as six films per second for a minimum of 5 seconds. This rapid filming does not permit a cooling time between exposures and therefore creates a large amount of heat (kilowatts) at the anode. The easiest way to decrease the heat at the anode is to increase the focal spot size. However, this is undesirable because it results in a decrease of radiographic quality. An alternate method employed to dissipate the heat at the anode is to rotate the anode at a higher speed than conventional radiography, which rotates at about 5000 revolutions per minute (rpm). The current high-speed anode rotation required for effective heat dissipation in angiography tubes is approximately 10,000 rpm. This prevents a localized buildup of heat in the anode and distributes the heat over the entire surface of the anode.

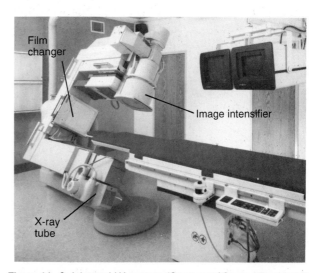

**Figure 11–3.** Advantx LUA system. (Courtesy of General Electric, Milwaukee, WI.)

## Magnification Tubes

Sometimes it is necessary to magnify an angiographic series. Magnification may be achieved in several ways. The most common method is to radiograph an image at a short source object distance and at a long object film distance. Unfortunately, image enlargement also results in a corresponding loss of radiographic quality. There are two primary methods used to counteract this loss. One method employs the line focus principle, which states that the effective focal spot size is smaller than the actual focal spot size (Fig. 11–4). This is usually achieved by decreasing the angle of the anode (Fig. 11–5). Most conventional radiographic x-ray tubes have an anode angle between 17 and 20 degrees. Angiographic x-ray tubes employ an anode angle between 7 and 10 degrees. A second method of increasing radiographic quality is to use a small actual focal spot. Most magnification x-ray tubes have a 0.3-mm focal spot, compared with conventional radiographic tubes, which have a 0.5- to 1.0-mm focal spot. As mentioned previously, serial filming does result in the production of large amounts of heat; therefore, it is impractical to reduce the size of the focal spot below 0.3 mm.

Although the decreased anode angle does increase radiographic quality, the size of the irradiated field is reduced. For example, at a 100-cm (40″) source image receptor distance, a 10-degree anode angle exposes a 36 cm × 36 cm (14″ × 14″) area. At the same source image distance, a 12-degree anode angle exposes a 36 cm × 43 cm (14″ × 17″) area.

## Transformers

To provide adequate power to the x-ray tube, a transformer similar to that used for conventional radiographic equipment is necessary. Radiographic generators are designed to operate at 480 V. However, x-ray tubes must operate at thousands of volts; therefore, it is necessary to have a transformer to increase the voltage. There are many transformers in the total x-ray circuit. The two major transformers are the autotransformer

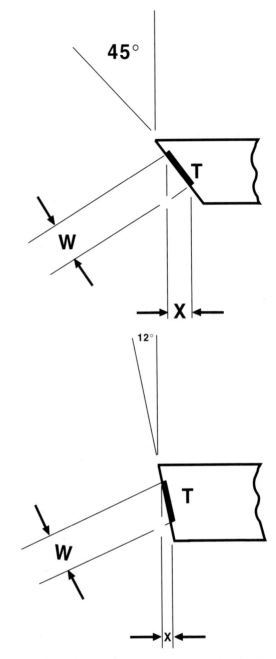

**Figure 11–5.** Effect of different anode angles on the effective focal spot size. T = target; W = width; X = effective focal spot.

and the high-tension (or step-up) transformer. The autotransformer preselects and maintains the voltage. The step-up transformer increases the voltage from hundreds of volts to thousands of volts. For the actual construction and operation of a transformer, the reader is advised to consult the references listed at the end of this chapter.

## Angiographic Tables

A variety of x-ray tables are commercially available. The type of table employed must meet the specific

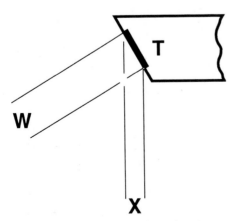

**Figure 11–4.** Line focus principle. T = target (actual focal spot); W = width (projected actual focal spot); X = effective focal spot.

needs of the imaging department. For example, if myelography or other procedures that require angling the patient are to be performed, then a tilt table should be used. Although procedures such as myelography may sometimes be performed, most angiographic room procedures usually do not require a tilting table. Thus, most angiographic rooms have tables that are stationary with a floating or movable top (Fig. 11–6). The tabletop should be capable of moving longitudinally and laterally. The degree of table movement should be such that the most extreme lateral and longitudinal areas of the patient may be positioned over the fluoroscope without repositioning the patient on the table. The controls for moving the table should be located on the side of the table and on a remote-control foot switch. The foot switch enables the angiographer to control the table movement during a procedure while maintaining sterile technique. If angiography of the extremities is to be performed, then the tabletop should also have a "stepping" capability, which allows for table movement at predetermined intervals and distances over the film changer. The "stepping" ability makes it possible to radiograph the abdomen, thighs, knees, and ankles during one injection of contrast medium. For further details, the reader is referred to the discussion of peripheral auxiliary equipment in Chapter 12, Serial Film Changers.

Angiographic rooms that do not use a C arm have an image intensifier located underneath or above the table. In instances where the image intensifier is under the table, the table must be high enough to accommodate the image intensifier underneath. The control for fluoroscopy should be located with the tabletop controls.

## Lighting

Because angiographic procedures require intermittent fluoroscopy, the room should contain both incandescent and fluorescent lights. Fluorescent lights are used during vessel puncture, patient preparation, and so on. The fluorescent lights should be connected to the fluoroscopic control so that when the fluoroscope is on, the fluorescent lights go off and when the fluoroscope is off, the fluorescent lights go on. Incandescent lights with dimming capability should be used during fluoroscopy. The incandescent lights should remain on at all times. Connecting the lights in this manner results in having both the fluorescent and incandescent lights illuminated for the vessel puncture and patient preparation, while during fluoroscopy, only the incandescent lights are on.

## Pickup Tubes

The majority of image intensifiers are connected to a pickup tube that changes the light produced by the output screen of the image intensifier to electrons (for specific details regarding this process, the reader is advised to consult the references at the end of this chapter). The electrons travel to the cathode-ray tube and produce a visible image (picture) on the screen. There are two types of pickup tubes available, the vidicon and the plumbicon. The vidicon is the simpler, smaller, and less expensive tube. The plumbicon has a different type of phosphor located on the target. It provides a better contrast and decreased lag time than the vidicon. However, the plumbicon pickup tube has an increased rate

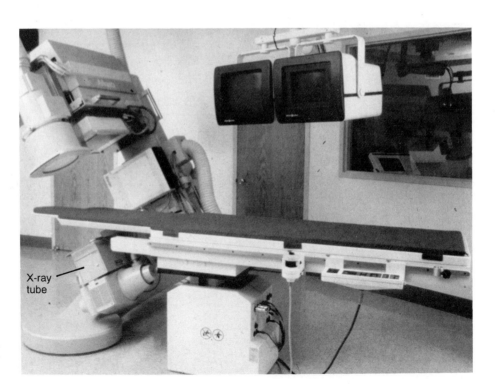

**Figure 11–6.** Angiographic table. (Courtesy of General Electric, Milwaukee, WI.)

of quantum mottle. Both tubes are compact (about 6″ in diameter and 10″ in length) and lightweight (weighs less than 10 pounds).

## Sink

A sink is of value for handwashing and reusable equipment that must be cleaned for resterilization. This is particularly important in imaging departments that autoclave their own equipment or when the central services department does not have the responsibility of cleaning the items before wrapping them for sterilization.

## Supplementary and Optional Equipment

Supplementary equipment is often stored in the angiographic room. If located in the room, catheters, guidewires, stopcocks, and other supplementary equipment are most conveniently hung from a wall (Fig. 11–7). Storing these items in the room facilitates the angiographic examination, prevents the items from being bent or torn, and allows constant visibility of the items. This facilitates maintaining the inventory because it enables the angiographer to observe which items are in short supply so that they can be reordered. Items kept in a separate storage room are often in the original boxes, which may be partially emptied, resulting in a miscalculation of the actual equipment available.

Optional items that may be located in an angiographic room are cineangiography equipment, video recorder, and cardiac catheterization equipment. The need for these items is determined by the procedures to be performed in the room. The reader is advised to consult the references at the end of this chapter for more specific information concerning these items.

## CONTENTS OF THE CONTROL ROOM

The primary equipment in the control room are the generators and program selectors (Fig. 11–8). The number of generators located in the control room depends on the number of x-ray tubes. It is possible for a generator to operate more than one x-ray tube. Although the generator may have the capacity to power more than one tube, such as fluoroscopic or radiographic tubes, it can only energize one tube at a time. To perform simultaneous biplane radiography, there must be two generators, one for each tube.

The generator, better known as the console panel, has various controls, for example, timer and milliampere knobs, which regulate the electrical supply. It is strongly recommended that the generator be three-phase and have a high milliampere setting. The three-phase circuits result in a more uniform heating of the anode and higher tube ratings than single-phase units. In addition, the voltage in a three-phase circuit is more constant than in a single-phase circuit. This permits higher energy x-ray production, reducing the exposure time required to produce a diagnostic radiograph. Short exposure times, measured in milliseconds, are desirable in angiography because of the need to obtain six radiographs per second. A second method of reducing exposure time is to employ a generator that has a high milliampere capacity. Angiographic generators should have a setting of at least 1000 mA.

Program selectors and computer consoles are also lo-

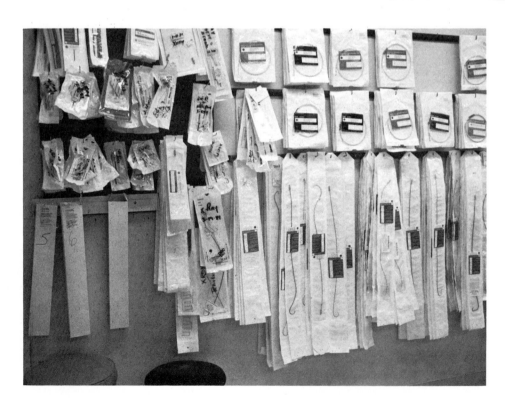

**Figure 11–7.** One method of supplementary equipment storage.

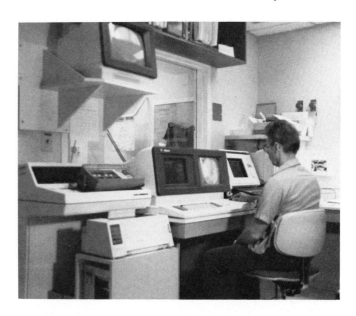

**Figure 11–8.** Control room equipment.

cated in the control room and may be mounted on the wall. They should be located in an area where personnel are not apt to run into them and that does not interfere with the operation of other equipment. The number of serial film program selectors depends on the number of film changers, with one program selector per changer. The reader is referred to the programming section of Chapter 12, Serial Film Changers, for more specific information regarding serial film program selectors. Another common type of console is a command control (Fig. 11–9). This unit can be connected to the electromechanical injector, serial film changer, and generator. The unit acts as the "brain" of the electric circuitry. It can be programmed to energize the electromechanical injector (to administer the contrast medium), start the serial film programmer, and initiate the exposures.

## CONTENTS OF THE PROCESSING AREA

### General Contents

The angiography processing area must contain the proper plumbing facilities for an automatic processor.

The automatic processor is identical to the type used in routine radiography. The additional equipment often found in an angiographic processing area is a duplication-subtraction unit (Fig. 11–10). Refer to Chapter 15, Digital Subtraction Angiography, for a discussion of subtraction.

### Optional Processing Area Equipment

If cardiac catheterization is performed in the angiographic room, additional equipment that may be needed are a processor for cineangiographic films and a cineangiographic projector.

## CONTENTS OF THE UTILITY ROOM

The utility room may have a variety of functions. The original concept of a utility room was for the resterilization of catheters, needles, guidewires, and so on, and for fabrication of catheters. With the advent of inexpensive, disposable needles and the large variety of catheter curves, lengths, and sizes, the importance of the utility room has decreased. However, if catheter

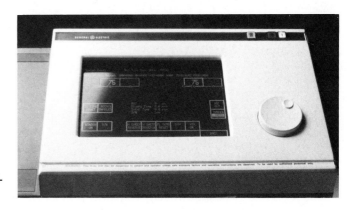

**Figure 11–9.** Command console. (Courtesy of General Electric, Milwaukee, WI.)

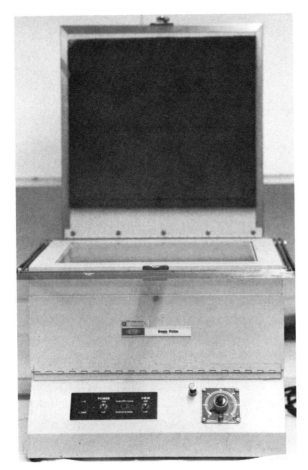

**Figure 11–10.** DuPont subtraction and duplication machine.

fabrication and resterilization of equipment are still performed, then the utility room should contain a workbench, a sink in which to clean equipment, and an autoclave to sterilize equipment. The workbench area should contain shelves to store catheter material, razors, water basins, and other equipment necessary for catheter fabrication. Currently most utility rooms are used to store the main stock of supplementary equipment.

## REVIEW QUESTIONS

1. An angiographic room should be located near ____.
   A. an exit
   B. the doctor's office
   C. the processing area
   D. computer facilities

2. The doors, walls, and floors of an angiographic room should be made of material that ____.
   A. is easy to clean
   B. reflects light
   C. is porous
   D. is dark-colored

3. Angiographic tubes differ from conventional x-ray tubes in ____.
   A. the angle of the anode
   B. weight
   C. the method of cooling
   D. the material used for the target

4. The approximate revolutions per minute of the anode for an angiographic tube is about ____.
   A. 6000
   B. 8000
   C. 10,000
   D. 12,000

5. The average focal spot size of an angiographic tube is ____ mm.
   A. 1.3
   B. 1.0
   C. 0.5
   D. 0.3

6. Angiographic tables should be capable of ____ movement.
   A. height (up and down)
   B. upright (90 degrees)
   C. longitudinal
   D. circular or arc

7. Tables employed for lower extremity angiography should have ____ capability.
   A. a 90-degree tilt
   B. a stepping
   C. a height adjustment
   D. stationary

8. Fluorescent lighting is useful in an angiographic room for ____.
   A. collimator light visualization
   B. cine filming
   C. fluoroscopy
   D. vessel puncture

9. Hanging catheters in an angiographic room ____.
   A. is not recommended
   B. prevents the wrapping from tearing
   C. increases contamination
   D. increases the sterility time

10. The minimum recommended milliampere setting of a generator for an angiographic room is ____.
    A. 400
    B. 600
    C. 800
    D. 1000

11. A cineradiographic unit is useful if ____ procedures are going to be performed in the room.
    A. cardiac catheterization
    B. renal angiography
    C. vascular interventional
    D. cerebral

## BIBLIOGRAPHY

Brinker, R and Skucas, J: Radiology Special Procedure Room. University Park Press, New York, 1973.

Ort, M, Gregg, F, and Kaufman, M: Subtraction radiography: Techniques and limitations. Radiology 124:65, July 1977.

Snopek, A: Fundamentals of special radiographic procedures. WB Saunders, Philadelphia, 1992.

Thompson, TT: A Practical Approach to Modern Imaging Equipment. Little, Brown & Co, Boston, 1985.

Tortorici, MR: Concepts in Medical Radiographic Imaging. WB Saunders, Philadelphia, 1982.

White, R: Fundamentals of Vascular Radiology. Lea & Febiger, Philadelphia, 1976.

Wojtowycz, M: Handbook of Radiology: Interventional Radiology and Angiography. Year Book Medical Publishers, Chicago, 1990.

# CHAPTER 12

# Serial Film Changers

*Marianne R. Tortorici, EdD, ARRT(R)*

Blood flow within vessels is extremely fast. Recording the arterial, capillary, and venous phases of the circulatory system requires a rapid filming sequence in which several radiographs are exposed within 1 second. Because conventional radiographic filming (manually changing cassettes) is too slow, rapid filming is accomplished by using an electromechanical device that can expose and transport film quickly. This device is appropriately called a rapid serial film changer.

The rapid serial film changer stores a minimum of 12 unexposed films in a supply magazine. Upon exposure, the unexposed films are transported (one at a time) toward the patient, exposed, and conveyed to a receiving magazine. The two major serial film changer categories are the cassette and cassetteless changers. As the names indicate, the primary difference between the two is that the cassette changer transports film in some form of cassette holder, while the cassetteless changer transports only the film. Cassetteless changers may transport film as cut film (sheets of film) or as a roll film (similar to that used in a photographic camera). Both categories of film changers work in conjunction with a programmer that regulates the rate of film exposure. Some changers are mounted on movable stands; others stand alone on the floor.

This chapter compares and contrasts the two categories of film changers, with an in-depth discussion of several types of cassetteless serial film changers. Also included is a discussion of programmers and different types of serial film changer stands. Several different product names appear throughout this chapter. Mentioning a product by brand name is designed to familiarize the reader with various types of equipment on the market and does not indicate an endorsement of that particular item.

## CASSETTE SERIAL FILM CHANGERS

The most common type of cassette serial film changer is the vacuum changer. One of the more popular vacuum changers is made by Picker-Amplatz. In this system a vacuum cassette is used to transport both the film and the intensifying screens. Because cassettes are heavier than film, during transportation the extra weight decreases the speed with which the film moves, resulting in an exposure rate slower than that of cassetteless changers. The maximum exposure rate for cassette changers is about four films per second. Additionally, the weight of the cassettes may cause vibration of the equipment during film transportation. This vibration may result in a blurred image on the film caused by the equipment motion.

Cassette changers have a good screen film contact. To achieve this good screen film contact on the Picker-Amplatz vacuum changer, the film and screen are placed in a black polyethylene bag and heat-sealed in a special vacuum unit. The heat-sealing unit is located in the developing section of the processing area and operates by placing the polyethylene bag with film and screen in the tray of the heat-sealing unit. When the processing area personnel or technologist closes the lid of the unit, the air is removed from the bag and the edges of the bag are sealed by heat. The bags may be loaded and stored up to 1 week without losing the vacuum seal. The vacuum changer can accommodate up to 21 cassettes.

The Picker-Amplatz changer employs the single-stage cassette changer principle (Fig. 12–1) for film transportation. In this method, the unexposed cassettes are stacked on a spring-loaded platform. The exposure is made directly over the stack. The cassettes beneath the top cassette are protected by the lead on the back of the top cassette. At the end of each exposure, the exposed cassette is moved to the receiving bin by a push bar, and the next cassette is ready for exposure.

The vacuum changer is no longer in production; however, because there are still many vacuum changers in use today, angiographers should be aware of the vacuum changer's existence.

## CASSETTELESS SERIAL FILM CHANGERS

Cassetteless changers may transport films individually (cut) or from a supply film spool (roll). Both systems can transport film equal to or faster than the cassette system, thereby increasing the exposure rate. Both roll and cut film changers use stationary intensifying screens. The screens separate during film transportation and close during film exposure. The primary problem with the continual opening and closing of the screens involves removing all of the air between the screens and film during the closing of the screens. Removing the air allows close film-to-screen contact.

Three different approaches have been used to solve the trapped air problem. The first approach is to have one of the screens slightly curved and the other screen straight. The curved plate makes contact with the straight plate in the center and then at the sides (Fig. 12–2A). This enables the trapped air to escape from the sides. The second approach is to mount the screens similarly to the way a book is made (Fig. 12–2B). The screens close at one end first, expelling the trapped air from the opposite end. The third and last approach is to use two curved screens (Fig. 12–2C). When the screens

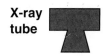

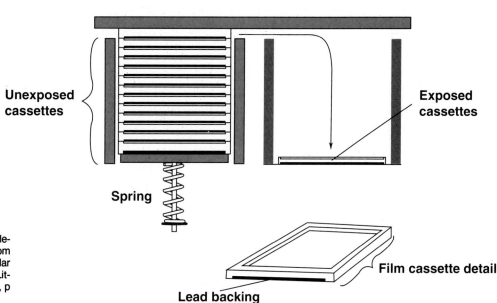

**Figure 12–1.** Diagram of a single-stage cassette changer. (From Abrams, H: Angiography: Vascular and Interventional, Vol 1, ed. 3. Little, Brown & Co., Boston, 1983, p 109, with permission.)

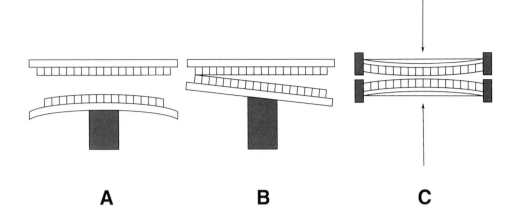

**Figure 12-2.** Various methods of screen closures. (*A*) Curved plate makes contact with center of straight plate; (*B*) plates close like a book; (*C*) curved plates make contact with each other in center. (From Abrams, p 109, with permission.)

close, they shut from the center first, forcing the air to be expelled at the peripheral edges.

Both cut and roll changers have advantages and disadvantages, which are explained in the following sections. Table 12-1 presents a summary of the characteristics of various changers.

## Roll Film Changers

The roll film changer operates on the same principle as a photographic camera. The unexposed film is rolled on a spool and placed on one side of the film changer. Film is threaded through the machine past the exposure area to another spool, which stores the exposed radiographic film (Fig. 12-3). Some roll changers are designed so that loading and unloading of the film must be performed in a darkened radiographic room. These types of changers present problems in radiographic rooms that cannot be made completely light-tight. Radiographic rooms that cannot be darkened may cause light fogging of the film during the loading or unloading of the film changer. Rooms that are not light-tight should have roll changers with a daylight loading capability. After the film changer is loaded, the unit is ready for use.

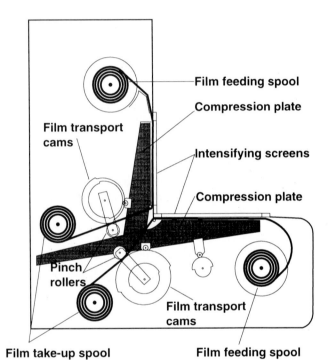

**Figure 12-3.** Cross section of a roll film changer. (From Abrams, p 117, with permission.)

Table 12-1. **Summary of Film Changer Characteristics**

| Factor | Type of Changer | | | | | |
| | Roll Film | Puck C | Puck CM | Puck 90M | AOT-S | Vacuum |
|---|---|---|---|---|---|---|
| Viewing radiographs | Difficult | Easy | Easy | Easy | Easy | Easy |
| Storing radiographs | Difficult | Easy | Easy | Easy | Easy | Easy |
| Film loading and unloading | Easy | Easy | Easy | Easy | Easy | Easy |
| Mechanical reliability | Excellent | Good | Good | Good | Good | Good |
| Film size availability | 14″ × 14″ | 14″ × 14″ | 14″ × 14″ | 14″ × 14″ | 10″ × 12″, 14″ × 14″ | 14″ × 14″ |
| Film-screen contact | Good | Good | Good | Good | Good | Excellent |
| Film capacity | 43 | 30 | 30 | 30 | 30 | 21 |
| Maximum film frequency (films/sec) | 12 | 4 | 6 | 4 | 6 | 4 |

The basic function of the roll changer is to move the film toward the patient, keep the film stationary during exposure, and transport the exposed film to the take-up spool as quickly as possible. Film exposure and transportation must be in sequence and are electromechanically controlled. The film is advanced by a serrated cam and pinch rollers (Fig. 12–3). These rollers serrate the film on the edges and move the film to the take-up spool. The speed at which the cam and the rollers rotate varies according to the selected filming rate. The maximum speed of a typical roll changer, for example, the Franklin roll changer, is 12 films or exposures per second. After the desired number of exposures have been made, the film is manually cut, unloaded into a light-tight carrier, and processed.

The simplicity of the roll film changer's mechanical drive results in easy film transportation and few film jams. The method of film transportation varies with the manufacturer. Both the Franklin and Elema roll changers employ the method described in the preceding paragraph.

After processing, the radiographs are viewed. Uncut film does not lend itself to easy viewing, unless a carousel-type viewer is available. Storage of roll film also presents problems. An alternate method is to cut the film between film images and store each one in a regular x-ray jacket. However, the advantages of leaving the roll in one piece (uncut) are that the radiographs are always in proper sequence and the loss of a single image is impossible.

The film for roll film changers is usually supplied in 50-foot lengths. Most changers expose a 14″ × 14″ (35 cm × 35 cm) area, allowing approximately 43 exposures per roll. Because of the number of radiographs required for each examination, often the last length of the film remaining in the changer is too short to record a subsequent examination. Therefore, this unexposed film is removed from the changer and a new roll of film is inserted. Consequently, the last few feet of film in a roll changer are unexposed and "wasted."

## Cut Film Changers

Cut film changers received their name because they use single or cut sheets of x-ray film for each exposure. The types of cut film changers discussed in the following paragraphs are the Puck film changers and the AOT-S film changer.

Three types of Puck film changers are the Puck CM, Puck C, and Puck 90M (Fig. 12–4). The Puck CM and C preceded the Puck 90M. The following is a brief description of the Puck CM's features. This unit has a fiberoptic, 100-character film-marking capability that displays patient information and examination data on two edges of the film. This information appears on the viewing side of the radiograph, making it easy to read. The receiving magazine can be removed by moving it to the right, left, or straight ahead (Fig. 12–5). This versatility in removing the magazine provides the user

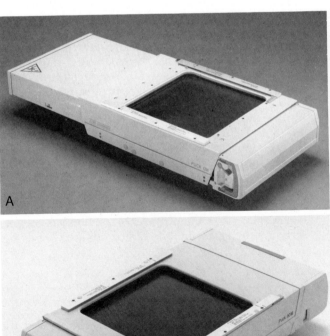

A

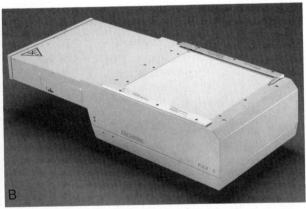

B

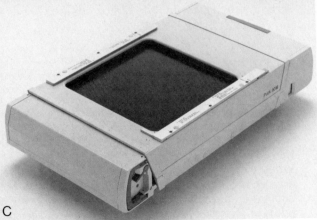

C

**Figure 12–4.** Puck film changers. (*A*) CM; (*B*) C; and (*C*) 90M. (Courtesy Elema-Schonander, Elk Grove Village, IL.)

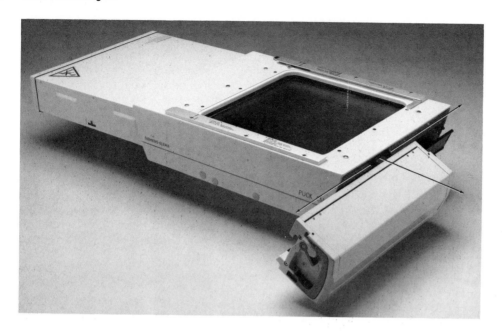

**Figure 12–5.** The Puck CM magazine may be removed by moving it to the left, right, or straight. (Courtesy Elema-Schonander, Elk Grove Village, IL.)

with alternate ways to detach the magazine when the changer is positioned near items that may be in the way of loading or unloading the changer. Another feature of the Puck CM is real-time viewing. This feature allows the changer to be positioned in front of the image intensifier. A small, radiolucent circular area allows radiation to pass through the changer to the image intensifier. This type of monitoring allows visualization of the catheter position and vessel filling during the examination and/or filming.

The Puck 90M succeeded the Puck CM changer. It contains all of the features of the CM. An advantage of the Puck 90M is that it is smaller than the CM, making it more versatile. Also, whereas the CM's supply magazine is interweaving (each film must be positioned between two metal or plastic dividers), the 90M supply magazine employs an S-stack loading magazine (has no dividers) and no interweaving. The S stack is loaded by using a film catch to pick up 30 films from the film bin

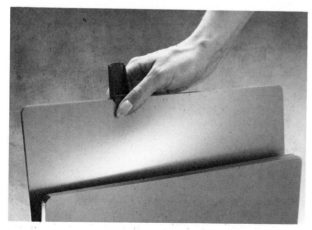

**Figure 12–6.** Film catch used to pick up 30 films for loading the Puck 90M. (Courtesy Elema-Schonander, Elk Grove Village, IL.)

(Fig. 12–6) with one grip, thus eliminating the need to count films.

The Puck C differs slightly from the Puck 90M and CM. It has the receiving magazine directly below the exposure area and is accessible from the same side as the loading (supply) magazine. Unlike the CM and Puck 90M, this design does not allow for real-time viewing. However, the advantage of the Puck C changer is that it is small enough to be used with a conventional radiographic and fluoroscopic unit.

The Siemens-Elema AOT-S is also a cut film changer. It can be computer programmed, can expose a maximum of six films per second, has a storage magazine with a 30-film capacity, allows daylight insertion and removal of the film magazine and receiving cassette, and marks patient identification and sequential numbering on each film frame. It is also available in 14″ × 14″ (35 cm × 35 cm) and 10″ × 12″ (24 cm × 30 cm) film sizes. The AOT-S loading magazine is a large, stainless steel container with a film capacity of 30. The upper third of the magazine has interlocking sliding lids. To load the magazine, the sliding lids are opened and the film is inserted between the wire dividers (Fig. 12–7A and B). After the film has been inserted in the magazine, the sliding lids are closed (Fig. 12–7C).

## STANDS

Film changers are attached to some type of stand, the simplest type being the mobile floor stand. In this system the changer is mounted on a frame with locking wheels. These stands are usually employed for the large film changers such as the AOT-S or Picker vacuum cassette changer. Although the changer can be wheeled around the room, its height cannot be adjusted. Some companies have improved the mobile stand to include hydraulics and an arm mount, which permit vertical or

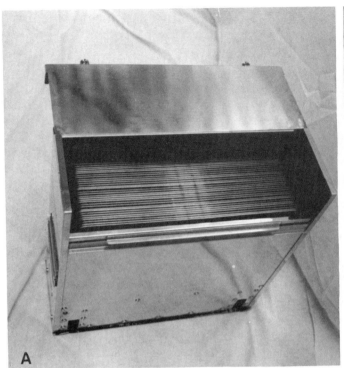

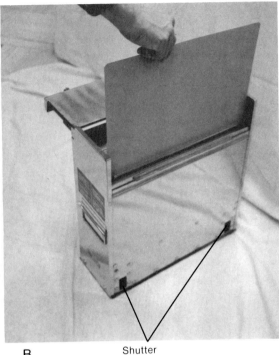

Shutter

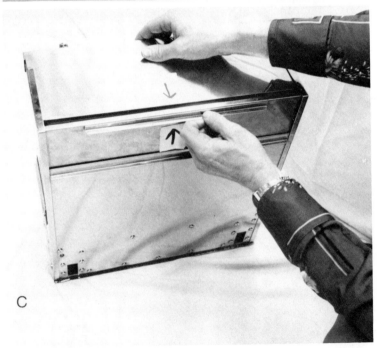

**Figure 12–7.** Loading AOT storage magazine. (*A*) Open magazine; (*B*) load magazine; (*C*) close magazine.

horizontal positioning and height adjustment of the changer (Fig. 12–8). Another common method of support for a film changer is a C-arm mount. This allows a variety of positions in which the changer may be placed.

## PROGRAMMING

### Types of Programming Systems

All of the changers previously mentioned use some form of computer programming to select the rate of

film exposure. Computer programming may be achieved through the use of a punched card, a panel, or a microprocessor console (Fig. 12–9). In the punched-card method, the angiographer programs the changer by using a stylet to punch the desired holes in a thin cardboard. Each row of the punched card gives the film changer a different command. Most cards contain a row, or rows, that must be punched to regulate the filming rate (including the ability to change the rate and have a pause between exposures), the injector operation, and the tabletop movement for units having auxiliary settings for peripheral angiography. The

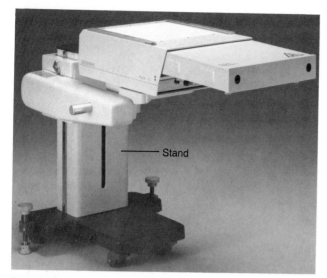

**Figure 12-8.** Puckwop stand. (Courtesy Elema-Schonander, Elk Grove Village, IL.)

punched card is inserted in a program selector that reads the card and performs the punched commands on the card.

The panel programmer is usually a wall-mounted solid-state unit that is often microprocessor-based. In these units, the angiographer uses knobs and switches on the panel to select the filming rate. Both the card and panel systems use lights to inform the angiographer which portion of the program the changer is operating. For example, in the Puck program selector, a bulb lights to inform the angiographer when the power is on; another light identifies that the film is in the exposure position; and still another light indicates when the x-ray apparatus is ready for use. Most of the lights and controls on the program selector are self-explanatory. It is strongly advised that the angiographer adopt the habit of checking and rechecking the light board to ensure that the proper steps for operation of the film changer have been completed.

The punched card and panel systems are rapidly being replaced by the microprocessor-based console. These units operate by either pressing keys on a keyboard or touching the screen. They are capable of storing frequently used programs for easy recall. All programmers have become sophisticated and often are capable of regulating and sequencing the injection,

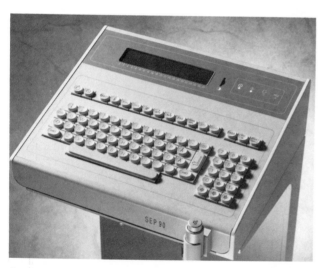

A

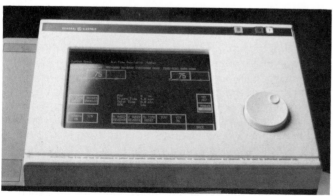

B

**Figure 12-9.** (*A*) SEP 90. (Courtesy Elema-Schonander, Elk Grove Village, IL.); (*B*) General Electric's Advantx program selector. (Courtesy General Electric, Milwaukee, WI.)

x-ray exposure, table movements, or film changer commands.

## Film Cycle Time

In all film changers, a certain amount of the film cycle represents the time the film is transported; the rest of the time the film is stationary (being exposed). The film is usually in motion 50 to 60 percent of the entire film cycle: this would mean that the film is stationary 40 to 50 percent of the time and is technically ready for exposure. However, because of certain electronic delays, not all of the film's stationary time is available for exposure. The two major electronic factors affecting the length of exposure time are the zero time and the phasing-in time.

### ZERO TIME

The film changer must signal the generator as to when an exposure should occur. The generator activates the shutter after a small delay. This delay is a constant for any given film changer and is a result of the closing of relay switches, increasing voltage, and so on. This period is called zero, or anticipation, time. Because zero time is a constant, it can be compensated for by presetting the exposure on the film changer. For example, if the zero time is 50 milliseconds (msec), then the signal for the exposure can be given 50 msec before the actual exposure should occur. The zero time is preset by the manufacturer. Generally speaking, modern solid-state generators have made zero time negligible.

### PHASING-IN TIME

The phasing-in time, or interrogation time, is a variable that changes depending on what part of the sine wave the film changer signals the generator to expose the film. The generator initiates the exposure when the sine wave is at zero. Thus, if the signal is given when the sine wave is at zero, then the exposure is made immediately, resulting in a phasing-in time of zero. However, if the signal is given after zero, then the exposure cannot be made until the sine wave reaches zero. On a single-phase 60-cycles/sec unit, the maximum amount of phasing-in time is 1/60 second, or 16.7 msec. Most generators operate on three-phase current. This means that a new phase begins every 120 degrees, or 2.77 msec. On a three-phase unit, the maximum amount of phase-in time is 1/360 second.

### MAXIMUM PERMISSIBLE EXPOSURE TIME

To determine the maximum permissible exposure time of a film, the maximum phasing-in time must be subtracted from the film's stationary time. The following is an example calculation using the maximum permissible exposure time of a film.

**Problem.** Given a filming sequence of five exposures per second, what is the maximum permissible exposure time per film?

*Calculation*

1. One second equals 1000 msec. Therefore, to determine how many milliseconds per film for a 5-exposure/sec sequence, divide by 5, or

$$\frac{1000}{5} = 200 \text{ msec}$$

2. If 200 msec is the time for each film cycle and 40 percent of the time the film is stationary, then by multiplying 40 percent by 200 msec, the time the film is available for exposure, or stationary time, can be determined.

$$0.40 \times 200 \text{ msec} = 80 \text{ msec}$$

3. Because the zero time is preset, it can be neglected; however, the phasing-in time is a variable. If the unit operates on a three-phase 60 cycles/sec setup, then the maximum phasing-in time is 1/360 second, or

$$\frac{1000}{360} = 2.77 \text{ msec}$$

Subtracting the maximum phasing-in time from the stationary time results in the maximum exposure time per film, or

$$80 \text{ msec} - 2.77 \text{ msec} = 77.23 \text{ msec}$$

## BIPLANE FILMING

Many angiographic procedures require anterior-posterior and lateral views. This may be accomplished by using one film changer and one radiographic tube to film each view separately or by employing two film changers and two tubes to radiograph both views simultaneously (Fig. 12–10). In the single film changer method, the film changer must be repositioned for each view. The single film changer has the advantage of excellent film quality. The disadvantages of the single changer are that the tube and changer must be repositioned for the second view and that two injections are required (one for each view).

In the two-film-changer method, only one injection is needed to obtain both views. This is accomplished by positioning one changer for the anterior-posterior view, with the other changer positioned for the lateral view. The filming of the patient may occur simultaneously, or the changers may alternate exposures. Both types of biplane filming create a problem of scatter radiation striking the unexposed film in the adjacent changer. One solution to this problem is to mount grids over the exposure area to absorb the unwanted secondary radiation. Another disadvantage of biplane filming is the need for a room large enough to accommodate two film changers and two x-ray tubes. Making the decision whether to use either the single or the biplane method of filming involves a combination of personal preference, available space, and money.

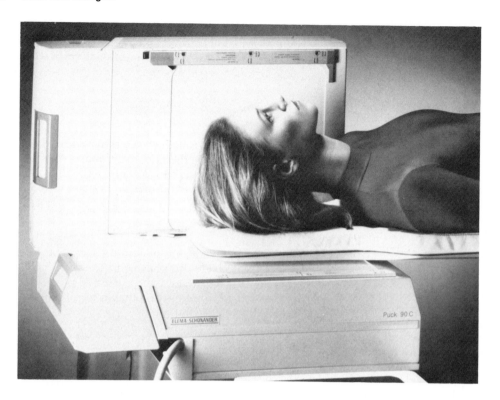

**Figure 12–10.** Setup for simultaneous bilateral filming. (Courtesy Elema-Schonander, Elk Grove Village, IL.)

## PERIPHERAL ANGIOGRAPHY EQUIPMENT

As mentioned previously, some film changer program selectors have the capability of moving the tabletop longitudinally for peripheral angiography of the lower extremities.

Peripheral angiography of the lower extremity includes filming of the pelvis, thighs, knees, and legs. This is accomplished by placing the film changer under the table and exposing the pelvis first. Then the table moves a predetermined distance so that the patient's thighs are over the film changer and a second exposure is made. This sequence is continued, exposing the knees and legs (Fig. 12–11). Because the thickness of the body varies, peripheral lower extremity angiography tabletop equipment allows the angiographer to preselect the kilovoltage for each exposure separately. The rate and amount of injection and filming are discussed in Chapter 26, Abdomen and Lower Extremity Angiography. However, it should be noted that the tabletop movement requires about 2 seconds, which must be taken into consideration when filming.

**Figure 12–11.** Peripheral tabletop movement. *1,* Position for exposing the pelvis; *2,* position for exposing the thighs; *3,* position for exposing the knees; *4,* position for exposing the legs.

## REVIEW QUESTIONS

1. Cassette serial film changers may cause _____ during the film transportation interval.
   A. fogging
   B. noise
   C. double exposure
   D. vibration of the equipment

2. The _____ serial film changer has the best film screen contact.
   A. Puck C     C. vacuum
   B. Puck CM     D. AOT-S

3. The _____ film changer heat-seals the film and screen.
   A. AOT-S     C. vacuum
   B. Puck 90M     D. Puck C

4. The primary problem with opening and closing intensifying screens for rapid film changers is _____.

A. removing the air
B. transporting the film
C. using a grid
D. synchronizing it with the exposure

5. In a roll film changer the cam and _____ are used to transport the film.
A. film feeding spool
B. film take-up spool
C. pinch roller
D. intensifying screens

6. A disadvantage of a roll film changer is that _____.
A. the film may not be in sequence
B. the last few feet of film are rarely exposed
C. it is easy to lose a film
D. film transportation is difficult

7. Real-time viewing of the Puck 90M allows for _____.
A. exposure of up to 7 films/sec
B. rapid transportation of film
C. the image intensifier to be over the changer
D. exposure of 1 msec

8. The Puck _____ uses an S-stack loading magazine.
A. 90M
B. C
C. CM

9. The most sophisticated type of programmer is the _____.
A. microprocessor-based console
B. panel
C. punched card

10. In rapid film processing, the film is usually stationary approximately _____ percent of the time.
A. 80 to 90
B. 60 to 70
C. 50 to 60
D. 40 to 50

11. _____ time is constant and represents the time the generator activates the exposure.
A. film cycle
B. zero

C. phase-in
D. stationary

12. The phase-in time for a three-phase unit is approximately _____ msec.
A. 1.03
B. 1.79
C. 2.77
D. 3.06

13. _____ msec is the approximate maximum-permissible exposure time per film on a 4-exposures/sec filming sequence using a three-phase unit with a film stationary time of 40 percent.
A. 46
B. 63
C. 85
D. 97

14. Using one film changer for biplane angiography has the advantage of _____.
A. excellent film quality
B. repositioning the changer
C. two injections
D. short zero time

## BIBLIOGRAPHY

Abrams, H: Angiography: Vascular and Interventional, Vol 1, ed 3. Little, Brown & Co, Boston, 1983.

Brinker, R and Skucas, J: Radiology Special Procedures Room. University Park Press, Baltimore, 1973.

Chesney, N and Chesney, M: X-ray Equipment for Student Radiographers, ed 3. Blackwell Scientific Publications, Oxford, 1984.

Grime, S: The programmed radiographic technique in direct angiography. Electromedica (Siemens Co) 41:162, 1973.

Hendee, W, Chaney, E, and Rossi, R: Radiologic Physics Equipment and Quality Control. Year Book Medical Publishers, Chicago, 1977.

Snopek, A: Fundamentals of Special Radiographic Procedures. WB Saunders, Philadelphia, 1992.

Thompson, T: A Practical Approach to Modern X-ray Equipment, ed 2. Little, Brown & Co, Boston, 1985.

Wojtowycz, M: Handbook in Radiology: Interventional Radiology and Angiography. Year Book Medical Publishers, Chicago, 1990.

# CHAPTER 13

# Electromechanical Injectors

*Marianne R. Tortorici, EdD, ARRT(R)*

During the early years of vascular radiography, all injections of contrast media were performed manually. Manual injection of contrast medium was most effective in small blood flow vessels. Manual injection was undesirable in large blood flow circulatory areas because it was impossible to introduce a large bolus of contrast medium in a short period of time. To compensate for the decreased bolus size in the vessel, it was necessary either to increase the amount of contrast medium injected or to increase the concentration of the medium. Both methods were discouraged because of the high toxicity of the medium. Therefore, to demonstrate large blood flow vessels of the circulatory system, a mechanical device (automatic injector) was needed to inject a large bolus of radiopaque contrast medium over a short period of time.

This chapter outlines electromechanical injector use and explains the various injector controls on the console (Fig. 13–1) and their function. Also included is a brief summary of the safety features and options of electromechanical injectors. Several different product names appear throughout this chapter. Products are mentioned to familiarize the reader with various types of equipment on the market and does not indicate an endorsement of that particular item.

## BRIEF HISTORY

The first automatic injector was introduced in the 1950s and was capable of injecting large quantities of contrast medium in a matter of seconds. It maintained a constant pressure during injection; thus, it was termed a constant-pressure injector. Although this injector was an improvement over manual injection, it presented the following disadvantages:

1. A fraction of a second was needed to deliver the required pressure.
2. Personnel had to be present in the radiographic room to initiate the injection.
3. It was impossible to initiate the injection when the heart was in diastole.
4. The syringe was covered in metal and could not be visualized to see if air bubbles were present in the barrel of the syringe.

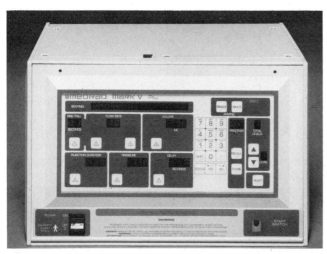

**Figure 13-1.** Medrad Mark V Plus console. (Courtesy of Medrad, Pittsburgh, PA.)

5. Catheter whipping could occur if there was too much pressure.
6. Too much pressure could result in vessel dissection.
7. The catheter could break if the pressure was set too high.

The first problem could be overcome by filling the catheter with normal saline solution. However, to solve the remaining problems, a new type of injector had to be designed.

As time progressed and injector manufacturers gained experience, the electromechanical flow rate injector was introduced. The increased capabilities of the electromechanical injector solved many of the problems of the constant pressure injector. These included using more pressure than the catheter could withstand, injecting the contrast medium too fast, lack of control of the injection of contrast medium to coincide with the heartbeat, and accidentally injecting air into the patient. Additionally, the numerous safety features built into electromechanical injectors helps prevent a mechanical malfunction, which could cause serious injury to the patient or damage to the equipment.

## FILLING THE SYRINGE

Electromechanical injectors have a syringe attached to a movable arm. Some injectors have a detachable arm that can be attached to the x-ray table. This is useful for examinations, such as lower extremity angiography, in which the patient and table move during x-ray exposure. Syringes may be disposable (plastic) or reusable (glass) and are available in varying sizes (Fig. 13-2). The reusable syringe requires maintenance, for example, cleaning the O rings. It is also difficult to remove all residual contrast medium or blood, which can cause cross contamination. The problems associated with the reusable syringe make the disposable syringe preferable because it is maintenance-free and eliminates cross contamination.

Filling a syringe with contrast medium requires ster-

ile technique, whether the syringe is used for an automatic or a manual injection. However, there is a difference in the method of filling a syringe attached to an automatic injector and a syringe used for manual injection. In the manual injection method of filling a syringe, an amount of air is injected into the vial and the same amount of contrast medium is withdrawn. In filling the syringe of an electromechanical injector, the seal and top of the contrast medium vial are removed and the medium is drawn up through a sterile extension tube.

Filling the automatic injector syringe is often performed while it is in a vertical position. This is useful when removing air after the syringe is loaded with the contrast medium. The controls that are used to fill the syringe and to prepare the injector are grouped together. The number and names of the controls vary slightly from injector to injector. In general, there are usually two controls, and these are most often labeled "load," "fill" or "reverse," and "unload" or "forward." For convenience, these controls are usually located on the movable arm rather than on the console.

To fill the syringe with contrast medium, the plunger must first be inserted completely in the barrel of the syringe. This is achieved by activating the "unload" or

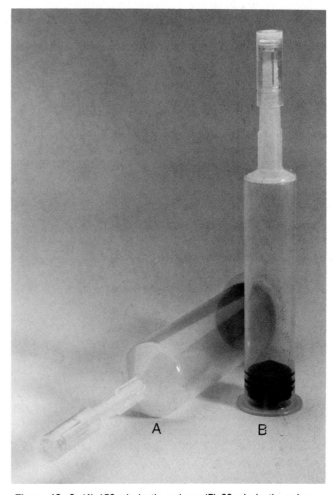

**Figure 13-2.** (A) 150-ml plastic syringe; (B) 60-ml plastic syringe. (Courtesy of Medrad, Pittsburgh, PA.)

"forward" control (Fig. 13–3A). After the plunger is inside the barrel of the syringe, an extension tube is attached to the end of the syringe (Fig. 13–3B). The opposite end of the extension tube is inserted into a contrast medium vial. The "fill," "unload," or "reverse" button is depressed to withdraw the desired amount of contrast medium (Fig. 13–3C). It is advisable to use a moderate load speed to avoid drawing air into the syringe. When the syringe is filled and before injection of the contrast medium, all air bubbles must be removed from the syringe and the extension tubing.

Removal of air bubbles is accomplished by slowly inserting the plunger into the barrel of the syringe until all of the air is eliminated (Fig. 13–3D). Most injectors have a manual knob that can be turned clockwise or counterclockwise to move the plunger slowly forward or backward. This knob is extremely useful since the plunger can be moved slowly without accidentally expelling the contrast medium. Other injectors have the ability to regulate the speed of the plunger movement. A slow speed is used when expelling the air from the syringe.

After the syringe is filled and all the air is removed, a "heater blanket" is attached to the plastic pressure jacket (Fig. 13–3E). The heater either is built into the syringe casing or is detachable. It is advisable to warm the medium prior to injection to approximate the human body temperature. This may be achieved by immersing the contrast vial in a special contrast medium warmer or warm water. Once the contrast medium is drawn into the syringe, the heating jacket aids in maintaining the temperature.

## DELIVERY OF CONTRAST MEDIUM

Electromechanical injectors are often referred to as flow-rate injectors. The name refers to the injector's ability to deliver a specific flow rate for a given time period. It is possible to determine flow rate by applying Jean Louis Marie Poiseuille's (a French physician, anatomist, and physiologist) formula. The formula for Poiseuille's law is

$$Q = \frac{\pi P r^4}{8nl}$$

Where $\pi$ = pi
$Q$ = milliliters delivered per second
$P$ = pressure in dynes per cubic centimeter
$r$ = radius of catheter in centimeters
$n$ = coefficient of contrast medium viscosity
$l$ = length of vascular catheter in centimeters

Assuming all other factors remain the same, the flow rate may be increased by increasing the radius of the catheter (r), increasing the pressure (P), decreasing the length of the catheter (l), or decreasing the viscosity of the contrast medium (n). Electromechanical injectors maintain the flow rate by increasing the pressure as required, up to a preprogrammed pressure limit.

For proper contrast medium delivery, the appropriate controls must be set. The number and names of the control switches vary from manufacturer to manufacturer. The amount and rate of contrast medium delivery are regulated by the volume control and the flow-rate control, respectively.

The most common units of measure for the volume of contrast medium delivered are milliliters (ml) or cubic centimeters (cm³). The most common rates for injection are milliliters or cubic centimeters per second (ml/sec or cm³/sec), milliliters or cubic centimeters per minute (ml/min or cm³/min), and milliliters or cubic centimeters per hour (ml/h or cm³/h). Dividing the volume of contrast medium delivered by the rate of injection determines the length of time of the injection. For example, if a volume of 10 ml of contrast medium is delivered at a rate of 5 ml/sec, then the length of time for the injection is

$$\frac{10 \text{ ml}}{5 \text{ ml/sec}} = 2 \text{ sec}$$

Some injectors have a built-in computer that allows the user to input data that affect the flow rate, for example, catheter length. The computer assesses the data and provides information on the predicted injection flow rate or the pressure limit for a specific flow rate. Also, some injector computers contain software that allow the user to program common injection protocols with the ability to store up to four flow rates in one injection.

In some instances, pathology, catheter placement, or other circumstances make it necessary to delay either the x-ray exposure or contrast medium injection. The exposure delay allows the injection of contrast medium to occur prior to filming, while injection delay initiates exposures prior to the contrast medium being delivered. There are two controls employed for x-ray or injection delays; they are the x-ray or injection delay control and the time delay switch. Energizing the x-ray delay switch postpones the initiation of the x-ray exposure. Selecting the injection delay control postpones the delivery of the contrast medium. The length of time the x-ray or injection is deferred is determined by setting the time delay switch.

After properly setting the controls, the injector is ready for use. The injection of contrast medium may be started automatically under the following conditions: when the injector is connected to the generator or when it is attached to a master control. The injection may be started manually by depressing the injection switch. Also, in most angiographic procedures, automatic initiation of the injection is preferred over manual initiation. Manual initiation of the injection often requires the use of a remote control to eliminate the need for an appropriate individual to be in the radiographic room to start the injection.

## SAFETY FEATURES

There are several safety features built into the electromechanical injector. The features are intended to prevent breaking the vascular catheter or the occur-

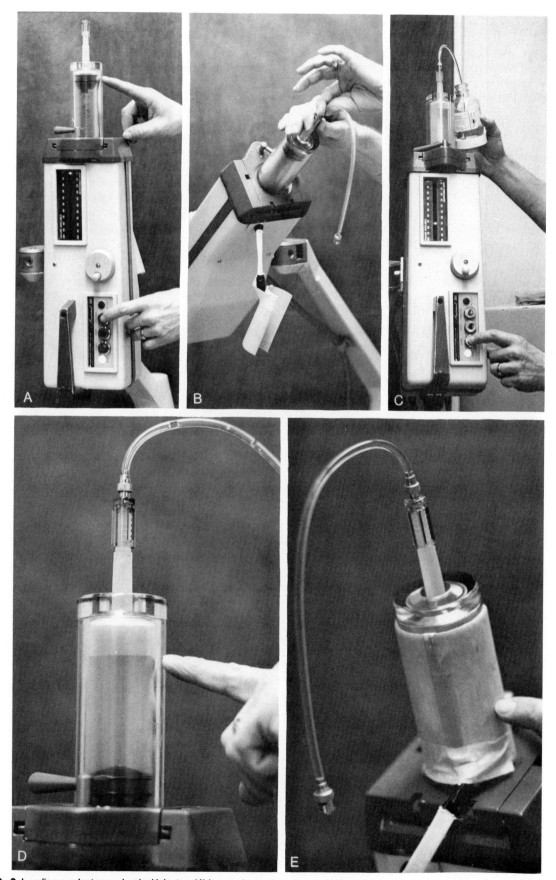

**Figure 13–3.** Loading an electromechanical injector. (*A*) Insert plunger in syringe; (*B*) place extension tube on syringe; (*C*) withdraw contrast medium; (*D*) remove air; (*E*) attach heater blanket.

rence of a mechanical malfunction or a "runaway" injection.

If too much pressure is employed during the injection, catheter whipping or breakage of the catheter may occur. To prevent an excessive pressure injection, electromechanical injectors have a pressure limit control. The unit for measuring the pressure is pounds per square inch (psi). The usual psi control range is from 100 to 1000. It is recommended that the pressure be set 100 psi below the lowest rating of the disposable catheter used during the procedure. The most common pressure control increments used are 400 and 500 psi.

Another safety feature is the rate rise control. By regulating the pressure during the injection, this control is designed to prevent a sudden, forceful injection. The rate rise control allows the pressure to begin at zero and slowly rise to the preset pressure limit measured in pounds per square inch. The rate rise control is incremented in tenths of a second. Thus, if the injector is set for 500 psi at a rate rise of 0.4 seconds, then the pressure begins at zero and rises to 500 psi in 0.4 seconds.

A third safety feature is a mechanical stop that controls the amount of contrast medium injected. The mechanical stop is designed to prevent a "runaway" injection. On some injectors, the mechanical stop is set automatically. On other models, the stop must be set manually. The mechanical stop is usually set for 2 or 3 ml greater than the volume set on the console. If the injection reaches the number of cubic centimeters set on the mechanical lock, then the injection is automatically terminated.

The last safety feature is designed to protect the pa-

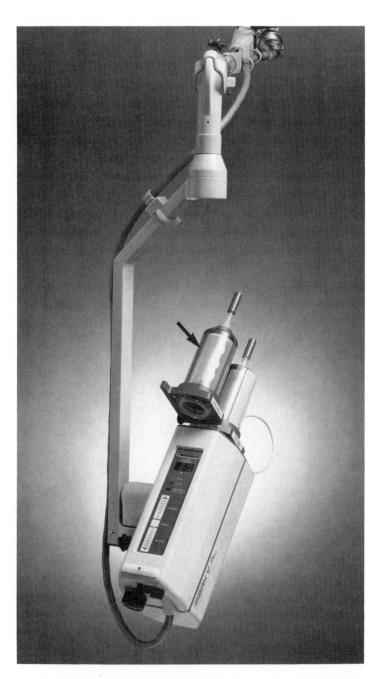

**Figure 13-4.** Clear plastic syringe pressure jacket. (Courtesy of Medrad, Pittsburgh, PA.)

tient and to prevent mechanical malfunctions. This major feature is the high-pressure plastic jacket around the syringe that prevents metal contact with the contrast medium, eliminating the possibility of an electric shock (Fig. 13–4).

## OPTIONS

Electromechanical injectors have several options. The most common options are multiple syringes (Fig. 13–5) and the electrocardiograph (ECG) monitor (Fig. 13–6). The multiple syringe injector has two syringes on the injector head. The two syringes allow the operator to change from syringe A to syringe B, eliminating the need to reload the syringe during the procedure. The Medrad V Plus system has two syringes of differing volume, a 60-cm³ and a 150-ml syringe. The smaller syringe is useful when performing low blood flow examinations, such as cerebral angiography, whereas the larger syringe is preferred for large blood flow vessel work, such as aortography. The ECG trigger option is designed to improve coronary angiography. The trigger is connected to an electrocardiograph that starts the injection at a preset time after the R cardiac wave impulse of the patient. Thus, the injection can be made during any cycle of the heart, diastolic or systolic. This

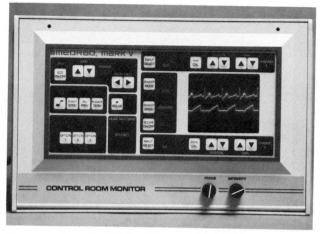

**Figure 13–6.** Medrad Mark V Plus electromechanical injector with ECG monitor. (Courtesy of Medrad, Pittsburgh, PA.)

synchronization is also useful in minimizing premature ventricular contractions (PVCs) and maintaining hemodynamic conditions.

## REVIEW QUESTIONS

1. A detachable syringe arm of an electromechanical injector is useful in _____ angiography.
   A. carotid
   B. pulmonary
   C. renal
   D. lower extremity

2. The _____ button is used to insert the plunger into the barrel of the syringe.
   A. load
   B. unload
   C. reverse
   D. fill

3. Flow rate of contrast medium may be increased by _____.
   A. decreasing the radius of the catheter
   B. decreasing the pressure
   C. increasing contrast medium viscosity
   D. decreasing the catheter length

4. A volume of 30 ml is to be delivered in 3 seconds; therefore, the rate of injection is _____ ml per second.
   A. 5
   B. 10
   C. 15
   D. 20

5. The pressure limit control should be set _____ PSI below the lowest rating of the catheter being used.
   A. 50
   B. 100
   C. 150
   D. 200

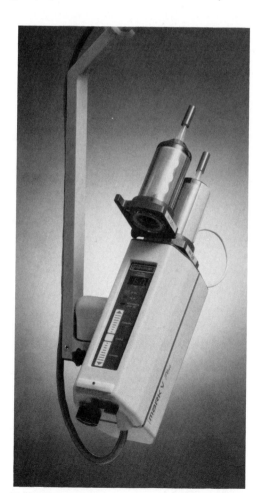

**Figure 13–5.** Multiple syringe. (Courtesy of Medrad, Pittsburgh, PA.)

6. The mechanical stop is designed to _____.
   A. stop catheter whipping
   B. prevent the catheter from breaking
   C. prevent a runaway injection
   D. regulate flow of contrast medium

7. List three disadvantages of constant-pressure injectors.

8. List two options on an electromechanical injector.

## BIBLIOGRAPHY

Abrams, HL: Angiography, Vol 2, ed 3. Little, Brown & Co, Boston, 1983.

Baltax, HA, Amplatz, K, and Levin, DC: Coronary Angiography. Charles C Thomas, Philadelphia, 1973.

Brinker, RD and Skucas, J: Radiology Special Procedure Room. University Park Press, Baltimore, 1973.

Chapman, G: The basic function and operation of high pressure angiographic injectors: A historical approach. Research paper presented as part of the degree requirements for the University of Nevada, Las Vegas, 1977.

Grollman, JH, Jr: Peripheral arteriography using the Medrad Universal Flow Module, Medrad, Inc.

Leslie, J, et al: A new simple power injector. AJR 128(3):381, March 1977.

Moss, G: Sequential, variable flow rate dye injector for arteriography. Journal of Association for the Advancement of Medical Instrumentation 5(4):212, July–August, 1971.

Schobinger, RA and Ruzicka, FF: Vascular Roentgenology. Macmillan, New York, 1964.

Snopek, AM: Fundamentals of Special Radiographic Procedures. WB Saunders, Philadelphia, 1992.

Thompson, TT: A Practical Approach to Modern Imaging Equipment, ed 2. Little, Brown & Co, Boston, 1985.

White, RI, Jr: Fundamentals of Vascular Radiology. Lea & Febiger, New York, 1976.

Wojtowycz, M: Handbook in Radiology: Interventional Radiology and Angiography. Year Book Medical Publishers, Chicago, 1990.

# CHAPTER 14

# Digital Imaging Techniques

*Marianne R. Tortorici, EdD, ARRT(R)*

In the early 1970s, computers were integrated into the field of medical imaging. Through the use of computers, data acquisition, manipulation, and display led to the introduction of new imaging modalities (e.g., computed tomography [CT]) and improvements in existing modalities (e.g., angiography). The use of computers in imaging required the development of a system to detect and convert remanent radiation into a digital computer image. A detection system is necessary to identify and assess the intensity of the radiation. When the detection system receives the data, it transmits the information to another component, the analog-to-digital converter, to change the analog information into a digital format. Once digitalized, the information is transferred to a central processing unit (CPU), where the image is processed. After the desired image is received, it may be printed, stored, displayed, manipulated, or sent to another area for viewing.

This chapter contains a brief summary of digital imaging, which is particularly useful in understanding Chapter 15, Digital Subtraction Angiography. The reader is referred to this chapter's bibliography for more in-depth information on computers and computer technology.

## THE DIGITAL IMAGE

### Image Acquisition

There are two common methods used to acquire information: (1) by performing several localized scans of an area of the patient, and (2) by using an array system in which a large area of the patient is scanned at one time. Both systems use detectors to identify the radiation intensity and transmit the information to an analog-to-digital converter. The detectors convert radiant energy to electricity and transmit this energy to the computer.

### Analog-to-Digital Converter

In general, information (data) is in either analog or digital format. Analog information is continuous, while

**129**

digital consists of discrete sets of data. The most typical analogy of digital data is a watch with a numeric display, which demonstrates discrete intervals of time. An analogy of analog data is a watch with a second hand that is continuously moving.

Information received from the detectors is analog. As such, the voltage varies in strength relative to its specific location on the continuum. These data must be changed to digital, or discrete, values. The analog-to-digital converter (ADC) changes the continuous voltage to a digital image by recording the potential at regular time intervals (Fig. 14–1). The computer allocates a digital value equal to the intensity of the voltage.

## Binary System

The binary system is a numeric system using base 2. In other words, the only acceptable values are 0 and 1.

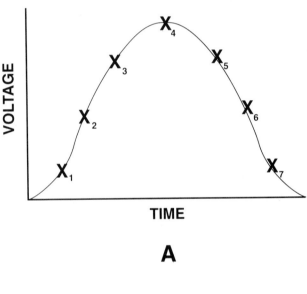

A single digit in binary is called a bit and is represented by 0 or 1. Eight bits equals a byte. The commonly used decimal system in the United States is base 10. Acceptable values in the decimal system are 0, 1, 2, 3, 4, 5, 6, 7, 8, and 9. In the binary system, as in the decimal system, the position of the number is the base value raised to a specific exponent. For example, the first digit to the right in the binary system is $2^0$; in decimal it is $10^0$. The next digit in binary is $2^1$, and $10^1$ in the decimal system. The total value of a number is determined by multiplying the digit by the position value and summing the products. For example, the binary number 0101 is

$$(0 \times 2^3) + (1 \times 2^2) + (0 \times 2^1) + (0 \times 2^0) =$$
$$(0 \times 8) + (1 \times 4) + (0 \times 2) + (1 \times 1) =$$
$$(0) + (4) + (0) + (1) = 5$$

The same is true of the decimal system. For example, the number 124 is

$$(1 \times 10^2) + (2 \times 10^1) + (4 \times 10^0) =$$
$$(1 \times 100) + (2 \times 10) + (4 \times 1) =$$
$$(100) + (20) + (4) = 124$$

## Image Matrix

The intensities obtained by the ADC are displayed in a matrix, which consists of rows and columns of cells. Each cell, called pixel for picture element, is located numerically by its row and column position (Fig. 14–2). Each pixel has a density relative to the intensity of the part imaged. A number is assigned to each pixel, representing the intensity or density of the image. The greater the intensity, the darker the pixel will be. The matrix, or group of pixels, results in an image that is very similar to a picture in a newspaper. Close inspection of a newspaper image reveals the small "dots" that make up the image. However, when observed from a distance, the dots "merge," creating a solid image.

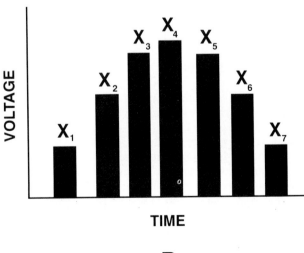

**Figure 14–1.** (*A*) Plot of analog information. (*B*) Digital plot of the analog information depicted in *panel A*.

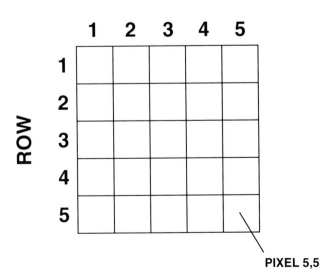

**Figure 14–2.** Image matrix with five rows and five columns.

## IMAGE CHARACTERISTICS

### Spatial Resolution

Spatial resolution is the ability to distinguish between two adjacent structures or areas on an image. Pixel size, in millimeters, and line pairs per millimeter (lp/mm) are used to measure spatial resolution. The smaller the pixel size and the greater the line pairs per millimeter, the better the spatial resolution. Pixel size is calculated by dividing the image size (in millimeters) by the number of pixels in a row or column (multiply the image size by 25.4 mm for units with image size measured in inches). For example, if the image size is 250 mm and the pixel row value is 512 (or a 512 × 512 matrix), the pixel size is 0.49 mm:

$$\text{Pixel size} = \frac{250 \text{ mm}}{512} = 0.49 \text{ mm}$$

Line pairs per millimeter are determined by using the following formula:

$$\text{lp/mm} = \frac{1}{2} \times \frac{1}{\text{pixel size}}$$

In the preceding example, for a 0.49-mm pixel size, the line pairs per millimeter are

$$\text{lp/mm} = \frac{1}{2} \times \frac{1}{0.49} = \frac{1}{0.98} = 1.02 \text{ lp/mm}$$

In the above example, for the same field of view (FOV), 250 mm, if the matrix were 1024 × 1024, the pixel size would be approximately 0.24 mm and the line pairs per millimeter would be 2.08. Thus, for the same FOV, the larger the matrix, the better the spatial resolution.

### Contrast Resolution

Contrast resolution represents the density difference between two pixels or the difference between two digital values. The number of gray scale steps and noise (see Noise section below) determines the contrast resolution. Since the computer uses the binary system, the number of gray scale steps is related to the binary system. For example, if the number of bits available to regulate the brightness is 2, then the number of gray scales is 4, or $2^2 = 4$. In an image having 8 bits, $2^8$, of information available for brightness, the number of gray scale steps is 256 (or 0 to 255). The frequency, or dynamic range, of an image is the total amount of contrast within the image.

### Noise

Noise is information that is detected but detracts from the image quality. There are several sources of noise. These include quantum, electronic, TV camera, ADC, and patient (superimposition of anatomy) noise. The total noise is the sum of the individual types of noise present. It is measured as the signal-to-noise ratio (SNR). SNR is the ratio of the output to the background noise. The higher the ratio, the better the image quality.

## MANIPULATING THE IMAGE

After the image has been stored, the operator may manipulate several factors, including density and contrast, to change the quality of the image. Among the more common manipulations are adjusting the window level or window width and filtering the image.

### Window

Most digital computers and their software are capable of displaying a large number of gray scale steps. The operator has the ability to control the range of image densities displayed, or window. The window represents a range of densities from white to black, known as the window width. Window level is the density level of the lower limit or center of the window. For example, if the window width is 600 and the center window level is set at 500 (for a 600 width, there are 300 levels above and below center), the range is 200 (500 − 300) to 800 (500 + 300). Notice in this example that the center window is still 500 and that the range is 600 (800 − 200). The window width regulates the image contrast. Reducing the window width increases image contrast. Window level controls density. Adjusting the window level to an upper limit of the window results in increased density.

### Filtering

Filtering is a mathematical function of the computer to remove unwanted data. This is usually accomplished by accentuating or suppressing selected frequencies received from the detectors. There are three types of filtering: low-pass, high-pass, and band-pass.

Low-pass filtering removes or amplifies all but the low frequencies. This is achieved by averaging each pixel's value with the adjacent pixels. Each pixel's value is replaced by the average value. This process, which is known as smoothing, is very useful in nuclear medicine studies. Low-pass filtering usually results in a reduction of image contrast.

High-pass filtering removes or amplifies all but the high frequencies. It may also be referred to as edge-enhancement filtering. The process of high-pass filtering is very similar to that of low-pass. The difference is that high-pass uses a weighted value to change the pixel values. High-pass filtering is useful in digital subtraction angiography and digital mammography. High-pass filtering tends to increase contrast.

Band-pass removes or amplifies all frequencies except those in a selected range or band. Band-pass is useful in delineating anatomic structures that have limited frequency bands.

# PICTURE ARCHIVING AND COMMUNICATIONS

Picture archiving and communications systems (PACS) is a method of computerizing and transmitting images. PACS may be applied to all types of imaging modalities, such as CT, magnetic resonance imaging (MRI), and digital subtraction angiography (DSA). To archive an image, it must be stored in the computer memory. Storing an image requires at least 1 to 6 megabytes ($10^6$) of memory. The actual storage capacity depends on the size of the storage medium and the type of modality. Examples of storage media available include, but are not limited to, laser memory cards, optical disks, and optical tapes. These media have a range of memory capacity from megabytes to gigabytes ($10^9$). Of the various modalities, nuclear medicine uses the least amount of storage space and digital radiography requires the greatest amount of memory.

Most computerized imaging systems can communicate or transmit the image to different locations for display or manipulation. Images may be sent anywhere from the next room to thousands of miles away. The system used to transmit images is called a network. A discussion of the specific types of network systems is beyond the scope of this text.

## IMAGE DISPLAY

There are several techniques that may be used to display the image. The most common is the cathode-ray tube (CRT) method. An example of a CRT is the typical TV monitor used with most computers. Although data for the image are stored in the computer memory, the image displayed on the CRT is temporary. Hard copies of an image may be made by transferring the data to an imaging medium. X-ray film is typically used to record the image and is processed by an automatic processor, which is similar to a conventional film processor.

## REVIEW QUESTIONS

1. A ____ is useful in obtaining the necessary information for image acquisition.
   A. ADC
   B. matrix
   C. network
   D. detector

2. The value of a single pixel represents the ____ of the image.
   A. contrast
   B. density
   C. gray scale
   D. edge enhancement

3. Select the answer below that provides the best spatial resolution. A $512 \times 512$ image with ____ mm pixel size.
   A. 0.50
   B. 0.45
   C. 0.40
   D. 0.35

4. For the same FOV, the ____ the matrix, the better the spatial resolution.
   A. smaller
   B. larger
   C. brighter
   D. more depth of

5. If the number of bits available to regulate brightness is 10, then the number of gray scale steps is ____.
   A. 64
   B. 256
   C. 512
   D. 1024

6. If the window width is 400 and the center window level is 500, then the range is ____.
   A. 300–700
   B. 200–600
   C. 100–500
   D. 500–900

7. List three types of filtering.

8. Actual storage capacity of a PACS system depends on the type of storage medium and ____.
   A. speed of the computer
   B. distance image must travel
   C. anatomy of part imaged
   D. type of modality

## BIBLIOGRAPHY

Bushong, SC: Radiologic Science for Technologists: Physics, Biology, and Protection, ed 5. Mosby, St Louis, 1993.

Carlton, RR and Adler, AM: Principles of Radiographic Imaging: An Art and a Science. Delmar Publishers, Albany, NY, 1992.

Curry, TS, Dowdey, JE, and Murry, RC. Christensen's Physics of Diagnostic Radiology, ed 4. Lea & Febiger, Philadelphia, 1990.

Hunter, TB. The Computer in Radiology. Aspen Publishing, Rockville, MD, 1986.

James, AE, Anderson, JH, and Higgins, CB. Digital Image Processing in Radiology. Williams & Wilkins, Baltimore, 1985.

Kelsey, CA: Essentials of Radiology Physics. Warren H Green, St Louis, 1985.

Kuni, CC. Introduction to Computers and Digital Processing in Medical Imaging. Year Book Medical Publishers, Chicago, 1988.

Tortorici, MR: Concepts in Medical Radiographic Imaging. WB Saunders, Philadelphia, 1992.

# CHAPTER 15

# Digital Subtraction Angiography

*Kathi A. Clark, BSBA, ARRT(R)(CV)*
*Marianne R. Tortorici, EdD, ARRT(R)*

Application of computer technology to radiology began during the 1970s. The initial imaging uses of computers included nuclear medicine, computed tomography, and ultrasound. The success in these areas led to integrating computers with angiographic procedures. The most common application of computers in angiography is that of digital subtraction angiography (DSA).

When DSA first evolved, it was predicted that it would replace many conventional procedures by performing them intravenously. Although DSA is very useful, economically efficient, and relatively safe, imaging problems and patient safety proved the original predictions to be false and intra-arterial access was still the preferred technique. As computer technology continues to evolve, many of the problems associated with DSA are being resolved.

This chapter is dedicated to providing information on the basic equipment needed for DSA, the types of DSA, advantages and disadvantages of DSA, and its application to angiographic procedures. The reader is referred to Chapter 14, Digital Imaging Techniques, for specific information on the technical aspects of digital imaging, including, but not limited to, analog-to-digital conversion, processing methods, manipulation techniques, and methods of displaying information.

## CONVENTIONAL SUBTRACTION

To facilitate the understanding of DSA, a discussion of conventional radiographic film subtraction is in order. There are three different methods of radiographic film subtraction. All methods require radiographs of the involved area, including a film *without* contrast medium (this film will be referred to as the initial radiograph) and a film *with* contrast medium (this film will be referred to as the contrast or angiographic film). It is critical that the patient's position be identical for both films. After the radiographs are obtained, subtraction is performed photographically in the processing area. The following sections are a brief discussion of the three methods of radiographic film subtraction.

## First-Order Subtraction

The first method, called the first-order subtraction, is the one most commonly employed. The process requires an initial radiograph (Fig. 15–1A) without contrast in the area of interest, a radiograph with contrast medium (Fig. 15–1B), and subtraction film. The first step is to make a mask of the initial radiograph by placing the initial radiograph on the emulsion side of a subtraction film and exposing both films with a subtraction unit. The mask (Fig. 15–1C) is a reversal of the initial image (the black areas are white and the white areas are black). The mask is then placed over the radiograph with contrast medium (Fig. 15–1D). Because the mask is a reversal of the initial radiograph, when the mask is superimposed over the radiograph having contrast medium, all images are blocked out except for the image of the contrast medium. These films are then placed on the emulsion side of a subtraction film, inserted in the subtraction unit, and exposed. The result is the subtracted print (Fig. 15–1E).

## Second-Order Subtraction

The second subtraction method is called second-order subtraction. In this method, a first-order mask is made (see the previous discussion). The mask is then superimposed over both the initial radiograph and a subtraction film and exposed in the subtraction unit. The result is a second-order mask. The subtraction print is made by superimposing the first-order mask, the second-order mask, and the contrast medium radiograph on the emulsion side of subtraction film. The films are placed in the subtraction unit and exposed. The subtraction film is developed and is termed the second-order subtraction print. A summary of the second-order subtraction method follows:

$$I + S = M_1$$
$$M_1 + I + S = M_2$$
$$M_1 + M_2 + C + S = P_2$$

where:

$I$ = initial radiograph
$S$ = subtraction film
$M_1$ = first-order mask
$M_2$ = second-order mask
$C$ = contrast radiograph
$P_2$ = second-order subtraction print

## Third-Order Subtraction

The third method of subtraction is called third-order subtraction. In this method, first-order masks are made of both the initial and contrast radiographs. An intermediate subtraction print is made by placing the initial radiograph over the first-order mask from the contrast radiograph. Both these films are placed over a subtraction film and exposed. The product is the intermediate subtraction print. The final subtraction print is made by superimposing the intermediate print, the contrast radiograph, and the first-order mask from the initial radiograph. All the films are placed on a subtraction film, inserted in the subtraction unit, and exposed. The developed subtraction film is the third-order subtraction print. A summary of the third-order subtraction method follows:

$$I + S = M_1$$
$$C + S = M_C$$
$$I + M_C + S = P_1$$
$$P_1 + C + M_1 + S = P_3$$

where:

$I$ = initial radiograph
$S$ = subtraction film
$M_1$ = mask of initial radiograph
$C$ = contrast radiograph
$M_C$ = mask of contrast radiograph
$P_1$ = intermediate subtraction print
$P_3$ = final third-order subtraction print

## EQUIPMENT

This section represents a summary of the types of equipment most commonly employed for digital subtraction angiography. To comprehend the contents of this section fully, the reader should be familiar with conventional radiographic equipment, for example, how a television (CRT) monitor works, and should have an understanding of the information provided in Chapter 14, Digital Imaging Techniques, prior to reading this section.

The type of equipment needed for DSA is very similar to that for conventional angiographic equipment. Because of cost restraints, many departments add the necessary computer equipment to a pre-existing angiographic room. However, obtaining high-quality DSA images requires more sophisticated equipment than the units associated with a routine conventional angiographic procedures room, especially if using DSA for the heart.

The basic apparatus for DSA includes, but is not limited to, an image processor, generator, image intensifier, x-ray tube, television and camera, and analog-to-digital converter. Refer to the respective sections in this chapter for a brief summary of each of these units.

A general summary of how these components integrate with one another follows. Figure 15–2 represents a diagram of DSA equipment integration. It is recommended that the reader correlate the diagram with the textual description that follows.

Since even slight movements by the patient create artifacts on the images, a C- or U-arm configuration connecting the image intensifier and x-ray tube is recommended. This allows the patient to remain supine, while the film and tube are manipulated to obtain oblique views.

The image processor is the "brain" for all the equip-

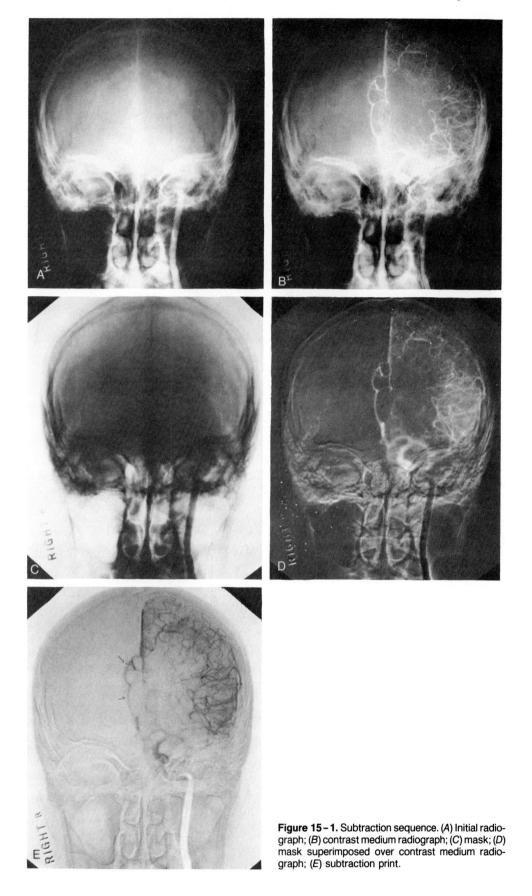

**Figure 15-1.** Subtraction sequence. (*A*) Initial radiograph; (*B*) contrast medium radiograph; (*C*) mask; (*D*) mask superimposed over contrast medium radiograph; (*E*) subtraction print.

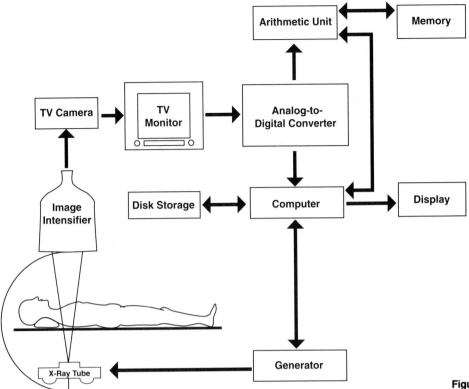

**Figure 15-2.** DSA equipment integration.

ment. The operator inputs instructions on the console of this unit to set the desired filming rate and processing instructions. The image processor is responsible for sending signals to the generator, which activates and deactivates the x-ray tube on command. The x-ray tube produces radiation, which passes through the patient and is detected by the image intensifier. The function of the image intensifier is to change the x-ray energy to light and transfer the light to the television camera. The television camera receives the light signal and directs it to the monitor. The signal also is sent through an analog-to-digital converter, where it is digitalized and forwarded to the image processor. The image processor receives the images and may perform one of many functions (see Image Processor section below).

## Image Processor

There are several types of image processors. The basic processor consists of a control console and a computer. The console usually consists of a keyboard and may contain knobs and a joy stick. The operator uses these items to input information or give commands to the computer. As previously stated, the computer is the primary brain of DSA. It performs several functions including digitizing, displaying, manipulating, and storing images (refer to Chapter 14, Digital Imaging Techniques, for more specific information on how the computer performs these functions).

The computer controls the generator initiation and termination of exposures. It also uses an arithmetic unit to store and retrieve images from memory. Another function of the computer is to display the image. The image may be displayed in several ways, for example, by video, by hard copy, and so on.

## Generator

The DSA generator serves the same purpose as in conventional x ray. However, unlike conventional units, a DSA generator must be capable of producing short exposures of equal intensity for all images and be able to operate at a high flux level. Equal densities resulting from equal intensities are essential in subtracting images. The time to prepare the tube for exposure (interrogation time) and the time to stop the exposure (extinction time) should be less than 5 msec. Also, because it takes about 33 msec for the computer to read an image, the exposure time must be less than 33 msec. If energy subtraction is used (see Types of Digital Subtraction section in this chapter), the generator needs to be able to switch kilovoltage rapidly.

## Image Intensifier

To visualize the entire field for many types of angiograms, the field size of the image intensifier should be 14″. Smaller field sizes, such as 9″, may require multiple injections of contrast medium and serial filming to demonstrate the area of interest.

The objective of an image intensifier is to change the

radiation striking the input screen to light and intensify it in proportion to the radiation intensity. The light exits the output part of the intensifier and is transmitted to the TV camera. Because the light produced by the image intensifier is much greater than the camera needs, a light diaphragm is placed between the output screen of the image intensifier and the TV camera. The diaphragm adjusts the light to a level the camera can use.

## X-Ray Tube

Because DSA requires multiple exposures at high technique, the x-ray tube must be able to withstand a great deal of heat. A suggested heat unit range for apparatus employed for DSA is 400,000 to 800,000. Higher heat units are required for cardiac catheterization. Some tubes may have the capability to use a compensating filter over areas of varying density, for example, part of a vessel may overlie tissue and another part may overlie bone. If energy subtraction (see Types of Digital Subtraction section in this chapter) is used in units adjusting energy level by filtration, a rotating filter is attached to the port.

## Television and Camera

The television and camera for DSA must be of higher quality than that used for routine angiography. To obtain an optimum image, the DSA setup should have a high signal-to-noise ratio, 1000:1. To avoid image noise, the camera needs to operate at the same "bit" as the analog-to-digital converter. The system may operate in the interlace or noninterlace mode. The pulse noninterlace mode is preferred. Employing a lead-oxide camera, called a plumbicon, results in a low lag time (fewer residue images or "ghosts") and improved digital image.

## Analog-to-Digital Converter

The function of the analog-to-digital converter (ADC) is to digitize the analog image from the TV to a digital format that the image processor can read. The converter must have a minimum $512 \times 512$ matrix and operate at 30 frames/sec. The dynamic range of the converter must match the computer. For example, an 8-bit converter ($2^8$, or 256) would have a range of 0 to 255.

## TYPES OF DIGITAL SUBTRACTION

As with conventional photographic subtraction, digital subtraction may employ one of several methods. Review of the literature indicates that the number and name of a specific technique vary. The four most commonly described methods discussed in this text are mask, time interval difference (TID), energy, and hybrid subtraction.

## Mask Subtraction

The mask subtraction method is the technique most closely related to conventional photographic subtraction. In this method, images are made both before and after contrast medium injection. The precontrast medium image, or mask, is subtracted from each postcontrast medium image. All images are stored and may be recalled at a later time. If the patient moves between images, the subtracted image is of poor quality. To compensate for image noise, the remask or integration technique may be employed.

In the remask method, a different image is used as the mask; it is used to subtract from the postcontrast medium image. The integration method combines several images to form the mask. The new mask is used to subtract the contrast medium image.

## Time Interval Difference Subtraction

Time interval difference subtraction (TID) is similar to mask subtraction. In this method the subtracted image is made from a different mask at fixed intervals of time. For example, the first subtracted image may be made from images 1 and 5 (interval = 4), the second image is made from images 2 and 6 (interval = 4), and so on. If the images do not superimpose correctly, it is possible to use reregistration or integration to adjust the images. In reregistration, the image is adjusted by manipulating, or moving, the position of the pixels so that the mask and follow-up images are superimposed. Unfortunately, the misalignment of pixels is rarely directly related. In other words, aligning one area of the image may misalign another.

## Energy Subtraction

Energy subtraction employs the concept of photoelectric interaction and is not dependent on contrast medium. In this method, the K-edge factor is employed. Recall that in the photoelectric effect, absorption decreases with an increase in energy. However, when an electron from the K shell is removed, there is a rapid increase in absorption, or K-edge, and then a decrease with an increase in energy. The K-edge for iodine is 33 kiloelectronvolts (keV) (Fig. 15–3). If two different energies are employed, before and after K-edge, then the difference between the two results in a high contrast image. Thus, by employing a beam of 32 keV and 34 keV, the difference between the two results in a high contrast image. Since the K-edges for soft tissue, bone, and contrast medium differ significantly, using 32 and 34 keV subtracts, or removes, soft tissue and bone from the image.

This method of subtraction is very difficult and expensive to obtain. One way to achieve energy subtraction is to alternate exposures using different kiloelectronvoltages. Another way to change the energy of the beam is to use two filters, for example, aluminum and

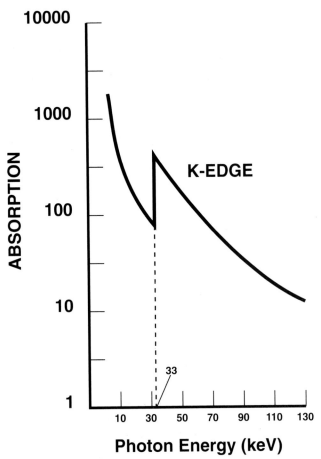

Figure 15–3. K-edge for iodine.

80 percent accuracy rate. The original concept of DSA was to reduce the number of direct arterial procedures by performing angiography intravenously. However, as the number of IV-DSAs increased, it was found that superimposition of vessels, misregistration artifacts, poor cardiac output, and renal toxicity limited its usefulness. It is most useful as a screening procedure for major vascular disease, especially atherosclerosis of the carotid arteries and the thoracic or abdominal aorta. Some common pathologies visualized with IV-DSA are renal artery stenosis, abdominal aorta atherosclerosis, aortic occlusion, aortic stenosis, and carotid atherosclerosis. Common pathologies demonstrated with IA-DSA are all of the above plus aortorenal vascular disease, hepatic arterial disease, portal vasculature, cerebral vascular disease, abnormal peripheral vasculature, aortic dissection, and intestinal ischemia and large A-V malformations.

### Preprocedural Care

Unlike conventional angiography, IV-DSA does not require premedicating the patient. However, it is important to perform an assessment of renal and cardiac function. Patients with a creatinine value of 3 mg/dl should not have an IV-DSA unless the clinical symptoms indicate that it is necessary. When creatinine levels are greater than 3 mg/dl, IV-DSA is contraindicated and should be performed only if no other alternative exists. IA-DSA is then the procedure of choice. Patients with congestive heart failure or poor cardiac output should not have an IV-DSA. IA-DSA requires the same patient preparation and premedication as conventional angiography.

copper, or a rotating filter with varying thickness or composition over the tube port.

### Hybrid Subtraction

Hybrid subtraction is a combination of mask and energy subtraction. In this method, the data and images are obtained using the mask technique. Recall that in mask subtraction, the mask is merged with a subsequent image. Also, energy subtraction uses two different energy levels. In hybrid subtraction a precontrast mask is created by combining a low-energy image with a high-energy image. A second mask is produced by combining a low-energy postcontrast image with a high-energy postcontrast image. Superimposing the pre- and postmask images results in a hybrid subtraction image.

### CLINICAL APPLICATIONS OF DSA

### Indications

There are two methods of performing digital angiography, intravenously (IV-DSA) and intra-arterially (IA-DSA). IV-DSA is a simple procedure that has about an

### Disadvantages

Although a single injection of contrast medium is significantly lower for DSA than for conventional angiography, multiple injections may be necessary to visualize the entire area, especially with IV-DSA or when a small image intensifier field size is employed. The maximum amount of contrast medium injected for a single procedure should not exceed 200 ml.

The most common disadvantage of DSA is motion artifacts. These artifacts may be a result of voluntary or involuntary patient movement. Even without artifacts, the decreased spatial resolution results in a poorer image compared to conventional angiograms.

When the anatomy of the part being examined has uneven absorption of the radiation, the image densities are unsatisfactory for subtraction. One method used to create even intensity on the image is to use a compensating filter at the port of the x-ray tube. The filter attenuates the x-ray beam, causing more even penetration of the object. Also, since IV-DSA demonstrates all vessels, sometimes overlapping or superimposition of vessels results.

DSA is not the procedure of choice for the study of small vessel disease or subtle abnormalities of the vessels, because these cannot be visualized on the image. IA-DSA or conventional angiography can be performed in these instances.

## Advantages

Intravenous digital subtraction angiography is advantageous because it is less traumatic to the patient than conventional angiography, is a safe procedure, and can be performed on an outpatient basis. IA-DSA employs less contrast medium than conventional angiography, uses a smaller-size catheter, decreases the length of time of the procedure, and enables the visualization of vessels without the need for selective catheterization. The reduced amount of contrast medium is especially helpful in patients with reduced renal function. Using a smaller catheter size, reducing the procedure time, and eliminating the need for selective catheterization are all instrumental in decreasing the trauma caused to the vessel. Another advantage of both types of DSA is that visualization of the image is immediate.

## Head and Neck DSA

Digital subtraction angiography of the head and neck area is the most common type of DSA procedure performed. The accuracy of IV-DSA of this area depends on both the ability to produce a quality image and the degree of pathology. Accuracy levels increase with an increase in image quality and pathology. Most artifacts that appear on the image, and decrease the quality, are caused by the patient swallowing or moving the eyelids. Swallowing often results from contrast medium irritation as it enters the body. It is possible to decrease the number of swallowing artifacts by having the patient hold the tongue between the front teeth. Eyelid movement may be decreased by having the patient keep the eyes closed during injection and filming.

The basic procedural methods for DSA of the head and neck are the same as for conventional angiography. The reader is referred to Chapter 22, Cerebral Angiography, for more information relative to the procedural methods. This section is dedicated to identifying the difference between conventional angiography and DSA of the head and neck.

Needle entry for IV-DSA may be via the cubital or the femoral vein. After needle insertion, a pigtail catheter is advanced into the superior vena cava, inferior vena cava, or right atrium for injection.

It is important that an aortic arch study be performed prior to any selective procedure. A volume of 20 to 40 ml of contrast medium is injected at a rate of 20 to 22 ml/sec. The filming rate begins 2 to 4 seconds after the injection for IV-DSA. A common filming sequence for the aortic arch area is 2 images/sec for 10 images and 1 image/sec for 4 to 8 images. The patient positions employed to demonstrate the arch and carotid bifurcation are 45- to 55-degree right and left posterior obliques (RPO and LPO). A large, 9" to 14" field should be

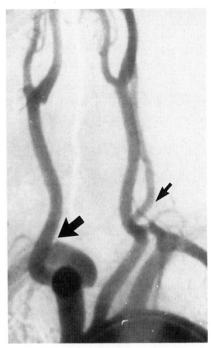

**Figure 15–4.** IA-DSA demonstrating an aortic arch steal. An obstruction of the right vertebral artery results in the left vertebral artery's stealing blood from the left brachiocephalic artery. This causes the left vertebral artery to enlarge and a decrease in blood flow to the left upper extremity. (Courtesy of Patti S. Foulds, General Electric Medical Systems, Milwaukee, WI.)

used. Figure 15–4 is an example of IV-DSA demonstrating arch steal.

Selective arterial DSA catheterization uses additional patient positions. An AP transorbital projection with a 20-degree cephalic angle is used to demonstrate the middle cerebral vessels. For visualization of the vertebrobasal vessels, an AP axial projection with a 30-degree caudal angle is employed. The carotid siphon is best demonstrated with a 20-degree off lateral angle.

IA-DSA of the head and neck is performed by puncturing the femoral artery. Unlike IV-DSA, the IA-DSA dilutes the contrast medium by one half or employs a lower concentration of contrast medium. Selective carotid angiography uses 8 to 10 ml of contrast medium injected at 8 ml/sec. The filming starts 2 to 3 seconds before injection and is at a rate of 2 to 4 images/sec. The amount of contrast medium employed for selective vertebral angiography is 6 to 8 ml. The filming rate is the same as for the carotid angiogram. Subclavian selection employs 15 to 18 ml injected at a rate of 8 ml/sec. Filming occurs at 2 to 3 images/sec. Figures 15–5 through 15–7 are images of selective vessels of the head and neck area. The positions for IA-DSA are the same as for IV-DSA. The field size for selective work is 6".

## Thoracic DSA

Digital subtraction angiography of the thoracic area is the least desirable study because of artifacts caused by normal heartbeat and breathing movements. Artifacts

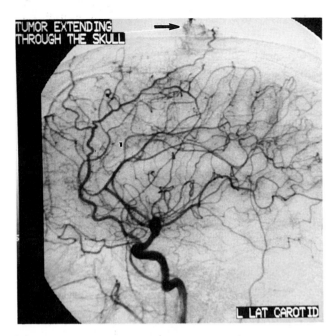

**Figure 15-5.** Left lateral carotid: tumor extending through skull. (Courtesy of Patti S. Foulds, General Electric Medical Systems, Milwaukee, WI.)

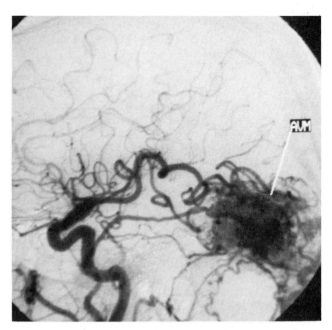

**Figure 15-7.** Left lateral carotid: IA-DSA of arteriovenous malformation. (Courtesy of Patti S. Foulds, General Electric Medical Systems, Milwaukee, WI.)

caused by heart movement may be decreased by triggering the injection to coincide with the electrocardiogram (ECG) of the patient. Also, the significant tissue density difference between the lung and mediastinum reduces image quality. It is possible to improve the image by using an attenuated x-ray beam to compensate for density differences over the lung area. The most common positions used for evaluation of the descending aorta (and to avoid superimposition of the heart) are the LPO and steep RPO. The reader is referred to Chapter 21, Thoracic Aortography, for more information about this procedure.

## Abdominal Aorta and Lower Extremity DSA

Breathing, peristalsis, and gas account for the majority of artifacts in abdominal DSA. Peristalsis may be slowed by injecting 1 mg of glucagon intravenously 1 to 2 minutes before the DSA. Using compression or positioning the patient prone is helpful in removing gas from the area of interest. Figures 15-8 through 15-10 are DSA images of the aorta.

Intra-aortic digital subtraction angiography is the method of choice for DSA of the abdominal aorta and

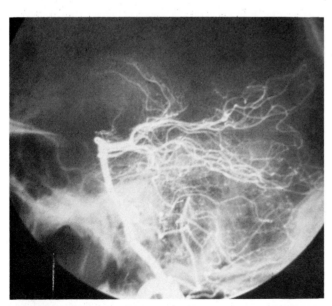

**Figure 15-6.** IA-DSA of left lateral vertebral. (Courtesy of Patti S. Foulds, General Electric Medical Systems, Milwaukee, WI.)

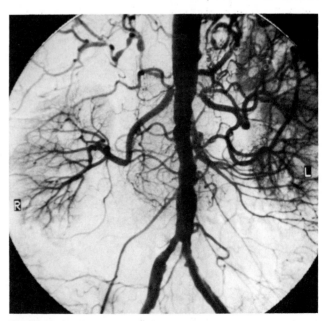

**Figure 15-8.** Abdominal femoral runoff. (Courtesy of Patti S. Foulds, General Electric Medical Systems, Milwaukee, WI.)

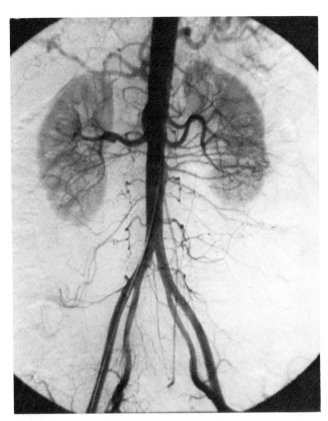

**Figure 15–9.** Anterior-posterior abdominal flush. (Courtesy of Patti S. Foulds, General Electric Medical Systems, Milwaukee, WI.)

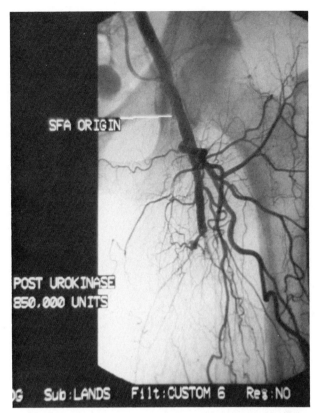

**Figure 15–11.** Superficial femoral artery (SFA) origin. (Courtesy of Patti S. Foulds, General Electric Medical Systems, Milwaukee, WI.)

lower extremity. Because the area is large and no stepping table is employed, multiple injections are often required. Patients with poor cardiac output are poor candidates for this procedure.

An injection volume of 15 to 20 ml of contrast medium at a rate of 8 to 10 ml/sec is common for abdominal aortography. Filming is usually 2 images/sec and may vary if blood flow is restricted. The common position used for filming is supine. Oblique positions may be employed to better demonstrate vessel branches. Figures 15–11 through 15–15 are images of the lower extremity vessels using IA-DSA.

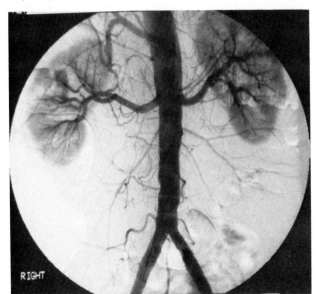

**Figure 15–10.** Anterior-posterior abdominal angiography. (Courtesy of Patti S. Foulds, General Electric Medical Systems, Milwaukee, WI.)

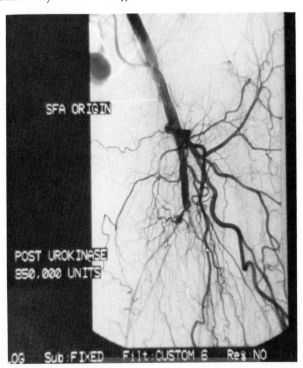

**Figure 15–12.** Superficial femoral artery (SFA) origin. (Courtesy of Patti S. Foulds, General Electric Medical Systems, Milwaukee, WI.)

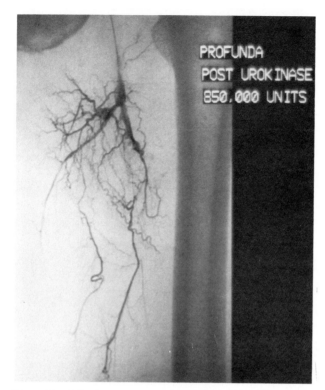

**Figure 15–13.** Profunda. (Courtesy of Patti S. Foulds, General Electric Medical Systems, Milwaukee, WI.)

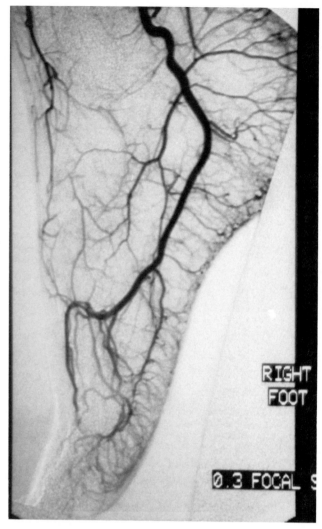

**Figure 15–14.** DSA of right lateral foot. (Courtesy of Patti S. Foulds, General Electric Medical Systems, Milwaukee, WI.)

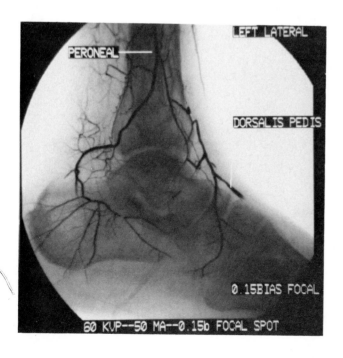

**Figure 15–15.** DSA of left lateral ankle. (Courtesy of Patti S. Foulds, General Electric Medical Systems, Milwaukee, WI.)

The amount of contrast medium and the injection rate for the lower extremities are the same as for abdominal DSA. However, the filming rate is slower at 1 image/sec. The quality of the vessels in the distal extremities by IA-DSA exceeds that of conventional angiography. Refer to Chapter 26, Abdomen and Lower Extremity Angiography, for specific information on this procedure.

## Selective Visceral DSA

Visceral DSA is best performed by IA-DSA. In angiography of the superior mesenteric and celiac vessels, 15 to 20 ml of contrast medium is injected at a rate of 5 to 7 ml/sec. A vasodilator, 25 mg of tolazoline, may be used for image enhancement. Filming rate is 1 image every other second for 12 to 15 images. Figures 15–16 and 15–17 are images of selective visceral catheterization.

Portography requires imaging over a large area. Therefore, several injections may be necessary to visualize the involved area. Although IA-DSA portography can be performed, the images may be inferior to conventional angiography because of the length of the run while breathing is suspended.

Renal procedures may be performed by IA-DSA or IV-DSA. Approximately 10 to 15 ml of contrast medium is injected for 3 to 4 seconds. Filming is at a rate of two to three images per second. The base positions used to demonstrate the renal arteries are the supine and slight RPO. IV-DSA does not demonstrate the renal branch arteries or small vessels well. IA-DSA or conventional angiography is preferred in these instances.

## Upper Extremity DSA

IA-DSA of the upper extremities is much less painful than conventional angiography because less contrast

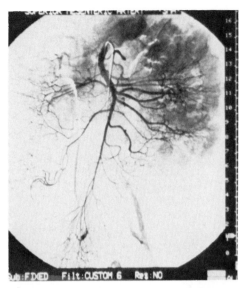

**Figure 15–17.** Superior mesenteric artery. (Courtesy of Patti S. Foulds, General Electric Medical Systems, Milwaukee, WI.)

medium is employed. As with all DSA imaging, patient immobility and cessation of respiration are extremely important. The catheter is positioned selectively into the artery of choice. Small injections of contrast medium ranging from 3 to 8 ml are made, and filming begins. Figures 15–18 through 15–21 are IA-DSA images of the hand.

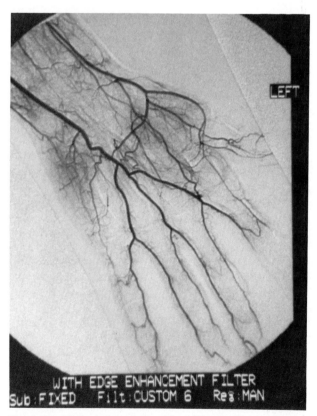

**Figure 15–18.** Posterior-anterior of the left hand with edge enhancement filter. (Courtesy of Patti S. Foulds, General Electric Medical Systems, Milwaukee, WI.)

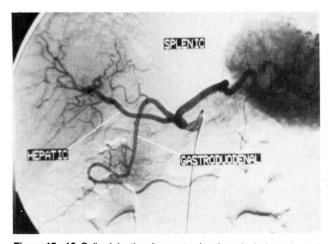

**Figure 15–16.** Celiac injection demonstrating the splenic, hepatic, and gastroduodenal arteries. (Courtesy of Patti S. Foulds, General Electric Medical Systems, Milwaukee, WI.)

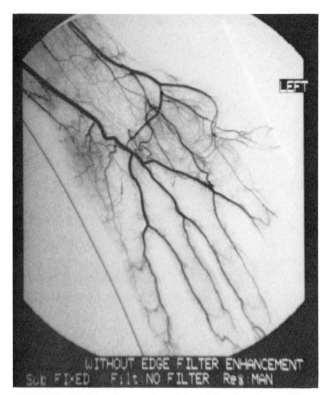

**Figure 15–19.** Posterior-anterior of the left hand without edge enhancement. (Courtesy of Patti S. Foulds, General Electric Medical Systems, Milwaukee, WI.)

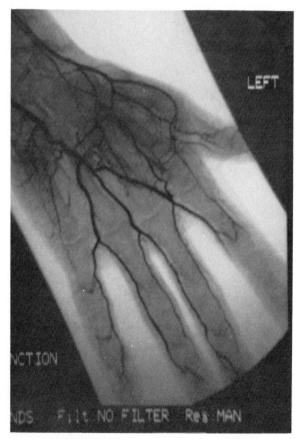

**Figure 15–20.** Posterior-anterior of the left hand, landscape function without filter. (Courtesy of Patti S. Foulds, General Electric Medical Systems, Milwaukee, WI.)

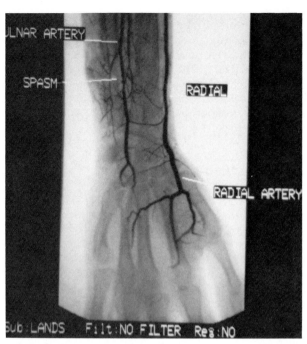

**Figure 15–21.** Posterior-anterior of the distal forearm. (Courtesy of Patti S. Foulds, General Electric Medical Systems, Milwaukee, WI.)

## Interventional Procedures with DSA

The basic methodology of interventional procedures is the same whether IA-DSA or conventional angiography is employed. However, using DSA for these procedures is advantageous because it decreases the length of time of the procedure, employs a smaller catheter, and utilizes less contrast medium than conventional angiography. This helps reduce trauma and discomfort to the patient. Also, road mapping is improved with DSA versus conventional angiography. Road mapping is a technique in which a static image of the contrast-filled vessel allows the radiologist to see the guide wire or balloon catheter.

## REVIEW QUESTIONS

1. In first-order subtraction the _____ is characterized by the reversal of images.
   A. initial radiograph
   B. mask
   C. angiographic film
   D. contrast film

2. To make a second-order subtraction print, the first-order mask, second-order mask, and _____ are placed over the subtraction film.
   A. initial radiograph
   B. intermediate print
   C. base film
   D. contrast film

3. _____ order subtraction employs an intermediate subtraction print.

A. First-
B. Second-
C. Third-

4. The _____ serves as the "brain" in DSA.
   A. image processor
   B. generator
   C. analog-to-digital converter (ADC)
   D. image intensifier

5. The generator receives information from the _____, which regulates the initiation and termination of the x-ray exposure.
   A. ADC
   B. image intensifier
   C. image processor
   D. x-ray tube

6. The exposure time for DSA should not exceed _____ msec.
   A. 18
   B. 17
   C. 21
   D. 33

7. The recommended field size of an image intensifier used for DSA is _____".
   A.  6
   B.  8
   C. 14
   D. 18

8. The x-ray tube for DSA should have a minimum heat unit capacity of _____.
   A. 100,000
   B. 170,000
   C. 280,000
   D. 400,000

9. The signal-to-noise ratio of a TV setup for DSA should be _____.
   A. 1000:1
   B.  800:1
   C.  500:1
   D.  200:1

10. The analog-to-digital converter is located between the _____ and _____.
    A. image intensifier, image processor
    B. image intensifier, TV
    C. TV, image processor
    D. generator, image intensifier

11. In mask subtraction, images are made _____ injection.
    A. before and after
    B. before
    C. after
    D. during

12. In the DSA _____ subtraction method, a different mask is made at fixed intervals of time.
    A. mask
    B. energy
    C. TID
    D. hybrid

13. _____ DSA subtraction employs the K-edge factor.
    A. Mask
    B. TID
    C. Hybrid
    D. Energy

14. The K-edge for iodine is _____ keV.
    A. 25
    B. 28
    C. 33
    D. 42

15. Hybrid subtraction is a combination of _____ and _____ subtraction.
    A. energy, mask
    B. TID, energy
    C. TID, mask
    D. first-order, energy

16. List two common pathologies visualized with IV-DSA.

17. DSA is contraindicated in patients with a creatinine level greater than _____ mg/dl.
    A. 0
    B. 1
    C. 2
    D. 3

18. The maximum amount of contrast medium injected in a patient for a single procedure should not exceed _____ ml.
    A.  50
    B. 100
    C. 150
    D. 200

19. The spatial resolution for DSA is _____ than(as) conventional angiography.
    A. better
    B. poorer
    C. the same

20. DSA uses a _____ catheter size than conventional angiography.
    A. smaller
    B. larger
    C. the same

21. The most common area to perform DSA is in the _____.
    A. upper extremity
    B. thorax
    C. head and neck
    D. abdominal aorta and lower extremity

22. To reduce the number of swallowing artifacts during a DSA of the head, the patient should be instructed to _____.
    A. hold the breath
    B. hold the tongue between the front teeth
    C. perform the Valsalva maneuver
    D. close the eyes

23. Filming for an IA-DSA study of carotid angiography begins _____ second(s) before injection.

A. 1
B. 2 to 3
C. 5 to 6
D. 7 to 8

24. A ___ field size should be used for selective carotid DSA.
    A. 4
    B. 6
    C. 9
    D. 14

25. ___ may be injected intravenously 1 to 2 minutes before abdominal aorta DSA to slow peristalsis.
    A. Tolazoline
    B. Glucagon
    C. Epinephrine
    D. Valium

26. The film rate for lower extremity DSA is ___ image(s)/sec.
    A. 1
    B. 2
    C. 3
    D. 4

27. ___ should not be used to demonstrate small renal vessel disease.
    A. Conventional angiography
    B. IV-DSA
    C. IA-DSA
    D. TID

## BIBLIOGRAPHY

Abrams, HL: Abrams Angiography Vascular and Interventional Radiology, ed 3, Vol 1. Little, Brown & Co, Boston, 1983.

Bushong, SC: Radiologic Science for Technologists, ed 5. Mosby-Year Book, St Louis, 1993.

Coulam, CM, et al: The Physical Basis of Medical Imaging. Appleton-Century, New York, 1981.

Curry, TS, Dowdey, JE, and Murry, RC: Christensen's Physics of Diagnostic Radiology, ed 4. Lea & Febiger, Philadelphia, 1990.

Hillman, BJ and Newell, JD: Symposium on digital radiography. Radiol Clin North Am 23(2):177, 1985.

Hunter, TB: The Computer in Radiology. Aspen Publications, Rockville, MD, 1986.

James, AE, Anderson, JH, and Higgins, CB: Digital Image Processing in Radiology. Williams & Wilkins, Baltimore, 1985.

Johnsrude, IS, Jackson, DC, and Dunnick, NR: A Practical Approach to Angiography, ed 2. Little, Brown & Co, Boston, 1987.

Kadir, S: Diagnostic Angiography. WB Saunders, Philadelphia, 1986.

Kruger, RA and Riederer, SJ: Basic Concepts of Digital Subtraction Angiography. GK Hall Medical Publishers, Boston, 1984.

Kuni, CC: Introduction to Computers and Digital Processing in Medical Imaging. Year Book Medical Publishers, Chicago, 1988.

Rouse, S: Clinical applications of digital subtraction angiography (DSA) and the radiographer's role. Radiographics 51(598):197, July/August 1985.

Sharma, RP, et al: Digital subtraction angiography of the abdomen: Henry Ford Hospital Experience. Henry Ford Hosp Med J 33(2 and 3):105, 1985.

Snopek, AM: Fundamentals of Special Radiographic Procedures, ed 3. WB Saunders, Philadelphia, 1992.

Thompson, TT: A Practical Approach to Modern Imaging Equipment, ed 2. Little, Brown & Co, Boston, 1985.

Tortorici, MR: Fundamentals of Angiography. CV Mosby, St Louis, 1982.

# CHAPTER 16

# Guide Wires and Vascular Catheters

*Marianne R. Tortorici, EdD, ARRT(R)*

Injection of a contrast medium into the circulatory system is most often accomplished through the use of a vascular catheter. The vascular catheter is introduced into a vein or artery and advanced until the catheter reaches the area to be examined. The catheter is most commonly introduced into the vessel by the Seldinger technique (see Chapter 19, Catheterization Methods and Patient Management). In this technique, first, the vessel is punctured with a needle; then a thin, stainless steel wire (guide wire) is inserted through the needle into the vessel; next, the needle is removed by slipping it over the guide wire; and, finally, the catheter is placed over the guide wire and inserted into the vessel using a twisting motion. The stainless steel wire guides the catheter for placement within the vessel and is appropriately called a guide wire. (It should be noted that some manufacturers refer to guide wires as wire guides. The terms are interchangeable.)

This chapter contains an in-depth discussion of the construction, use, and precautions in the use of guide wires and vascular catheters. It is possible to purchase vascular catheter material in bulk, which would allow angiographers to fabricate their own catheter sizes, shapes, and lengths. However, commercially produced catheters are available in so many varieties that fabrication of catheters by angiographers is essentially nonexistent. Therefore, fabrication of catheters is not included in this text.

Catheters and guide wires may be used for diagnostic or interventional procedures. There are significant differences between diagnostic and interventional guide wires and catheters. This chapter concentrates on diagnostic guide wires and catheters. Interventional catheters or guide wires are discussed in the respective interventional chapter.

## GUIDE WIRES

### Construction

Guide wires may be constructed as solid stainless steel (or other metal alloy) wires or as thin stainless steel cores around which more thin stainless steel is wrapped. Both types of guide wires have one end that is rigid, with the opposite end flexible. The flexible tip is introduced into the blood vessel first so that if the tip of the guide wire strikes a vessel wall, it will bend, preventing damage to the vessel.

The solid guide wire and the wrapped guide wire each have advantages and disadvantages. The advantages of the solid guide wire include reducing the possibilities of catheter tip flaring, blood clotting on the guide wire, abrasion of the vessel wall, and the danger of unraveling. One disadvantage of this type of guide wire is its lack of versatility. The wrapped guide wire can be constructed so that it has a movable core, making it more versatile than the solid stainless-steel guide wire. However, with the wrapped guide wire, the possibilities of catheter tip flaring, blood clotting on the guide wire, abrasion of the vessel wall, and unraveling do exist.

As previously mentioned, the wrapped guide wire can damage the vessel or the catheter. To reduce the likelihood of injury, the wrapping may be Teflon-coated or heparin-coated. The Teflon-coated guide wire lowers the coefficient of friction between the guide wire and the vessel wall, reducing the possibility of vessel damage. The Teflon coating also reduces the friction between the lumen of the vascular catheter and the guide wire, allowing easier passage of the catheter over the guide wire. The heparin-coated guide wire reduces the possibility of blood clotting, which could eventually result in an embolism in the patient's vessel. The inner core is responsible for the degree of rigidity of the guide wire. It is usually tapered at the distal end, and it stops several centimeters before reaching the tip of the guide wire (the actual distance varies with the type of guide wire).

## Cores

Guide-wire cores may be fixed or movable (Fig. 16–1). A fixed core allows the guide wire to keep its original shape. The fixed core is used in normal vascular systems for diagnostic angiography and in interventional angiography. Movable cores have a handle (also referred to as a mandril) for adjusting the position of the core within the guide wire. The movable-core guide wire is advantageous for use in tortuous vascular structures. The insertion or withdrawal of the handle of a movable-core guide wire varies the amount of tip flexibility. As the core is inserted into the guide wire, there is a decrease in the flexibility of the guide-wire tip. Withdrawing the core increases the tip's flexibility (Fig.

16–2). The ability to control tip flexibility makes the movable-core guide wire more versatile than the fixed-core guide wire. Solid-core guide wires are fixed. Wrapped guide wires may be fixed or movable.

The diameter of the core affects the "stiffness" of the guide wire. Large-core diameters are more rigid than small-core widths. Stiff guide wires may have fixed or variable (movable) cores.

## Torque

Torque refers to the response of the guide wire or catheter to twisting and turning. For example, when the proximal end of a guide wire or catheter is rotated 90 degrees, the distal end also rotates 90 degrees and the guide wire or catheter is said to have good torque control. However, if the proximal end of the guide wire or catheter is rotated 130 degrees for the distal end to rotate 90 degrees, then the guide wire or catheter has poor torque. The better the torque, the more efficiently the angiographer can control the direction of the catheter in the vessel.

Some guide wires have a movable torque vise (Fig. 16–3) that may be placed anywhere on the shaft. Rotation of the torque vise turns the distal end of the guide wire the desired degrees. Other guide wires may use a deflector handle (Fig. 16–4) that is attached to the proximal end of the guide wire to adjust the degree of stiffness and subsequent torque. The torque device is used to direct the guide wire toward the desired arterial branch that the angiographer is attempting to catheterize.

## Tip Configurations

There are two tip configurations available for guide wires, the straight tip and the J-shaped tip (Fig. 16–5). In wrapped guide wires, both types of tip configurations can be used in conjunction with a fixed or movable core (movable cores are not available with solid-core construction). Thus, it is possible to have a straight tip with a fixed core, a J-shaped tip with a fixed core, a straight tip with a movable core, or a J-shaped tip with a movable core.

The length of the flexible straight tip on a guide wire may differ from one wire to another. The length of flexible tip is measured in centimeters. Most fixed-core straight guides have a 3-cm flexible tip, whereas most movable-core straight guides have a 10- to 15-cm flexible tip. There are a variety of commercially available

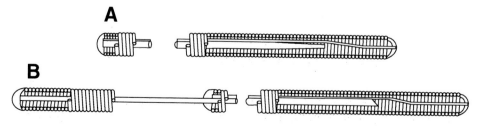

**Figure 16–1.** (*A*) Cross section of a fixed-core guide wire; (*B*) cross section of a movable-core guide wire.

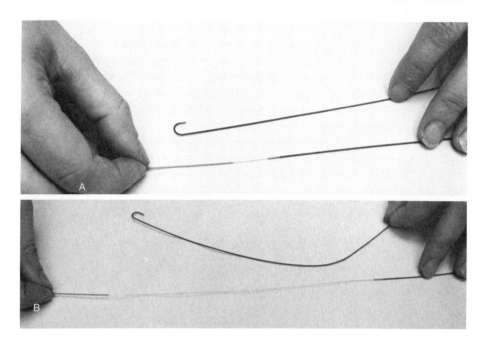

**Figure 16–2.** Movable-core guide wire. (*A*) Inserted; (*B*) retracted.

flexible tip lengths. Angiographers may order the type of tip configuration and flexibility length most suitable for their needs.

Unlike the straight tip, the J-shaped tip is measured by radius and not by length. Manufacturers offers a variety of radii. The most common J-shaped radius for both the fixed and movable core is 3 mm; however, the radius can be as large as 3 cm.

Some guide wires have two flexible ends. These guide wires are only available with fixed cores. The difference in the ends is in the configuration of their tips. For example, one end may have a 3-mm-radius J tip, and the other end may have a 3-cm straight tip (Fig. 16–6). Because both ends are flexible, either end may be used for entry into the vessel. These types of guide wires are used in certain vessels that require two types of tip configurations in order to advance the catheter in the vessel.

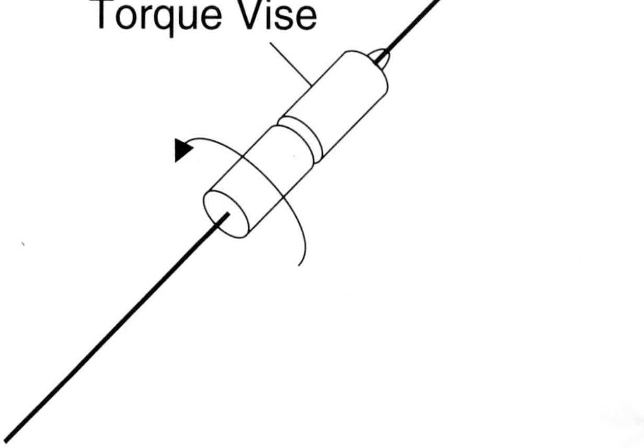

## Lengths

Guide-wire length varies from 30 to 260 cm. The shorter guide wires, 30 to 50 cm long, are usually used for percutaneous or direct vascular punctures. The average guide wire employed for adults undergoing selective angiography is approximately 100 to 150 cm in length. The 260-cm guide wire is used when interchanging vascular catheters. The extra length of wire allows the catheter to be changed without losing the position of the guide wire in the vessel.

## Diameters

The diameters of guide wires are measured in fractions of an inch, or millimeters. The range is 0.014″ (0.35 mm) to 0.052″ (1.32 mm). The most common diameters used for adults are 0.035″ (0.89 mm) and 0.038″ (0.97 mm). There are several factors that must be taken into consideration when selecting the proper diameter size. These factors include needle gauge, vessel size, and size of the lumen of the vascular catheter (Table 16–1).

Needle gauge is a significant factor when introducing the guide wire through the needle because it is impor-

**Guidewire**

**Torque Vise**

**Figure 16–3.** Torque vise. (Courtesy of Medi-tech, a division of Boston Scientific Corporation, Watertown, MA.)

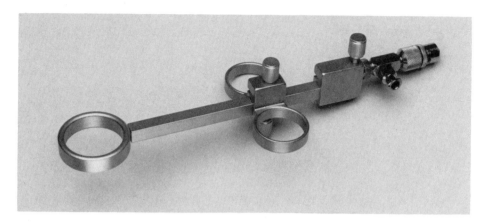

**Figure 16–4.** Deflector handle. (Courtesy of Cook Incorporated, Bloomington, IN.)

tant that the guide-wire diameter be large enough so that blood cannot flow back through the cannula of the needle. A backflow of blood over a given period of time can result in significant blood loss, leading to a decrease in the patient's blood pressure and possible shock. If there is a noticeable backflow of blood, an increase in guide-wire diameter is indicated.

It is impossible to introduce a guide wire that is too large for the lumen of the needle. It is possible, however, for a guide wire that is too large for a vessel to be introduced through a needle. Thus, the second factor to be considered when selecting the proper guide-wire diameter is the size of the vessel. The diameter of the guide wire should be small enough that it does not obstruct the flow of blood when inside the vessel. The blood must continue to flow freely, even after the vascular catheter has been placed over the guide wire. Obviously, any obstruction of blood flow can cause serious complications, such as a stroke or an infarction. Restricted blood flow becomes increasingly important when the catheter and the guide wire are in vital areas, such as the carotid or coronary arteries. The actual vascular structure of the patient determines the diameter of the guide wire.

The third factor in the selection of proper guide-wire diameter is the size of the lumen of the vascular cath-

eter. When the vascular catheter is inserted over the guide wire, each must move independently of the other. Therefore, care should be taken to select a guide-wire diameter that allows independent movement without the loss of blood through the catheter. An indication that the guide-wire diameter is too large is that there is difficulty in advancing either the guide wire or the catheter.

## Safety Tests

After selecting the type of guide wire (for example, a movable-core, 3-mm J tip, 150 cm long) for the examination, three tests should be performed to determine the safety of the guide wire. The first test is to determine the flexibility of the tip by bending the tip 180 degrees. If the tip does not bend freely, it is too rigid and should not be used. A rigid tip will not yield to the fragile vascular structure and may cause severe damage to the vessel. The damage may vary from a slight abrasion to a punctured vessel wall. The degree of injury depends on the stiffness of the tip and the amount of force used to advance the guide wire in the vessel. The more rigid the tip and the more force employed to advance the guide wire, the more severe the vascular damage.

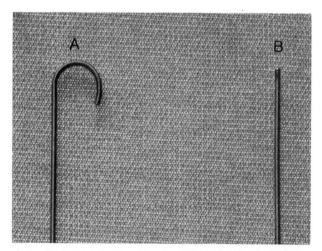

**Figure 16–5.** (A) J-tipped guide wire; (B) straight-tipped guide wire.

Table 16–1. **Suggested Needle and Catheter Sizes for Guide Wire Diameters**

| Guide-Wire Diameter | | Suggested Needle | Suggested Catheter |
|---|---|---|---|
| Inches | Millimeters | Size (gauge) | Size (French) |
| 0.018 | 0.46 | 21 thin wall | 3 or 4 |
| 0.021 | 0.53 | 20 thin wall | 4 or 5 |
| 0.025 | 0.64 | 19 thin wall | 4 or 5 |
| 0.028 | 0.71 | 19 thin wall | 5 or 6 |
| 0.032 | 0.81 | 18 thin wall | 5 or 6 |
| 0.035 | 0.89 | 18 thin wall | 5 or 6 |
| 0.038 | 0.97 | 18 thin wall | 6 or 7 |
| 0.045 | 1.14 | 16 thin wall | 6 or 7 |
| 0.047 | 1.19 | 16 thin wall | 7 or 8 |
| 0.052 | 1.32 | 15 thin wall | 7, 8, or 9 |

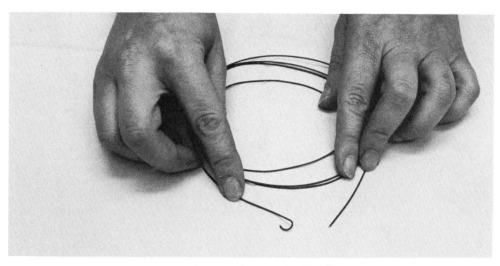

**Figure 16-6.** Double flex-tipped guide wire.

The next safety test for a wrapped guide wire is a visual inspection of the junction of the stiff core and the external coils at the distal tip. The coils should not be deformed. A deformed coil may result in a rough outer coating of the guide wire, which can cause abrasions to the vessel. Any kinks or bends in the wire may weaken the guide wire. If the guide wire is weakened, it is easily broken; furthermore, a broken piece may free itself from the core of the guide wire. As long as the broken piece flows with the blood, there is no danger to the patient. However, if the piece becomes lodged or caught in the vessel, the broken part may act as an embolus, causing a stroke or an infarction.

The last safety test is a check of the core, accomplished by giving the guide wire a slight twist and tug. The core should not kink or break. If the core demonstrates weakness, the guide wire should not be used. After the guide wire has passed these three safety checks, it is ready for use.

## Proper Guide-Wire Use

The vascular structure of the patient determines the type of guide wire to be used in an angiographic examination. Selecting the wrong guide wire can result in certain serious side effects, such as abrasions or emboli. Therefore, it is important to know the limitations of the guide wire and to use it appropriately.

The normal vascular system has vessels that are reasonably straight and do not have sharp bends or curves. The lumina of normal vessels are reasonably large and contain no plaques; therefore, it is not difficult to position a catheter within a normal vessel. Because of the relative ease with which the catheter can be positioned, the straight-tip guide wire is used in vessels that are relatively straight. This type of guide wire should not be employed in tortuous or atherosclerotic vessels. Tortuous vessels have many curves, turns, and twists. Atherosclerotic vessels have lipid deposits and plaques in the intima (almost always present in middle-aged and

elderly individuals) with a consequent reduction in the size of the vessel lumen. In attempting to advance a straight-tip guide wire through an atherosclerotic vessel, the guide wire to be directed into the subatheromatous space may loosen plaques (Fig. 16-7), causing an embolism. In such cases a J-shaped guide wire should be used.

The J-shaped fixed-core guide wire is usually able to negotiate most moderately tortuous and atherosclerotic vessels (Fig. 16-8). However, when extremely tortuous vessels are encountered, it may be necessary to resort to a J-shaped tip with a movable-core guide wire. On reaching an extremely tortuous region, the core is withdrawn, increasing the length of flexible tip by 10 to 15 cm. This increased length of flexible tip should be sufficient to allow the guide wire to advance through the tortuous region. Once the tortuous area has been passed, the core is inserted back into the tip and the normal advancement of the guide wire is resumed (Fig. 16-9).

## Precautions

There are certain precautions that must be taken when using a guide wire. These precautions include care in advancing the guide wire, position of the needle bevel, cleaning the guide wire, and using a new guide wire.

If the guide wire is not advancing smoothly, the reason for difficulty should be evaluated. Force should never be used if the guide wire meets resistance. Such force may result in serious damage to the vessel (abrasions, emboli, perforation, and so on). Most resistance encountered when advancing the guide wire may be attributed to tortuous vessels. If this is the case, then a change of the type of tip configuration, the core, or both may resolve the problem. However, other reasons for difficulty may include the position of the needle or the position of the bevel of the needle. If the needle is not properly positioned in the center of the vessel, the

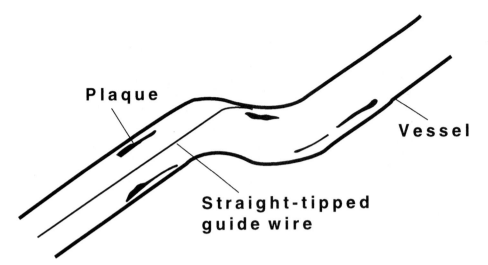

Plaque

Vessel

Straight-tipped
guide wire

**Figure 16–7.** Straight-tipped guide wire in atherosclerotic vessel. (Reprinted from Cook publication WG 4/11-74, Cook Incorporated, Bloomington, IN.)

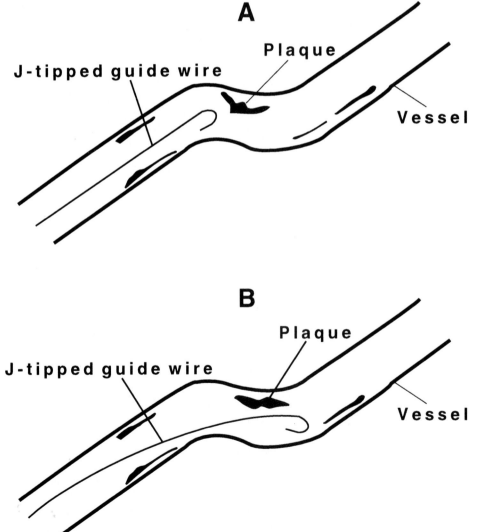

**A**

J-tipped guide wire

Plaque

Vessel

**B**

J-tipped guide wire

Plaque

Vessel

**Figure 16–8.** Fixed-core J-tipped guide wire in tortuous vessel. (A) Prior to tortuosity; (B) beyond tortuosity. (Reprinted from Cook publication WG 4/11-74, Cook Incorporated, Bloomington, IN.)

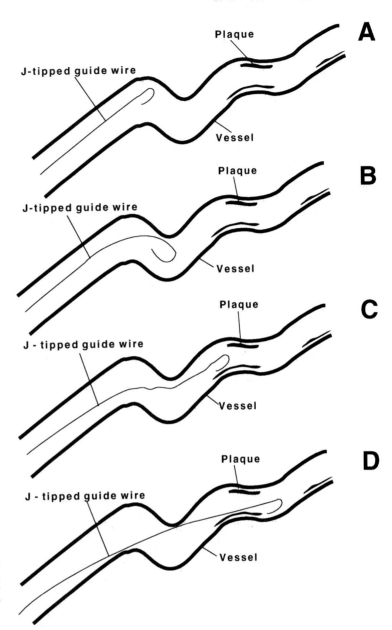

**Figure 16-9.** Movable-core J-tipped guide wire in tortuous vessel. (*A*) Prior to tortuosity, core inserted in guide wire; (*B*) handle of guide wire and core withdrawn; (*C*) guide wire moves through tortuosity; (*D*) handle of guide wire and core inserted. (Reprinted from Cook publication WG 4/11-74, Cook Incorporated, Bloomington, IN.)

guide wire may encounter the wall of the vessel. Therefore, any attempt to advance the guide wire could be dangerous (Fig. 16-10).

The bevel should be facing upward. If it is angled downward, the advancement of the guide wire is difficult, and any force applied to the guide wire may cause the sharp edge of the needle to sever the guide wire (Fig. 16-11). Any damage to the guide wire increases the risk of complications to the patient.

In addition to being alert to any resistance to the guide wire and bevel position, care should also be taken to avoid cleaning the guide wire too often. Although it is necessary to clean the guide wire during the examination, saline solution of a high concentration can start stress corrosion of the stainless steel wire at room or elevated temperatures. This condition is most noticeable with movable-core guide wire because rust or corrosion hinders the movement of the core.

Complete internal cleaning of the guide wire is impossible; for this reason, all guide wires should be discarded after use. Any reuse of guide wires increases the possibility of complications caused by contamination from the residue of blood from the previous examination.

## VASCULAR CATHETERS

A large percentage of angiographic procedures require the selective or superselective catheterization of a vessel. Selective refers to catheterizing a vessel that branches off the main vessel. Superselective refers to catheterizing a vessel that branches off a selective vessel. These types of catheterizations are performed by introducing a catheter into a main blood vessel and manipulating it to the desired artery or vein. A catheter

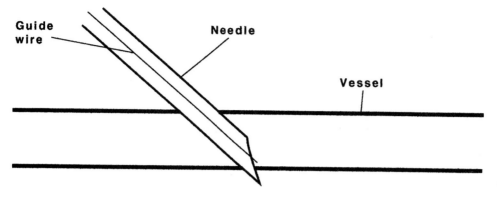

**Figure 16–10.** Improper position of needle in vessel.

is a long, hollow, thin tube with one to several holes at its distal end. The catheter serves as a pipeline through which contrast medium is injected. In the early history of angiography, a ureteral rubber catheter was employed for selective angiography. Since that time the advancement of plastics has resulted in a variety of other types of catheter material. The most common materials are Teflon, polyethylene, and polyurethane.

## Material

The type of catheter material chosen is based on its ability to be manipulated within the vessel. It is important that the angiographer be able to control the direction in which the catheter moves inside the vessel. Manipulation of the catheter depends on the skill of the angiographer, the memory of the catheter, and the

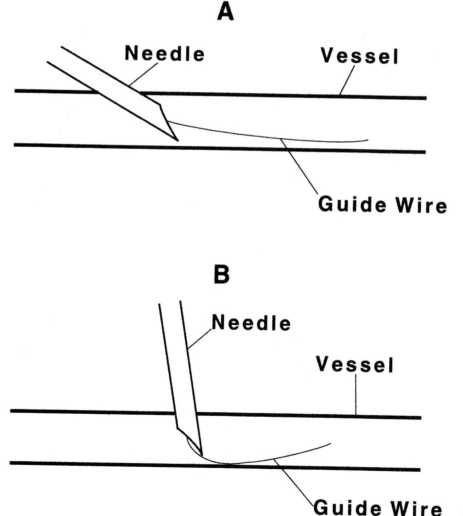

**Figure 16–11.** Direction of bevel in vessel. (*A*) Upward (correct); (*B*) downward (incorrect).

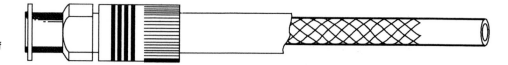

**Figure 16-12.** Cross section of braided catheter.

torque of the catheter. The type of material used in the catheter has a direct effect on the memory and torque.

Memory is the capacity of the catheter to retain its original shape. This is important, as it directly affects the ability to catheterize a vessel.

Torque refers to the response of the catheter to twisting and turning. Some catheter materials may be braided (Fig. 16-12) to increase torque control and radiopacity.

A catheter may be radiopaque or radiolucent. It is suggested that radiolucent catheters be employed for visualization of air bubbles. Location of radiolucent catheters in a vessel is obtained by fluoroscoping the guide wire positioned within the catheter lumen. Most angiographic procedures employ radiopaque catheter material. These catheters may have lead, bismuth salt, or barium salt added to the plastic material for radiopacity. A radiopaque catheter may be readily visualized under fluoroscopy, facilitating catheter placement.

Of the three major types of catheter material (Teflon, polyethylene, and polyurethane) Teflon has the lowest coefficient of friction, which facilitates the movement of the catheter in the vessel. Other characteristics of Teflon include excellent memory and the ability to withstand high temperatures. The excellent memory is a result of a rigid catheter tip; however, rigid tips can damage a vessel. Teflon can withstand high temperatures; therefore, it can be autoclaved for reuse.

Polyethylene has a medium coefficient of friction and is softer than Teflon. It may be sterilized with cold or hot gas.

Polyurethane contains many of the same characteristics as polyethylene. Both materials have about the same memory, softness, and sterilization requirements. Some authors believe that polyurethane has better torque control than polyethylene.

If proper sterilization techniques are followed, catheters can be reused. However, because it is nearly impossible to remove all the blood from the catheter, contamination can occur. Therefore, reuse of catheters is strongly discouraged.

## Sizes

Catheter size is most commonly expressed in the French scale, which refers to the size of the outer diameter of the catheter. The French number was developed by a French instrument maker named Charrière. The French scale has increments of approximately 0.33, or 1/3, mm; thus, 1 French (1F) is equal to 1/3 mm, or 0.33 mm; 2F is equal to approximately 2/3 mm, or 0.67 mm; 3F is equal to 3/3 mm, or 1 mm; and so on. Scales that convert French sizes to millimeters and inches (Fig. 16-13) are commercially available. The

smaller French sizes are generally employed for children; adults usually require a 4 or 5 French catheter.

## Tip

The distal end of the catheter has a specific shape and number of holes. The shape chosen depends on the vessel being catheterized. There are a multitude of catheter shapes available. Common catheter shapes are illustrated in Fig. 16-14.

The number and location of holes at the end of the catheter are chosen in relation to the vessel being examined. The more holes at the end of the catheter, the more contrast medium delivered. Thus, in the larger vessels (e.g., the aorta) catheters with multiple holes are used. The smaller vessels (e.g., the carotid artery) require a catheter with only an end hole.

The majority of catheters used in angiography have an end hole; others have side holes in addition to the end hole. Catheters with only end holes are used for selective angiography. Injections through these catheters emit a strong stream of contrast medium that can damage a vessel. In addition, high pressure injections through a catheter with only an end hole may result in transient narrowing of the vessel just beyond the catheter tip.

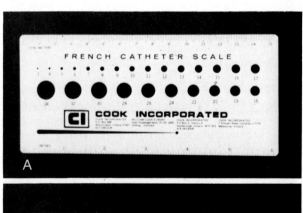

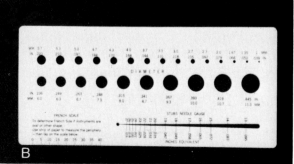

**Figure 16-13.** Conversion ruler. (*A*) French scale; (*B*) English scale.

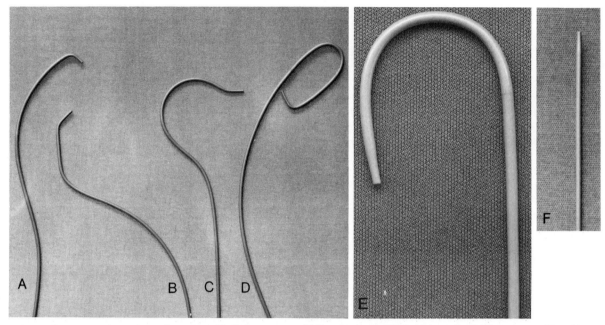

**Figure 16–14.** Common catheter tip configurations. (*A*) Right coronary; (*B*) Headhunter 1; (*C*) Headhunter 3; (*D*) left coronary; (*E*) multipurpose J—visceral; (*F*) straight catheter—visceral. (Courtesy of Cook Incorporated, Bloomington, IN.)

The combination of an end hole and several side holes reduces the trauma to the vessel and enhances the mixing of contrast medium with the blood. A multiple-holed catheter also reduces any recoil (catheter whipping) caused by the jet effect of a high-pressure injection. Multiple-holed catheters have the disadvantage of increased blood clotting potential; therefore, it is important to flush the catheter often to reduce the possibility of blood clot formation on the catheter, which may dislodge and become a thrombus or cause an embolus.

Catheters with side holes and no end hole are also available. These catheters are useful in intracardiac and pulmonary artery injections. The jet effect and recoil are greatly reduced with catheters having only side holes. Because the catheter has no end hole, a guide wire cannot be employed. Introduction of the side-hole catheter in the vessel is accomplished by inserting the catheter through a sheath placed in the vessel beforehand.

Regardless of the shape or number of holes, all catheter tips must be tapered. A tapered end facilitates entrances into the vessel and reduces the possibility of trauma to the vessel.

Many catheter tips are designed to retain their original shape. Others may allow the user to vary the shape of the tip (Fig. 16–15). These catheters employ a handle attached to the proximal end of the catheter, which changes the direction of the tip.

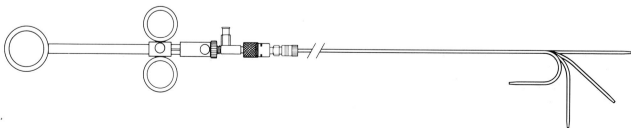

**Figure 16–15.** Deflecting catheter tip. (Courtesy of Cook Incorporated, Bloomington, IN.)

# REVIEW QUESTIONS

1. The _____ of a guide wire is introduced into the blood vessel first to prevent vessel damage.
   A. rigid end
   B. core
   C. flexible tip
   D. handle

2. A solid guide wire has the disadvantage of _____.
   A. lack of versatility
   B. increasing blood clotting
   C. increasing vessel abrasion
   D. catheter tip flaring

3. Coating a guide wire with heparin _____.
   A. lowers the coefficient of friction
   B. increases friction
   C. increases flexibility
   D. reduces possibility of blood clotting

4. As the core of a guide wire is _____, the flexibility _____.
   A. inserted, increases
   B. withdrawn, remains the same
   C. withdrawn, decreases
   D. inserted, decreases

5. Torque of a guide wire or catheter refers to _____.
   A. flexibility
   B. twisting or turning
   C. diameter
   D. the type of configuration

6. A _____ guide wire is useful in vessels that require two types of tip configurations to advance the catheter in the vessel.
   A. J-tip
   B. 5-cm straight flexible tip
   C. solid-core
   D. two flexible end

7. The _____ cm guide wire is employed when interchanging vascular catheters.
   A. 80
   B. 150
   C. 220
   D. 260

8. Employing the correct catheter and guide wire results in _____.
   A. a backflow of blood
   B. a free flow of blood
   C. blood clotting on guide wire
   D. blockage of blood flow

9. A _____ tip _____ core guide wire is recommended for extremely tortuous vessels.
   A. J-, movable-
   B. J-, fixed-
   C. straight, movable-
   D. straight, fixed-

10. _____ of a vascular catheter refers to its ability to retain its original shape.
    A. Torque
    B. Memory
    C. Configuration
    D. Degree of flexibility

11. Some vascular catheters may be _____ to increase torque control and radiopacity.
    A. braided
    B. cooled
    C. flushed with saline
    D. coated with plastic

12. A 3 French catheter is _____ mm in diameter.
    A. 1
    B. 2
    C. 3
    D. 4

13. Large vessels generally employ a catheter with _____.
    A. side and end holes
    B. end hole only
    C. side holes only

14. Catheters with _____ hole(s) are usually employed in selective angiography.
    A. side and end
    B. an end
    C. a side

15. Catheter recoil is most common with catheters having _____ hole(s).
    A. side and end
    B. an end
    C. a side

16. List three safety tests that should be performed prior to employing a guide wire.

17. Identify three precautions that must be taken when using a guide wire.

# BIBLIOGRAPHY

Abrams, HL: Angiography, Vol 1, ed 2. Little, Brown & Co, Boston, 1971.

Abrams, HL: Angiography, Vol 1, ed 3. Little, Brown & Co, Boston, 1983.

Ayella, RJ: A new device for cleaning guide wires in angiography. Radiology 97:686, December 1970.

Butto, F, et al: New-duty exchange guide wire. Radiology 163:276, April 1987.

Cardiovascular catheters and accessories, vascular prostheses, embolectomy, thrombectomy, irrigating catheters for cardiology, radiology and surgery. Ballston Spa, NY, 1977, Universal Medical Instrument Corp.

Carpenter, PR, et al: Compliance characteristics of angiographic guide wires. Radiology 118(3):719, March 1976.

Chen, PS: A simple method of cleaning a clotted catheter. Radiology 107:463, May 1973.

Cook angiography and interventional catalogue. Bloomington, IN, 1976, Cook Incorporated.

Cordis Guide Wire 1992 catalog.

Diagnostic and intervention products for the radiologist, cardiologist and surgeon. 1976–77 catalog. Bloomington, IN, 1976, Cook Incorporated.

Hawkins, IF, Jr and Kelley, M, Jr: Benzalkonium heparin coated angiographic catheters. Radiology 109:589, December 1973.

Instruments and accessories catalog, section 4. Glens Falls, NY, 1977, United States Catheter and Instrument Corp.

Johnsrude, IS, Jackson, DC, and Dunnick, NR: A Practical Approach to Angiography, ed 2. Little, Brown & Co, Boston, 1987.

Kandarpa, K: Handbook of Cardiovascular and Interventional Radiologic Procedures. Little, Brown & Co, Boston, 1989.

Medi-Tech angiography and interventional catalogue. Watertown, MA.

Miller, RE and Ng, AC: Forming teflon catheters during angiography. Radiology 97:340, November 1970.

Ouitt, TW, et al: Guide wire thrombogenicity and its reduction. Radiology 111:43, April 1974.

Ravin, CE and Koehler, P: Re-use of disposable catheters and guide wires. Radiology 122:577, March 1977.

Roberts, GM et al: Thrombogenicity of arterial catheters and guide wires. Br J Radiol 50:415, 1977.

Robertson, JD, et al: A new torque guide wire. Radiology 165:572, November 1987.

Snopek, A: Fundamentals of Radiologic Special Procedures. WB Saunders, Philadelphia, 1992.

White, RI, Jr: Fundamentals of Vascular Radiology. Lea & Febiger, New York, 1976.

Wojtowycz, M: Handbook in Radiology: Interventional Radiology and Angiography. Year Book Medical Publishers, Chicago, 1990.

Yashire, N, et al: Development of multi-purpose catheter for visceral arteriography. Radiat Med 7(6):278, November-December 1989.

# CHAPTER 17

# Supplementary Catheterization Equipment

*Marianne R. Tortorici, EdD, ARRT(R)*

The introduction of a catheter into a vessel requires the use of accessory equipment. Some of the equipment, for example, the needle, is used for puncturing the vessel. Other accessory equipment, such as stopcocks and vessel dilators, facilitates the introduction of the vascular catheter or allows for the introduction of pharmaceuticals into the vessel. The accessory equipment discussed in this chapter is limited to percutaneous needles, adapters, stopcocks, manifolds, and vessel dilators.

## PERCUTANEOUS NEEDLES

All angiographic procedures require the insertion of a percutaneous needle into the vessel. The length, gauge, and shape of the needle depend on the vessel to be punctured. Discussion here is limited to the percutaneous arterial needles used for diagnostic angiographic work. Specialized needles, such as translumbar or interventional needles, are discussed in the chapters relative to those angiographic procedures (Chapters 19, 28, 29, and 30).

There are two major parts of a percutaneous entry needle—the cannula and the hub (Fig. 17-1). The cannula may have a cutting edge that is sharp enough to puncture the tissues and the vessel, or it may be blunt or pointed. The cannula is a long, hollow tube through which the contrast medium, blood, guide wire, or other materials pass. The cannula may protrude through the hub, facilitating free blood flow and decreasing the chance of coagulation. The hub permits the attachment of a syringe or other equipment to the needle. The inner lumen of the needle may be tapered to facilitate guide-wire entry.

Most needles have a baseplate attached to the hub. The baseplate facilitates the puncture by permitting the angiographer to grasp the needle more securely. There are two types of baseplates—the half and the full (Fig. 17-2). When positioned properly, the half baseplate indicates that the bevel of the needle is up-

**159**

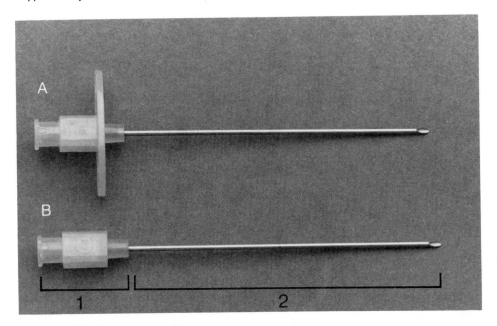

**Figure 17–1.** (*A*) Arterial needle with baseplate; (*B*) arterial needle without baseplate and showing parts: 1, hub, 2, cannula. (Courtesy of Cook Incorporated, Bloomington, IN.)

ward (Fig. 17–3). If the bevel of the needle is in the downward position, the guide wire may be damaged on entry into the vessel or the guide wire may be directed toward the vessel wall. In both instances, vessel injury may occur.

Some needles also include a stylet and an obturator (Fig. 17–4). The stylet is solid, has a cutting edge, and is inserted into the cannula of the needle. The end of the stylet may be flush with the cannula or it may protrude slightly. Both the cannula and the stylet are used during the vessel puncture. After the puncture, the stylet may be removed and the obturator may be inserted into the needle cannula. The obturator is made of solid metal and prevents the backflow of blood through the needle.

Needles are available in various sizes and shapes (Fig. 17–5). The size is identified by gauge number. The higher the gauge number, the smaller the inner diameter of the needle lumen. It is important to match the guide-wire diameter to the needle gauge (Table 17–1). The guide-wire diameter should be large enough to prevent the backflow of blood through the needle lumen and small enough to move freely within the needle lumen.

Needles are described by length and cannula thickness as well as by gauge. Needle length is measured from the tip of the cannula to the point where the cannula meets the hub. Most needles are measured in inches. The average lengths of arterial needles are 2⅛″ and 3¼″.

The cannula thickness may vary. Most needles are identified as either thin wall or regular. The difference between a thin-wall needle and a regular needle with the same gauge is in the thickness of the needle wall (the distance from the outer surface of the cannula to the lumen). The thin-wall needle is thinner or has a smaller distance than a regular needle.

When ordering needles, a combination of gauge, length, or cannula thickness is available. For example, it is possible to order an 18-gauge 2½″ thin-wall needle (18T) or an 18-gauge 3¼″ regular needle (18 gauge).

Most percutaneous needles are disposable and are used only once and then discarded. Reusable needles are commercially available; however, they must be thoroughly cleaned and sterilized before they are reused. Reuse of needles is greatly discouraged because it is impossible to remove all residue blood, which is

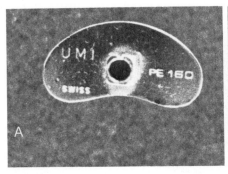

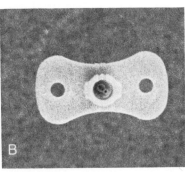

**Figure 17–2.** View of needle looking into the hub. (*A*) Half baseplate; (*B*) full baseplate.

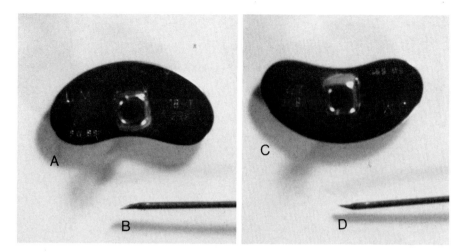

**Figure 17 – 3.** Relationship of half baseplate and bevel position. (*A*) Half baseplate resulting in (*B*) the bevel-up position (proper position); (*C*) half baseplate down resulting in (*D*) the bevel-down position (improper position).

conducive to cross-contamination. Also, constant re-sterilization of needles dulls the cutting edge.

## ADAPTERS

In order to connect syringes or other instruments to catheters or other accessory equipment, the ends of the items to be connected must be compatible. The ends of catheters or syringes often have an adapter for connecting one instrument to another.

Adapters may be constructed of metal or plastic. Metal adapters are generally stronger and provide a more secure connection than plastic adapters. Plastic adapters may be opaque or transparent (Fig. 17 – 6). Transparent adapters make it easy to determine whether air bubbles are present. Adapters are classified as male or female. The male adapter may be connected only to a female adapter and vice versa.

The end of an adapter may have a Luer-Lok or a rotating lock, or it may be tapered (Fig. 17 – 7A – D). The Luer-Lok and rotating lock provide a screw connection and are not likely to be accidentally disconnected. Luer-Loks and rotating locks are used for connecting two metallic-tipped instruments, for example, a syringe and a needle. The tapered-end adapter is used for connecting tubing to another instrument, for example, a syringe.

A Tuohy-Borst adapter is a special type of connection often made between a Luer-Lok and side-arm adapter (Fig. 17 – 7E). A side-arm adapter is used to enable the angiographer to inject contrast medium or other solutions into the patient while the catheter and guide wire are positioned in the patient. One end of the side arm is attached to the catheter or guide wire, and the other end is used to connect to a syringe for solution injection. The Tuohy-Borst may be turned clockwise or counterclockwise. The objective of a Tuohy-Borst adapter is to prevent the backflow of blood or the injected solution.

## STOPCOCKS AND MANIFOLDS

Stopcocks function similarly to water valves in that they control the flow of fluid from one area to another. In angiography, stopcocks are connected to some form of fluid reservoir. An example is a bottle of saline solution, with an intravenous tubing, attached by a stopcock to a catheter.

The fluid flow in a stopcock is controlled by a lever attached to a valve (Fig. 17 – 8). By rotating the lever, the valve opens or closes, controlling the flow of fluid. A valve is considered opened when the hole is parallel with the lumen of the adapter. When the hole is perpendicular to the lumen, the flow is stopped (the valve is

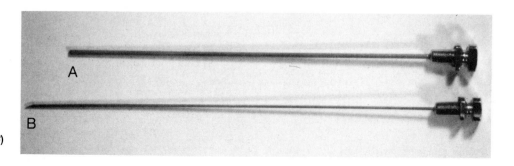

**Figure 17 – 4.** (*A*) Obturator; (*B*) stylet.

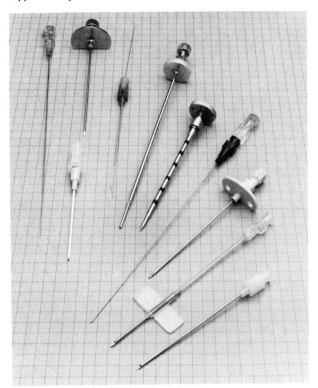

**Figure 17–5.** Assorted needles. (Courtesy of Cook Incorporated, Bloomington, IN.)

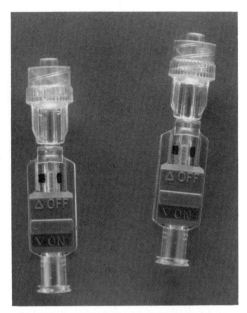

**Figure 17–6.** Transparent adapters. (Courtesy of Medi-tech, a division of Boston Scientific Corporation, Watertown, MA.)

considered closed). The valve may be made of metal or plastic. Metal valves tend to rust or oxidize. Once a metal valve has been oxidized, it will "freeze" and is no longer functional. Plastic valves do not oxidize, reducing the possibility of "freezing," but they cannot withstand high temperatures. Therefore, care should be taken when sterilizing a plastic stopcock not to melt the valve.

Two common types of stopcocks are the two-way and three-way. The two-way stopcock allows the flow of fluid to and from two items (Fig. 17–9A). A three-way stopcock allows the flow of fluid to and from three items (Fig. 17–9B).

As with adapters, the ends of stopcocks are classified as either male or female (Fig. 17–10). It is possible to have any combination of ends, for example, female and male or male and male. Often it is necessary to have more than one item connected to the patient. In this instance a manifold is employed. A manifold is a series of stopcocks attached to one another.

The stopcocks may be placed in a linear position or in a Y formation (Fig. 17–11). The linear manifold allows individual adjustment of each stopcock, whereas the Y manifold does not allow for the individual adjustment of the stopcocks.

Reusable stopcocks and manifolds are designed so that they may be disassembled. When cleaning a stopcock or manifold, it is advisable to remove the valve and clean all of its parts. It is also suggested that the valve be lubricated to prolong the life of the stopcock or manifold. Some stopcocks and manifolds have O rings to prevent leaks. These rings should be checked during cleaning and replaced when necessary. Manifolds and stopcocks may be made of reusable metal or disposable plastic. However, it is recommended that disposable manifolds and stopcocks be used whenever possible to avoid cross-contamination.

## VESSEL DILATORS

After the puncture of a vessel, a guide wire is introduced into the artery or vein. The guide wire has an outer diameter measured in hundredths of an inch and is used to guide the catheter. The diameter of the catheter is measured in French (F) sizes (1 French = $\frac{1}{3}$ mm). To facilitate the introduction of the catheter over the guide wire, vessel dilators are first introduced into the punctured artery or vein.

Table 17–1. **Suggested Guide-Wire Size for Various Needle Gauges**

| Needle Gauge (thin-wall) | Recommended Guide-Wire Diameter | |
| --- | --- | --- |
| | **Inches** | **Millimeters** |
| 21 | 0.018 | 0.46 |
| 20 | 0.021 | 0.53 |
| 19 | 0.025–0.028 | 0.64–0.71 |
| 18* | 0.032–0.038 | 0.81–0.97 |
| 16 | 0.034–0.047 | 1.14–1.19 |
| 15 | 0.052 | 1.32 |

*Most commonly used.

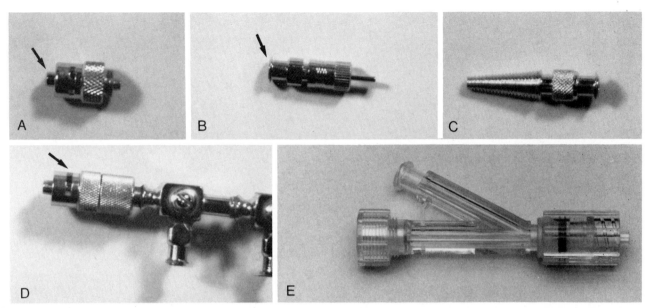

**Figure 17–7.** Adapters. (*A*) male Luer-Lok; (*B*) female Luer-Lok; (*C*) tapered end; (*D*) rotating male Luer-Lok; (*E*) clear body Tuohy-Borst with rotating male side arm. (*E* courtesy of Cook Incorporated, Bloomington, IN.)

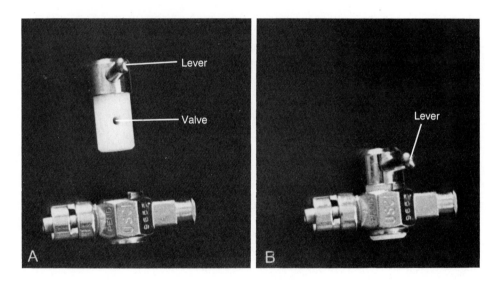

**Figure 17–8.** (*A*) Stopcock with valve removed from casing; (*B*) valve inserted in casing.

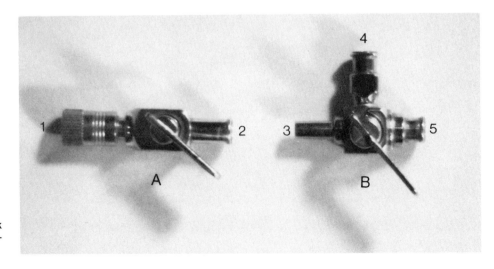

**Figure 17–9.** (*A*) Two-way stopcock (fluid flows at 1 or 2); (*B*) 3-way stopcock (fluid flows at 3, 4, or 5).

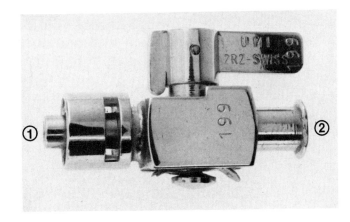

**Figure 17–10.** Two-way stopcock: 1, Male end; 2, female end.

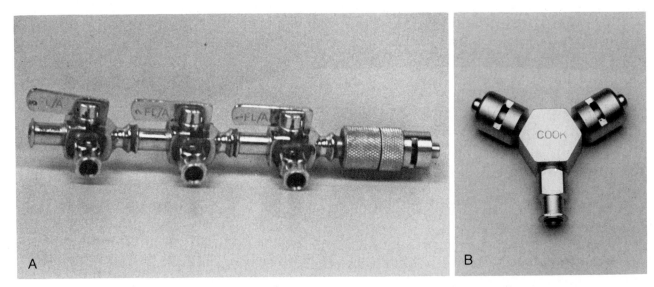

**Figure 17–11.** Manifolds. (*A*) Linear; (*B*) three-way Y. (*B* courtesy of Cook Incorporated, Bloomington, IN.)

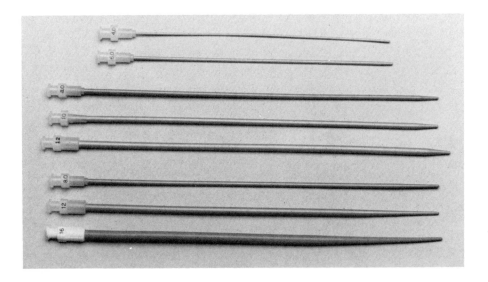

**Figure 17–12.** Vessel dilators displaying French size on hub. (Courtesy of Cook Incorporated, Bloomington, IN.)

A vessel dilator is placed over the guide wire and introduced through the puncture site. Vessel dilators are measured in French sizes (Fig. 17–12). They are usually 5″ to 6″ in length and have a tapered end. A 5 French vessel dilator may have a measurement range of 4.5F to 5F.

If an angiographer is going to use an 8F catheter for a procedure, it may be necessary to dilate the vessel first. This is performed by first introducing the smallest-size vessel dilator, for example, 4F. The small dilator is removed and a vessel dilator of the next-larger size is introduced, for example, 5F. This process is continued until the vessel is dilated to the desired size. The maximum-size vessel dilator should be equal to the size of the catheter to be used. Care should be taken not to dilate the vessel larger than the catheter, as this will result in bleeding around the catheter.

## REVIEW QUESTIONS

1. The inner lumen of a needle may be tapered to _____.
   A. reduce the backflow of blood
   B. facilitate guide wire entry
   C. increase contrast medium flow
   D. ensure a close fit with the stylet

2. When positioned properly, the half baseplate needle _____.
   A. prevents puncturing the outer wall of the vessel
   B. decreases the chance of coagulation
   C. indicates the position of the bevel
   D. permits easy attachment of the syringe

3. A needle obturator is used to _____.
   A. prevent the backflow of blood
   B. indicate bevel position
   C. facilitate guide wire entry
   D. decrease coagulation

4. The higher the needle gauge, the smaller the _____.
   A. outer diameter of the obturator
   B. stylet diameter
   C. inner diameter of the needle lumen
   D. hub

5. An 18-gauge thin-wall needle has the(a) _____ lumen diameter as (than) an 18-gauge regular needle.
   A. same
   B. smaller
   C. larger

6. When the hole of the valve of a stopcock is perpendicular to the lumen of the adapter, _____.
   A. the fluid flow is stopped
   B. the valve is opened
   C. fluid flows through the valve

7. The _____ manifold does not allow for the individual adjustment of the stopcocks.
   A. linear
   B. female end
   C. tapered end
   D. Y

8. Vessel dilators are used over _____.
   A. needles
   B. guide wires
   C. stylets
   D. catheters

9. If a 5 French catheter is employed for an angiogram, the maximum size vessel dilator to be used is _____.
   A. 3
   B. 4
   C. 5
   D. 6

## BIBLIOGRAPHY

Cardiovascular Catheters and Accessories, Vascular Prostheses, Embolectomy, Thrombectomy, Irrigating Catheters for Cardiology, Radiology and Surgery. Universal Medical Instrument Corp., New York, 1975.

Catalog. Cook Incorporated, Bloomington, IN, 1986.

Cordis Guide Wire Catalog. Cordis Laboratories, Inc., Miami. FL, 1977.

Instruments and Accessories Catalog, sec 4. United States Catheter and Instrument Corp., Glens Falls, NY, 1977.

Johnsrude, I, Jackson, D, and Dunnick, NR: A Practical Approach to Angiography, ed 2. Little, Brown & Co, Boston, 1987.

Medi-Tech: 1991 Angiography and Interventional Catalogue. Medi-Tech Corporation, Watertown, MA, 1991.

Snopek, A: Fundamentals of Radiographic Special Procedures. WB Saunders, Philadelphia, 1992.

Wojtowycz, M: Handbook in Radiology: Interventional Radiology and Angiography. Year Book Medical Publishers, Chicago, 1990.

# METHODOLOGY OF APPROACH

## CHAPTER 18

# Sterile Technique

*Marianne R. Tortorici, EdD, ARRT(R)*

Prior to the middle of the nineteenth century, the death rate among patients in hospitals was extremely high. Around the year 1850, English surgeon Joseph Lister (1827–1912) hypothesized that deaths caused by infection were the result of unsterile technique. To test his hypothesis, Lister employed antiseptics to clean wounds. As a result of Lister's use of antiseptics, deaths attributed to infection decreased substantially. Unfortunately, although Lister proved the importance of sterilization, proper sterile technique methods are often neglected. This still represents the leading cause of infection in hospitals today. This chapter contains a brief summary of how infection is spread and addresses the proper sterile technique practices applicable to an angiographic room. The reader is advised to refer to a patient care text for more specific information on sterile technique.

## INFECTION

Infection is spread from one area to another when a source of the infecting organism (pathogen), a means of transmission of the organism, and a susceptible host are all present. Sources of the infecting agent may be patients, visitors, employees, or objects that have become contaminated. In angiography, the primary sources of infection are the angiographers, instruments, and equipment. By wearing sterile gloves and gowns and employing sterile instruments, the rate of infection is greatly reduced.

## PATHOGEN TRANSMISSION

### Method of Transmission

There are four main methods for transmitting pathogens: contact, airborne, vehicle, and vector-borne. The contact method is the transmission of infection by direct contact (physical transfer of an infectious agent from an infected person to a host), indirect contact (personal contact between infected objects and a host), or droplet contact (infectious agents come in contact with the patient's nose or mouth). Airborne transmission occurs when infected droplets (or evaporated droplets suspended in air) or infected dust particles are inhaled by the host. Droplet contact differs from airborne contact in that the transfer of pathogens by the droplet method requires close association with the agent, for example, 3 feet. The vehicle route of transmission applies to diseases transmitted through contaminated media such as food, water, drugs, or blood. The vector-borne transmission is spread of disease through an insect or animal. An example of a vector-borne disease is malaria, which is transmitted by mosquitoes. Proper sterilization and sterile technique minimizes the transmission of infection. Of the four methods of transmitting infectious agents, the contact and airborne methods predominate in the angiographic room.

## Preventing the Spread of Infection

Infections may be prevented by eliminating the infecting agent or by eliminating the mode of transmission. The major sources of infecting agents during angiography are the individuals performing the procedure and the instruments and equipment used. To avoid possible transmission of infection from the angiographer to the patient, the angiographer should wear sterile gloves and a sterile gown. While masks are strongly recommended, especially if the angiographer has a cold, wearing them as part of the sterile protocol varies from institution to institution. To prevent the transmission of infection by needles, syringes, and other supplementary equipment, it is important that the instruments be sterilized. As a protection to the angiographer, some form of eye protection, for example, plastic glasses, should be worn. Adhering to these simple procedures can prevent a large percentage of postangiographic infections.

## BASIC PRINCIPLES OF STERILE TECHNIQUE

Contamination can be avoided by following the basic principles of sterile technique. These principles include the following:

1. If in doubt about the sterility of an object, consider it unsterile. An unsterile object should be removed, covered, or replaced.
2. Sterile persons should avoid unsterile areas.
3. Anything below the level of the table or the waist is considered unsterile. Items that fall below this area must be considered contaminated.
4. Gowns are considered sterile on the sleeves and the front from the waist up. The back of the gown and below the waist are considered unsterile.
5. Persons dressed in sterile gowns and gloves must pass each other back to back.
6. A sterile person touches only what is sterile.

7. Unsterile persons should not reach above or over the sterile field.
8. Sterile materials must be kept dry; moisture permits contamination. Packages that become wet must be resterilized or discarded.
9. If a solution soaks through a sterile field to a nonsterile field, the wet area should be redraped.
10. Hands covered with sterile gloves should be kept in sight and above waist level.

Angiography requires an invasive procedure, for example, catheterizing a vein or an artery. Although these invasive procedures do not require major surgery, it is essential that proper sterile technique be employed. Sterile technique includes the proper opening of sterile packages, careful handling of sterile instruments, proper drawing of drugs, correct gowning and gloving, proper skin preparation, and proper draping of the patient. Improper practice of any one of these procedures may result in postangiographic infection.

## OPENING STERILE PACKAGES

Angiographic instruments, especially items used for catheterization, are packaged in sterile containers. It is essential that the instruments remain sterile during use in the angiographic procedure. To prevent contamination, appropriate steps must be followed in opening sterile packages and handling sterile instruments. Some instruments are wrapped in cloth or paper (with or without a plastic covering), while many other items are only sealed in a see-through package. Items that are wrapped must be opened differently from sealed equipment.

To open a wrapped item, the package should first be positioned so that the top flap opens away from the individual opening the package. The next two flaps should open to the sides, and the last flap should open toward the individual opening the package (Fig. 18–1). After all four flaps have been opened, the sterile items are exposed and should only be handled by an individual who is wearing sterile gloves and a sterile gown.

Once the package has been opened, the sterile radiographer or nurse sets up the instrument tray in the manner preferred by the radiologist. Items such as guidewires and catheters are sealed in a see-through package and are not found on the tray. These items must be extended toward the sterile individual by the unsterile person. To properly hand an item in its package, for example, a syringe, to a sterile person, the unsterile person places both hands together and grasps the edges of the package. Turning the hands outward and downward, the unsterile person breaks the seal opening the package. Care should be taken to avoid touching the inside of the package with the hand, which would contaminate the item. The opened end of the package is extended toward the sterile individual, who removes the item from the wrapping, being careful not to touch the outside, unsterile, part of the wrapping (Fig. 18–2).

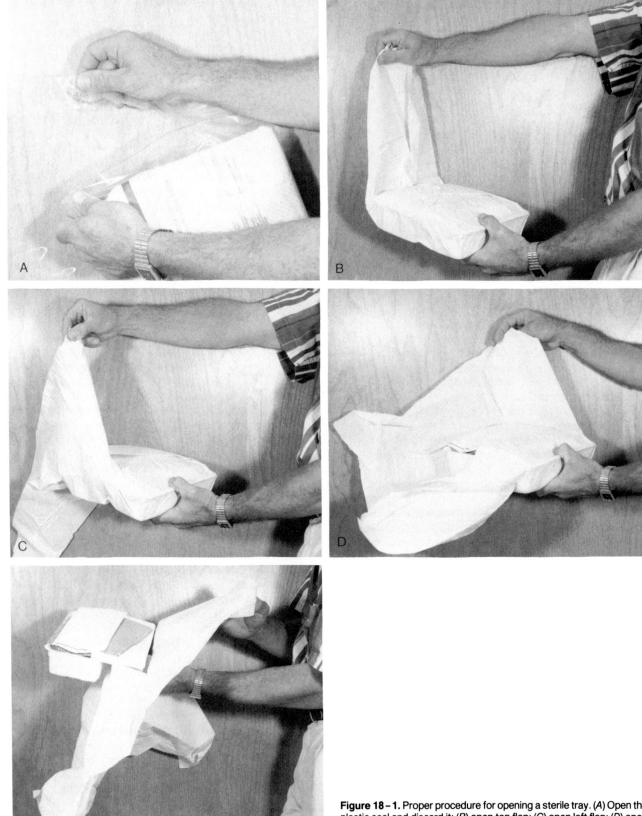

**Figure 18‑1.** Proper procedure for opening a sterile tray. (*A*) Open the plastic seal and discard it; (*B*) open top flap; (*C*) open left flap; (*D*) open right flap; (*E*) open bottom flap.

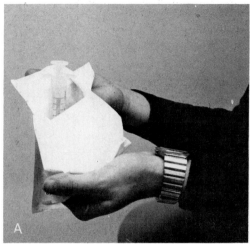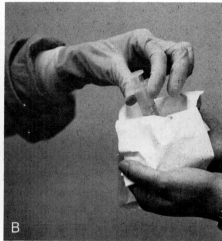

**Figure 18–2.** Proper procedure for handling sterile package. (*A*) Peel away package; (*B*) hand to sterile person.

## DRAWING UP DRUGS

Liquid drugs may be bottled in a vial or an ampule. A vial usually contains multiple doses; an ampule contains a single dose (Fig. 18–3). Vials usually have a rubber self-sealing stopper. The rubber stopper enables a needle to be inserted into the vial several times without contaminating the drug. The solution in the vial is in a vacuum, so injecting 10 ml of air into the vial will draw 10 ml of the drug back into the syringe.

When assisting a sterile person drawing up a drug from a vial, the unsterile person handles the vial. If the vial is new (Fig. 18–4*A*), the unsterile person opens the top by pulling the aluminum tab and breaking the seal (Fig. 18–4*B*). Once the vial is opened, the rubber stopper is exposed. Because the vial is new, there is no need to disinfect the rubber stopper. After the top is opened, the unsterile person holds the vial firmly with the label up so that the sterile person can read the label and verify the contents. The sterile person attaches a needle to a syringe and pulls back the plunger of the syringe to the desired measure of solution they wish to draw up (Fig. 18–4*C*). The unsterile person inverts the vial so that the sterile person can insert the needle into the rubber stopper to inject air into the vial (Fig. 18–4*D*) and withdraw the desired amount of the drug (Fig. 18–4*E*). After the drug is drawn up, the sterile worker withdraws the needle from the vial.

Ampules have long, thin tops with the neck of the ampule top weakened by the manufacturer to facilitate opening it (Fig. 18–5*A*). To assist a sterile person in drawing up a drug from an ampule, the unsterile person opens the ampule by wrapping a piece of gauze around the top of the ampule, curling one index finger around the body of the ampule and the other index finger around the top of the ampule, and placing the thumbs on the neck of the ampule (Fig. 18–5*B*). The neck of the ampule is then broken by applying pressure on the weakened portion in a direction away from the body (Fig. 18–5*C*). When opening the ampule, care

should be taken to prevent cutting oneself or allowing small pieces of glass to fall into the ampule.

The unsterile person holds the ampule firmly with the label up. The sterile person holds the syringe with the plunger fully inserted (Fig. 18–5*D*), then inserts a needle into the ampule, and withdraws the drug by pulling back on the plunger of the syringe (Fig. 18–5*E*). Often it is necessary for the unsterile person to reposition the ampule so that the sterile person can keep the lumen of the needle in the solution while withdrawing the drug from the ampule. When the drug is withdrawn, the sterile person removes the needle from the ampule.

In both the vial and ampule methods of drawing up drugs, it is important that the sterile person not touch

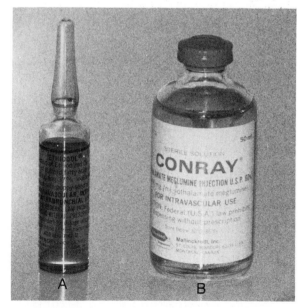

**Figure 18–3.** (*A*) Ampule of Ethiodol; (*B*) vial of Conray.

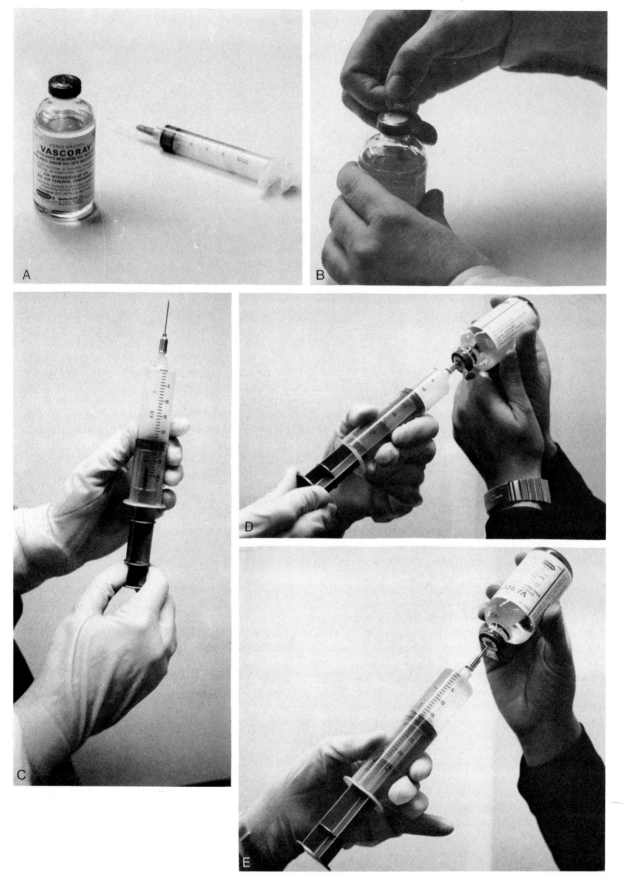

**Figure 18–4.** Withdrawal of contrast medium from vial. (*A*) Sealed vial; (*B*) open top of vial; (*C*) withdraw plunger of syringe; (*D*) inject air in vial; (*E*) withdraw contrast medium.

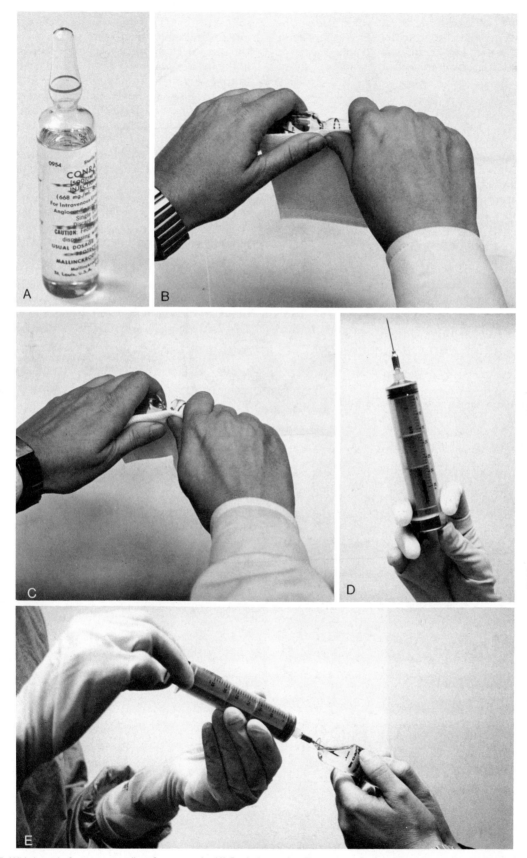

**Figure 18–5.** Withdrawal of contrast medium from ampule. (*A*) Sealed ampule; (*B*) grasp neck of ampule with gauze; (*C*) break neck of ampule (away from body); (*D*) insert plunger in syringe; (*E*) withdraw contrast medium.

the side of the bottle with the needle when attempting to insert the needle into the bottle. If the needle touches the bottle, the needle should be considered contaminated and be replaced by another sterile needle.

## GOWNING

To drape the patient in preparation for the examination, sources that may cause infection must be eliminated. It is important, therefore, that the angiographer wear a sterile gown. Usually radiographers gown themselves first, then drape the patient, then assist the radiologist with gloving and gowning.

### Self Gowning

To gown oneself, unwrap the package containing the gown, then stand about 12″ from the sterile area and pick up the gown by its folded edges, inside of gown

(Fig. 18–6A). To avoid touching the wrapper, lift the gown directly upward from the package. Make sure that no objects are near the gown; then grasp the gown at the inside of the neckband, hold at arm's length, and unfold (Fig. 18–6B). It may be necessary to gently shake the gown so that it opens freely. The inside of the gown should be facing you. To put on the gown, hold it by the inside shoulder seams, raise your arms upward, and slip them into the sleeves (Fig. 18–6C). An unsterile worker should stand behind you and adjust the gown by reaching inside the sleeves, grasping them, and pulling gently (Fig. 18–7A). The unsterile worker may pull the sleeve over the gownee's hand or just until the gownee's fingertips are visible. The distance that the unsterile person pulls the sleeve depends on whether the open or closed gowning method is used (see Gloving section). If the open method is used, then the sleeves should be pulled over the hands. If the closed method is employed, then the sleeves should be pulled so that only the fingertips are visible. After the sleeves are adjusted, the unsterile worker fastens the back of the gown (Fig. 18–7B through F) and ties the waistband, if applicable.

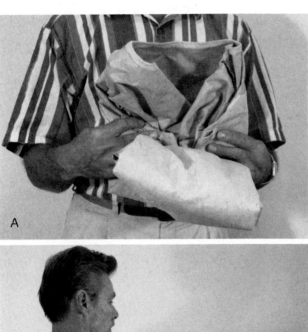

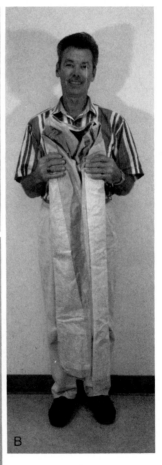

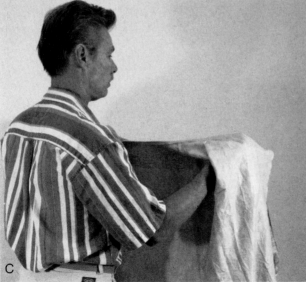

**Figure 18–6.** Self gowning. (A) Grab gown from inside; (B) unfold gown; (C) slip arms in gown.

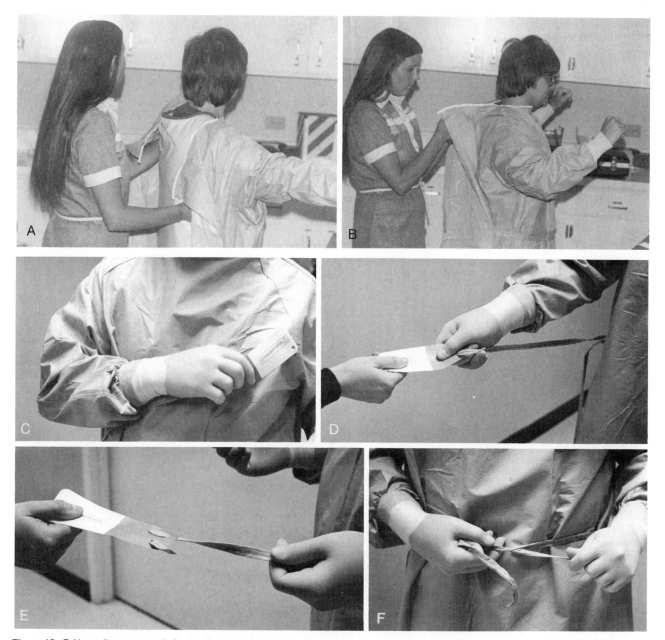

**Figure 18–7.** Unsterile person assisting sterile person in gowning. (*A*) Unsterile person adjusts sleeves and (*B*) secures neckband; (*C*) and (*D*) sterile person hands unsterile person waist belt; (*E*) unsterile person returns waist belt to sterile person after wrapping belt around gown; (*F*) sterile person ties waist belt.

## Gowning Another Person

The radiologist usually enters the room after the sterile tray has been set up and the patient is draped. The radiologist performs the catheterization and, therefore, must also be gowned. Because there is already a sterile person in the room to facilitate the procedure, the sterile person assists the radiologist in gowning.

To assist another person in gowning, the sterile person, who is already gowned and gloved, should pick up the gown by the neckband, hold it at arm's length, and let it unfold. The gown should be held by the outside shoulder seams so that the outside of the gown is facing the sterile person (Fig. 18–8). The assistant protects his or her sterile gloves by placing both hands under the gown at the top shoulder seam, making a cuff that covers the gloves; this also exposes the sleeves to the person being gowned. The gownee slips his or her arms into the sleeves in a downward motion (Fig. 18–8) until the hands emerge from the sleeves. Unsterile hands should not touch the sterile person during this process. Once the person being gowned has slipped both arms into the sleeves, the sterile person pulls the gown over the gownee's arms and shoulders. The gown is secured by an unsterile person as in the self-gowning technique.

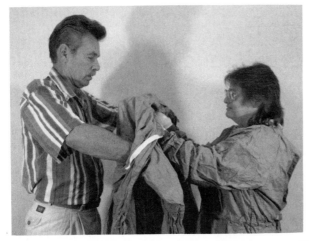

**Figure 18–8.** Assisting person in gowning by holding gown open with gloves covered while gownee slips hands into sleeves.

## GLOVING

Gloving should be done after the gown has been put on and properly adjusted. All jewelry should be removed from the fingers and wrists before gloving to avoid tearing the glove. There are two methods of

gloving: the open and closed methods. Although the open gloving method predominates, the closed method reduces the possibility of contamination. Regardless of which method is employed, the glove package should be opened and placed in front of the glovee so that the right glove is on the glovee's right side and the left glove is on the glovee's left side. Most gloves have talcum powder inside the glove to facilitate slipping the glove over the hand. If the gloves do not have talcum powder inside, powder may be put on the hands before slipping on the gloves. It should be noted that if a glove tears, the talcum powder may fall out of the glove onto the sterile area. For this reason, some individuals prefer not to use talcum.

## Closed Gloving Method

To put on gloves using the closed gloving method, the hands of the individual gloving are covered by the gown. As an example, to glove the right hand, pick up the right glove with the sleeved left hand (Fig. 18–9A) and place the palm of the right glove on the covered palm of the right hand (Fig. 18–9B). If this is performed properly, the fingers of the glove are facing the right elbow and the thumb of the glove is directly over the thumb of the glovee's hand. Grasp the bottom part

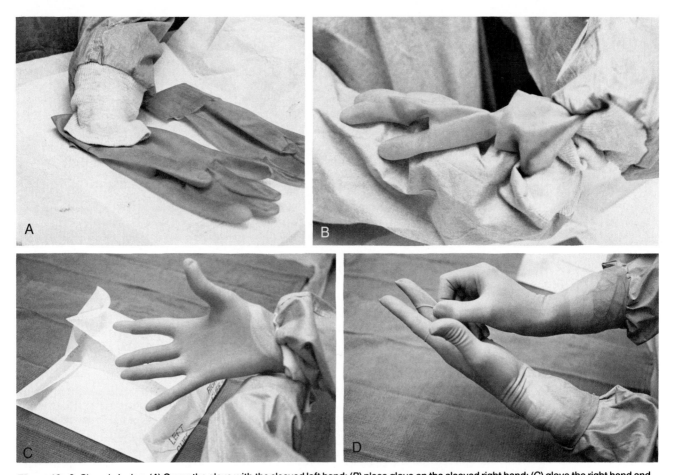

**Figure 18–9.** Closed gloving. (A) Grasp the glove with the sleeved left hand; (B) place glove on the sleeved right hand; (C) glove the right hand and repeat steps A, B, and C for the left hand; (D) adjust fingers.

of the cuff of the glove with the fingers of the right hand, and with the left hand grasp the top part of the cuff and pull it over the back of the right hand, slipping the fingers into the appropriate holes while pulling the glove over the hand (Fig. 18–9*C*). Repeat the procedure for the other hand. Adjust the fingers of the glove so they are comfortable (Fig. 18–9*D*).

## Open Gloving Method

For the open gloving method, the hands of the individual gloving are visible through the sleeves. Open the glove package as described previously. With the nondominant hand, grab the cuff of the glove to be placed on the dominant hand (Fig. 18–10*A*). Although touch-

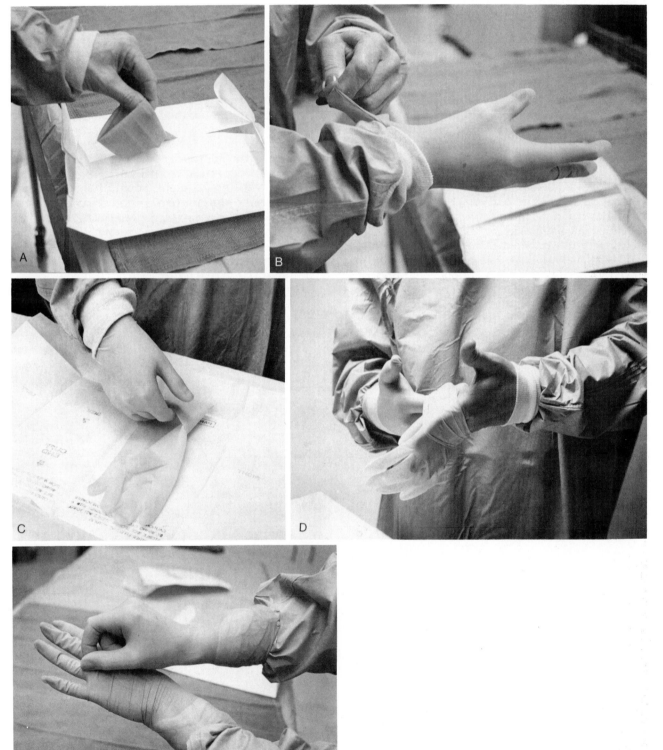

**Figure 18–10.** Open gloving. (*A*) Grab glove by cuff; (*B*) glove hand; (*C*) grab other glove by inside cuff; (*D*) glove hand; and (*E*) adjust fingers.

ing the cuff with the hand contaminates it, the cuff is folded over so the hand makes contact with the inside of the cuff, which, in any case, is against the skin. Avoid having the fingers of the nondominant hand touch the outside of the glove, place the dominant hand in the glove, and pull the glove over the hand with the nondominant hand (Fig. 18–10B). Usually the glove does not fit perfectly and will need adjusting, but this should not be done until both hands have been gloved. To glove the nondominant hand, pick up the glove by placing the sterile hand under the folded cuff of the glove (Fig. 18–10C). Put the nondominant hand in the glove and pull the glove over the hand with the sterile gloved hand (Fig. 18–10D). Avoid having the sterile hand touch the skin of the nondominant hand. When both hands are gloved, adjust the gloves so that they fit the hands comfortably (Fig. 18–10E). The cuff may be adjusted over the sleeve of the gown by inserting the fingers of the opposite hand in the folded portion (outside part of glove) and pulling the cuff over the sleeve. Care should be taken not to touch the contaminated part of the cuff (inside portion).

To glove another person, the sterile glove package should be opened previously. Always inform the individual being gloved whether the right hand or the left hand is to be gloved first. The sterile person picks up a glove by inserting the fingers of one hand under the folded cuff. The fingers of the other hand are inserted under the cuff opposite the first hand, and the glove is stretched open so that the thumb of the glove faces the glovee (Fig. 18–11A). The thumbs of the sterile person's hands are held away from the glove to avoid possi-

ble contact and contamination by the glovee's hand during insertion into the glove. To put on the glove, the unsterile individual places the hand in the glove, using a downward motion, while the sterile person pulls the glove up over the hand (Fig. 18–11B). This procedure is repeated for the other hand. When both hands are gloved, the glovee may adjust the gloves for comfort.

## PATIENT PREPARATION

After sterile packages have been opened and the radiographer has gloved and gowned, the patient is prepared for the procedure. This preparation includes cleaning and draping the puncture site.

To clean the skin, all of the hair in the involved area must be removed. This procedure should be performed by the appropriate personnel the day before the examination. However, if it is necessary to shave the patient in the angiographic room, it should be performed by the unsterile person. After shaving, the area is cleaned with an antiseptic solution using circular motions, starting in the center and rotating outward (Fig. 18–12). The skin is cleaned at least twice, using the same circular motions. A new sponge is used for each cleaning cycle so that no area will be cleaned twice with the same sponge. After the antiseptic is administered, a sterile gauze may be used with the same circular motions to remove the excess liquid. Once the area is clean, the patient is draped by the sterile person.

The most common puncture sites for angiographic

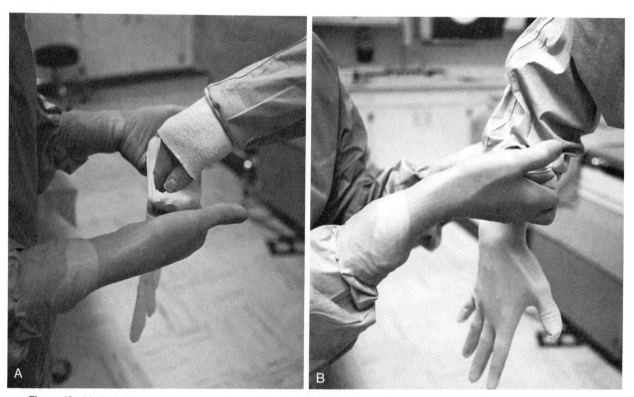

**Figure 18–11.** Assisting person in gloving. (A) Hold glove open, thumbs out; (B) move glove upward as person inserts hand.

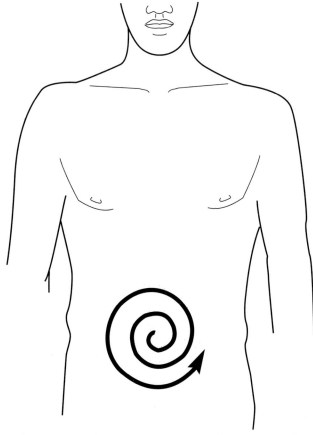

**Figure 18–12.** Clean skin in circular motions, inside to outside.

procedures are the groin, neck, antecubital area, and axilla. Most angiographic departments use disposable rather than cloth drapes. Disposable drapes are more advantageous than linen drapes because the disposable drapes are nonabsorbent and self-adhesive, prevent slippage, and are lint-free. The draping routine will vary over time as new materials and ideas evolve. Regardless of the draping materials employed, four basic principles should be followed:

1. Handle drapes so that the gloved hands are covered.
2. Drape front to back.
3. Consider anything below table level unsterile.
4. Never use drapes that are torn or have worn spots.

## REVIEW QUESTIONS

1. _____ transmission occurs when infection droplets or infected dust particles are inhaled by the host.
   A. Contact
   B. Vehicle
   C. Airborne
   D. Vector-borne

2. Anything _____ is considered unsterile.

   A. in front of the gown
   B. on the sleeves of the gown
   C. at the x-ray table level
   D. below the waist

3. Persons dressed in sterile gowns pass each other _____.
   A. front to back
   B. side to side
   C. back to back
   D. front to front

4. When opening a wrapped package, the top flap is opened _____ the individual.
   A. toward
   B. to the dominant side of
   C. to the nondominant side of
   D. away from

5. If one would like to draw up 15 ml of a drug from a vial, _____ ml of air is injected into the vial.
   A. 15
   B. 20
   C. 25
   D. 30

6. When self gowning, to avoid contamination, the gown is unfolded _____.
   A. while standing near the sterile table
   B. while holding it at arm's length
   C. by the unsterile person
   D. from the outside of the gown

7. When cleansing the patient's skin for needle puncture, it is important to _____ for each cleaning cycle.
   A. resoak the sponge
   B. reverse the circular motions
   C. squeeze the sponge
   D. use a new sponge

8. List two reasons disposable drapes are preferred over cloth drapes.

9. List at least two sources of infection often found in an angiographic room.

10. List two methods of gloving.

## BIBLIOGRAPHY

Berry, E and Kohn, M: Operating-Room Technique, ed 3. McGraw-Hill, New York, 1966.
Chesney, D and Chesney, M: Care of the Patient in Diagnostic Radiography, ed 4. Blackwell Scientific Publications, Oxford, 1975.
Du Gas, B: Introduction to Patient Care, ed 2. WB Saunders, Philadelphia, 1972.
Ginsberg, F: Manual of Operating Room Technology. JB Lippincott, Philadelphia, 1966.
Isolation Techniques for Use in Hospitals, ed 2. Department of Health, Education and Welfare, Washington, DC, 1975.
Johnsrude, I and Jackson, D: A Practical Approach to Angiography. Little, Brown & Co, Boston, 1979.
Powell, N: Handbook for Radiologic Technologists and Special Procedures Nurses in Radiology. Charles C Thomas, Springfield, 1974.
Wood, L: Nursing Skills for Allied Health Services, vol 3. WB Saunders, Philadelphia, 1977.

# CHAPTER 19

# Catheterization Methods and Patient Management

*Marianne R. Tortorici, EdD, ARRT(R)*
*Patricia A. Messmer, RN, CCRN*
*Jeanne L. Neuman, ARRT(R) (CV)*

The human circulatory system is a closed system. Blood leaves the heart through the arteries and returns to the heart via the veins. The blood vessels serve as the pathway for the circulation of the blood from one area to another. Because the circulatory system is closed with vessels branching or extending one from another, it is possible to selectively catheterize a vessel. For example, the renal artery may be catheterized through a variety of approaches such as the brachial artery, the femoral artery, or the aorta. The approach employed by the angiographer is usually determined by the area to be examined, the patient's condition, the patient's age, or the angiographer's personal preference.

This chapter describes the various angiographic methods of catheterization and the related patient management techniques. Included are brief summaries of preangiographic care, intraprocedural care, postangiographic care, and complications that may occur with angiographic catheterization.

## ANGIOGRAPHY TEAM

It is recommended that an angiographic team consist of a minimum of five people. These include the radiologist, a scrub technologist or nurse, a circulating technologist, a nurse, and a patient advocate (either nurse, physician, or technologist). Perhaps it is also appropriate to list the patient, whose cooperation is often the key to limiting procedural complications, as a member of the team.

The primary tasks of the radiologist are to perform the catheterization and to be responsible for overseeing all the medical aspects of the procedure. The scrub person assists the radiologist in the catheterization process. The circulating technologist is responsible for the technical aspects of the procedure, which include setting up equipment, filming, and so on. The nurse provides patient care practices, especially medications. The patient advocate's responsibilities are to oversee the safety and comfort of the patient and to free the scrub person from patient care duties.

Mutual respect and rapport among the angiographic team are essential for the successful completion of any procedure. Trust and ease among team members are evident to the patient and his or her family and create an environment of comfortable, efficient, and professional care.

## PREANGIOGRAPHIC CARE

### Patient History

Most angiographic examinations are scheduled for, and are performed on, individuals who have had a previous diagnostic examination. Thus, the clinical histories of the majority of angiographic patients are known. A radiologist's review of the patient's clinical history and consultation with the patient's physician are recommended as the first steps in preangiographic care. In consultation with the patient's physician, the radiologist should determine, first, if there is a need to perform the examination and, then, the specific type of angiography needed. It is possible that, after the radiologist has consulted with the attending physician, an alternate procedure may be indicated.

If the decision is made to perform the procedure, the radiologist reviews the patient's medical history. In assessing the patient's condition, the radiologist should review the patient's pulmonary, cardiovascular, neurologic, and renal functions. In addition, the patient's medication history, including allergies, types of reactions, and medications the patient is currently taking, is noted. Of special importance is heparin, warfarin sodium (Coumadin), or aspirin therapy, or a history of hypersensitivity to contrast media. Heparin, Coumadin, and aspirin "thin" the blood and can promote excessive bleeding during the angiographic procedure. Patients with a history of hypersensitivity to contrast media must be assessed as to the nature of the previous episode. A premedication protocol may be ordered for patients with previous serious reactions (see Chapter 3, Contrast Media).

Review of laboratory analyses includes blood chemistry, particularly blood urea nitrogen (BUN) and creatinine levels to determine renal function. Hemoglobin, hematocrit, platelets, prothrombin time, and partial thromboplastin time are used to evaluate the clotting ability so that the angiographer may anticipate and avoid any bleeding problems likely to occur. Arteriography should be avoided if the protime or activated partial thromboplastin time (APTT) is more than one and a half times the control time or if the patient has fewer than 50,000 platelets per cubic millimeter. Ultimately, the decision to proceed or not lies with the radiologist and attending physician.

High risk patients include those who have anuria, heart failure, impending or recent myocardial infarction, impending cardiovascular accidents or blood dyscrasia, or those who have had previous severe reactions to contrast media. The irony of these high risk situations is that often these conditions are the reasons for performing the angiogram. Once it is determined that the patient's condition is conducive to undergo the procedure, the patient is informed of the decision, the procedure is explained to the patient, a limited physical assessment is performed, and appropriate medications are prescribed.

### Physical Assessment

An accurate assessment of the patient's mental and physical preprocedural status is essential as a baseline against which subsequent intraprocedural and postprocedural events are judged. Evaluation of the mental status of the patient occurs during patient consultation. The assessment reveals the level of consciousness, confusion, comprehension, stress, and anxiety, and the patient's mental state. This information is best obtained by interviewing the patient.

Evaluating the patient's physical status requires a limited physical examination. The results are useful in establishing the necessary baselines to determine any change in the patient's physical condition through the procedure and in anticipation of any interventions that may be required.

Assessment of the neurologic status of the patient includes evaluating the pupillary response, determining if any sensory or motor deficits such as those of the hand grasp and dorsoplantar flexion are present, assessing the strength and equality between the extremities, and determining the degree of speech clarity. It is important to note any existing paralysis or deficits, especially when planning on neuroangiography or neurointerventional procedures, where the possibility of exacerbating or inducing neural deficits is high.

Cardiopulmonary status is important to assess because many complications involve these areas. Obtaining baseline lung sounds (clarity or otherwise) and heart tones (rhythm and characteristics) are the essential components of assessment.

Appraisal of the vascular system is essential because of the direct invasion of this system by needles, introducers, and catheters. The peripheral pulses of all extremities are evaluated to determine vascular access and any pre-existing deficits. Assessment of the lower extremities includes recording the bilateral femoral, posterior tibial, and dorsalis pedis pulses. In the upper extremity, bilateral axillary, brachial, and radial pulses are recorded. If neither upper nor lower extremity pulses can be obtained, Doppler ultrasound should be used to determine the status.

### Patient Consultation

Discussing the procedure and explaining it to the patient is one of the most important aspects of preangiographic care. The patient interview should be approached from the perspective of involving the patient as a participant rather than as an object of study. For inpatients, the consultation should take place in the privacy of the patient's room. In the case of outpatient angiography, preprocedural discussion between the patient and radiologist should occur at the time the patient arrives for the procedure. Include any family members who may be present in the discussion. Consulting with the patient and family members helps alleviate the patient's fears and anxieties and aids in building a good "patient-caregiver" rapport.

During the interview, the patient's level of stress and anxiety is evaluated along with his or her mechanisms of coping with stress. In the majority of cases, much of the anxiety can be minimized with a thorough discussion of the procedure, giving the patients some level of control over the procedure and a vested interest in the successful outcome. A patient who is calm and has confidence in the medical personnel can help facilitate the procedure and perhaps reduce the occurrence of complications.

The interview includes a step-by-step explanation of the procedure in a language the patient understands. In addition to the technical aspects of an examination, physical and emotional aspects are discussed. Examples include explaining the experience of the introduction of a local anesthesia, contrast medium, conscious sedation, and angiographic introducer. Descriptions of risks and complications inherent to the procedure are also presented during the consultation. It is incumbent upon each angiography–interventional radiology department to investigate the respective institution's risk management policy and procedures regarding who may and may not discuss these risks and complications and to follow policy guidelines. Some institutions allow nurses and technologists to describe risks to patients, while others grant that responsibility only to physicians.

The culmination of the consultation leads to the granting of permission by the patient, or family member, to proceed with the examination. This is accomplished in the form of a written informed consent (refer to Chapter 2, Medical-Legal Implications, for more information on informed consent). The original document is kept with the patient's medical records chart, and a copy is retained for the radiology files. After the patient signs the informed consent, preangiographic medication and diet are prescribed.

## Premedication and Diet

The type and amount of preangiographic medication prescribed depend largely on the patient's condition or the type of angiographic procedure. For example, patients with severe pulmonary diseases are prone to respiratory depression after barbiturate administration; therefore, care should be taken when prescribing preangiographic medication for these patients. The most common preangiographic prescriptions include the following:

1. An injection of 0.4 to 1.0 mg of atropine administered intramuscularly to protect against vasovagal reaction.
2. An injection of 50 to 100 mg of meperidine hydrochloride (Demerol) administered intramuscularly. (Meperidine hydrochloride should not be administered to cardiac patients having a cardiac or brachiocephalic study because hypotension may aggravate an already-compromised circulation.) Demerol serves as a narcotic analgesia.
3. An injection of 5 to 10 mg of diazepam (Valium) administered intramuscularly, or 50 to 100 mg of sodium secobarbital administered intramuscularly. This helps decrease patient anxiety.
4. Hydroxyzine (Vistaril), 25 to 100 mg administered either orally or intramuscularly to decrease anxiety and serve as an antiemetic.
5. Premedications may be prescribed for patients with a previous history of reaction to contrast media. Refer to Chapter 3, Contrast Media, for the recommended protocol for these cases.

Anticoagulants (or heparin) are withheld for at least 4 hours before the procedure. Administration of these drugs may be safely resumed 6 hours after the procedure; however, to reduce the possibility of bleeding at the puncture site, it is recommended that administration not be resumed until 24 hours after the procedure. If this is not possible, protamine sulfate may be administered as a slow intravenous injection at a dosage of 10 mg per 1000 units of heparin being neutralized. Coumadin should be stopped several days before arteriography. If immediate arteriography is necessary, fresh frozen plasma can be used to replenish the hepatic coagulation factors affected by Coumadin.

Although not a common practice, 10 grains of aspirin may be administered the night before the examination. The aspirin is useful in diminishing platelet adhesiveness.

Conscious sedation (Table 19–1) is defined as the administration of pharmacologic agents producing a depressed level of consciousness but allowing the patient to retain the ability to independently maintain a patent airway and respond appropriately to physical and/or verbal stimuli. In angiography, conscious sedation is used to maintain a level of comfort during procedures likely to induce high levels of discomfort. It also has the added advantage of producing varied levels of amnesia when the medication mix includes benzodiazepines, such as Valium or Versed. According to a position statement from numerous professional nursing organizations, it is within the scope of practice of a registered nurse to manage the care of the patient receiving intravenous conscious sedation. This professional responsibility must follow the guidelines of state laws and institutional policy and procedure. Key points of policy should include:

1. The physician selects and orders the medications.
2. Guidelines for the types of monitoring and time intervals are established.
3. The professional administering conscious sedation has the responsibility for the management and care of that patient.

4. The professional administering conscious sedation has the knowledge and skills to assess, diagnose, and intervene in the event of complications and to institute interventions in compliance with orders or institutional protocols.
5. Documentation exists to qualify caregivers for administration of conscious sedation and periodic review of competency according to institutional policy.
6. Essential monitoring and accessories include, but are not limited to:
   a. continuous ECG
   b. continuous pulse oximetry
   c. blood pressure
   d. assessment of patient's respiratory rate and level of consciousness
   e. continuous IV access
   f. supplemental oxygen
   g. emergency cart with defibrillator

It is incumbent on the professional administering conscious sedation to be knowledgeable of the pharmacology of the medications being used. Because few radiologic technologists have this knowledge, most angiography suites have registered nurses perform these functions.

When administering these medications, a sufficient amount of time must elapse before increasing dosage to allow the medication to reach its peak effectiveness. Failure to wait before increasing dosage may result in oversedation of the patient, requiring unnecessary interventions to return to the physiologic baseline. The professional administering the sedation continually assesses the patient and informs the physician of the patient's physiologic status and level of consciousness.

Some of the commonly used sedative agents, as well as their properties, dosages, actions, and reversal agents, are listed in Table 19–1. The two primary sedative categories listed in Table 19–1 are opioids and benzodiazepines.

Opioids are strong respiratory depressants, requiring supplemental oxygen and monitoring of oxygenation levels. The respiratory depressant effect may not be noticed for several minutes; thus, it is important for the medication to reach its peak effect before administering a second or further dose. Opioids potentiate (add to the effect of) and are potentiated by sedative-hypnotic agents. Some common adverse reactions to both classes of opioids are hypotension, bradycardia, nausea, vomiting, physical dependence, constipation and paralytic ileus, dizziness, and blurred vision. Naloxone (Narcan) is a useful agent used to reverse the effects of opioids. It may be administered intravenously, intramuscularly, or subcutaneously. The usual dose is 0.1 to 0.2 mg for intravenous administration at 2- to 3-minute intervals until the desired effect is obtained. It is important to monitor patients receiving Narcan because the duration of the sedative's effect may exceed the effect of Narcan.

Benzodiazepines also are strong respiratory depressants. Patients should be monitored for underventilation or apnea, which can lead to hypoxia or cardiac arrest unless effective countermeasures are initiated. Concomitant use of barbiturates, opioids, or other central nervous system (CNS) depressants increase the

**Table 19–1. Properties of Common Sedative Agents**

| Type | Name | Method of Administration | Adult Dosage | Comment |
|------|------|--------------------------|--------------|---------|
| Opioid | Meperidine (Demerol), synthetic opioid | Intramuscular, intravenous | 12.5–25 mg | Patients with allergy to opioids are not always allergic to meperidine |
| Opioid | Morphine sulfate—true opioid | Intramuscular, intravenous | 5–10 mg, intravenously | Dosage depends upon patient response and tolerance; patients allergic to meperidine may tolerate morphine |
| Opioid | Fentanyl citrate (Sublimaze); alfentanil (Alfenta, sister drug to Sublimaze), synthetic opioid | Intravenous | Individualized | Fentanyl is 50 to 100 times more potent than morphine |
| Benzodiazepines | Diazepam (Valium) | Sublingual, oral, and intravenous | 5–10 mg for sublingual and oral; intravenous doses are individualized | Onset is faster with sublingual than oral. Intravenous dose is given slowly, 1 min per 5 mg or 1 ml. Avoid small veins, intra-arterial injection, and extravasation. Do not mix with other solutions. |
| Benzodiazepines | Midazolam hydrochloride (Versed) | Intravenous | Titrated to desired level | Maximum dose 2.5 mg/2 min with a 2-min pause before administering more to evaluate effect of preceding dose |

risks and may contribute to profound or prolonged drug effect. The common adverse reactions to benzodiazepines are similar to opioids and include drowsiness, hypotension, bradycardia, nausea and vomiting, and blurred vision. A reaction particular to Versed is the partial or complete impairment to recall for several hours following administration. Versed is three to four times more potent than Valium, but its period of effectiveness is shorter. Also, patients on Versed tend to be more alert after it wears off. Paradoxic reactions to benzodiazepines include acute hyperexcited states, hallucinations, increased muscle spasticity, and insomnia. An antagonist to benzodiazepines is flumazenil (Mazicon), which is usually administered intravenously at a dose of 0.2 mg. If the desired level of consciousness is not obtained after 45 seconds, another 0.2 mg can be injected and repeated at 60-second intervals up to a maximum total dose of 1 mg. The patient must be continuously monitored for resedation because the effects of benzodiazepines may outlast the effects of Mazicon. In the event of resedation, repeat doses may be administered at 20-minute intervals. However, no more than 1 mg should be administered at any one time, with no more than 3 mg administered in 1 hour.

Dietary requirements of the patient include fasting for 4 to 8 hours before the examination. Patients with chronic renal disease should be given fluids orally or intravenously to reduce the possibility of renal failure during the angiographic procedure.

## INTRAPROCEDURAL CARE

It is not unusual for the sedative administered to the patient to decrease the patient's alertness and response time. For this reason and others, the patient is attended by a person who acts as caregiver and advocate (a nurse, technologist, or resident radiologist) whose primary responsibility is for the comfort, safety, and care of the patient during the examination. The most important function of the advocate is maintaining communication. Simple conversation has a calming effect and distracts the patient from dwelling on the physical or emotional discomfort of the procedure. The advocate advises the patient about impending events such as needle sticks, reviews the procedure agenda, and reassures the patient. The patient is made as comfortable as possible within the confinements of the procedure. This includes extra padding at pressure points, a pillow or sponge under slightly flexed knees, sponges placed to maintain required obliquity, and covering to maintain modesty and warmth. Besides emotional comfort, the caregiver offers maintenance of physical comforts, such as small changes in position to relieve pressure points and muscle strains. If the patient is required to change position dramatically, then the caregiver assists in the change.

Prior to the procedure, the patient is positioned on the imaging table and attached to an electrocardiograph (ECG), noninvasive blood pressure (NIBP) monitor, and pulse oximeter. These devices are used to obtain baseline values and monitor the patient's vital signs throughout the procedure.

The electrocardiogram is monitored continuously for any changes that may occur. Deviation from baseline rhythm is brought to the attention of the radiologist. Oxygen saturation is maintained at a level above 90%. If the saturation declines and maintains a level below 90%, oxygen by nasal cannula or mask is administered to augment the patient's respiratory status in a flow necessary to maintain adequate saturation. Blood pressure readings are taken at intervals of approximately 5 minutes, or more frequently if necessary. Several readings are assessed for hypotension or hypertension. Because respiratory monitors are unreliable, it is best to assess the patient's respiratory status by direct visualization with a correlation to the pulse oximeter. Assessing the patient's status and tolerance of the procedure is ongoing. Documenting the patient's condition and vital signs is easily accomplished with a flow sheet (refer to Chapter 2, Medical-Legal Implications). Monitor printout sheets are also good reference sources for charting a patient's progress.

During any invasive procedure, the angiography team must be prepared to handle any emergency that may occur. This may range from patient anxiety to cardiopulmonary arrest. Life-threatening conditions may require using oxygen, defibrillation, suction, artificial respiration equipment, intubation equipment, and any medications necessary to alleviate the life-threatening reactions. All angiography personnel should be certified in cardiopulmonary resuscitation (CPR). It is also recommended that personnel obtain Advanced Cardiac Life Support (ACLS) certification.

## SELDINGER TECHNIQUE

All selective angiographic percutaneous methods, except the cutdown and translumbar techniques, employ the Seldinger technique (Fig. 19–1) for catheter introduction into the vessel. This technique was developed by Sven Seldinger in the 1950s and is a simple, safe method of puncturing and catheterizing a vessel. In this method, to select a puncture site, the pulses and blood pressures of both extremities are recorded. A weak pulse may indicate a problem proximal to the puncture site. Arterial murmurs may signify partial occlusion. In both these instances, puncturing the vessel should be discouraged. Once a puncture site has been selected, the peripheral vessels are palpated and their pressures recorded. These vessels are repalpated at the end of the procedure and their postprocedural pressures compared with the preangiographic record. A decrease in pressure may be a sign of a problem, for example, a clot or a vascular spasm.

To perform the actual puncture, the site is cleaned and the area draped. The physician administers a local anesthetic in the perivascular tissues; this anesthetizes the tissues and prevents vasospasm. A small incision of about 2 mm is made in the skin approximately 1 to 2 cm

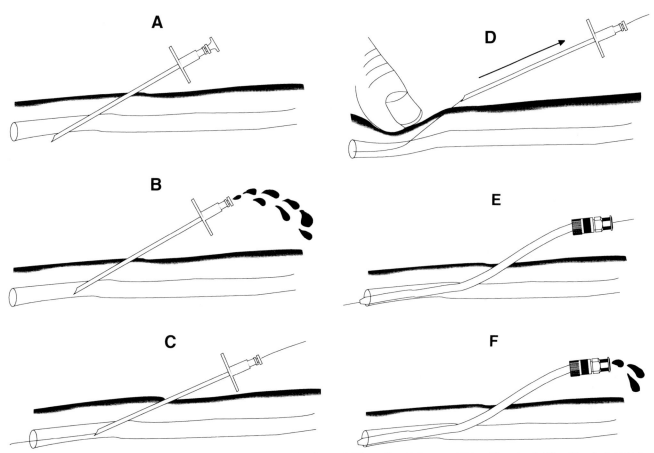

**Figure 19–1.** Seldinger technique. (*A*) Needle punctures both walls of vessel; (*B*) needle withdrawn until blood flows back; (*C*) guide wire inserted; (*D*) needle removed; (*E*) catheter placed over guide wire; (*F*) catheter inserted in vessel, guide wire removed.

below the intended puncture site. The needle is placed in the incision. Pulsations felt against the needle enable the physician to locate the artery. The pulsations should be felt in a to-and-fro motion. If the pulsations are felt on the right or the left side of the needle, the needle is located to the side of the vessel and must be repositioned. When the needle is centered on the artery, the needle is advanced, puncturing both walls of the vessel. If the needle has a stylet, this is removed after the vessel walls are punctured.

To place the needle in the lumen of the artery, the needle is angled so that it is parallel to the skin and is slowly withdrawn until there is a blood backflow. The blood flow pattern is observed. A forceful but irregular flow may indicate a stenosis. A dripping or slight flow may mean that the patient has severe hypotension or occlusive disease or that the needle is located subintimally. In the first instance, the needle is removed and a new site is found. In the case of a subintimal puncture, the needle is reinserted into the incision to relocate the needle properly in the vessel. When a steady flow is obtained, the flexible end of the guide wire is inserted through the needle and advanced at least 6 to 10 cm in the vessel. The needle is removed over the guide wire while pressure is applied to the puncture site to prevent hematoma formation. After cleaning the guide wire

with a gauze soaked in saline solution, a vessel dilator, which is at least 2 French sizes smaller than the catheter to be used, may be placed over the guide wire and inserted in the artery. To facilitate catheter insertion, a vessel dilator may be used to enlarge the tissue "tract" leading to the vessel and lumen of the vessel. The vessel dilator is removed and, if necessary, a larger dilator is inserted. Care should be taken never to dilate the vessel larger than the size of the catheter.

After the vessel has been dilated, the guide wire is cleaned with gauze soaked in saline and the catheter is slipped over the guide wire and brought near the vessel. The catheter is inserted in the vessel using a forward rotating movement. When both the guide wire and the catheter are in the vessel, the catheter may be positioned using fluoroscopic visualization. The guide wire must always precede the catheter in the vessel. Once the catheter is in the desired location, the guide wire is removed, leaving only the catheter in the vessel.

## APPROACHES

Angiography is performed by introducing a catheter into one of several different vessels. It is desirable to enter a vessel that is large, has no, or little, tortuosity, and is least likely to cause complications. There are two types of approaches: the percutaneous and the cutdown. Both of these approaches may be performed on a variety of vessels. The percutaneous approach is more desirable than the cutdown. Of the various percutaneous vessel sites, the femoral artery is the most desirable. Other percutaneous locations include the brachial, axillary, abdominal aorta, and carotid (for information on percutaneous carotid puncture, refer to Chapter 22, Cerebral Angiography).

## Percutaneous Femoral

Puncturing the femoral artery is the most common catheterization approach. The femoral artery is easily accessible, is fairly large, and has the lowest statistical complication rate. It arches over the pectineus muscle in a posterior medial direction and becomes the external iliac artery. The femoral artery is lateral to the femoral vein and beneath the inguinal ligament (Fig. 19–2), which attaches to the anterior superior iliac spine and pubic tubercle. Body habitus plays a role in locating

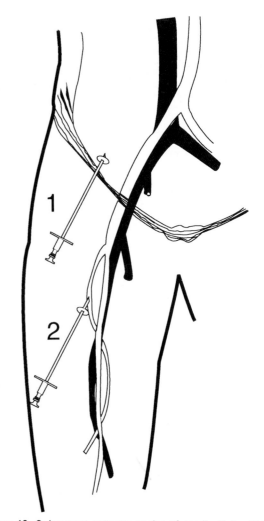

**Figure 19–3.** Incorrect entrance angles of needle: *1,* too high and misses artery; *2,* too low and punctures deep femoral artery.

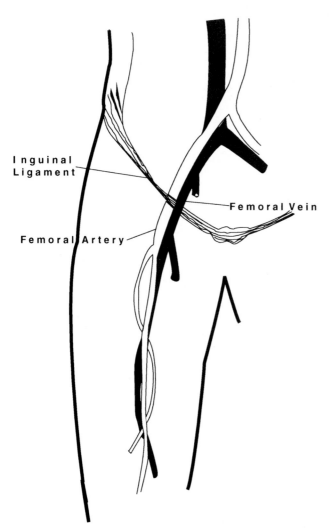

**Figure 19–2.** Anterior view of femoral artery.

the inguinal ligament. For example, both slim and obese patients present difficulty in locating the inguinal ligament.

Once the inguinal ligament is located, the pulse of the femoral artery is palpated about 1 cm below the inguinal ligament. If it is difficult to find a pulse, for example, on an obese patient, an ultrasound transducer can be placed inside a sterile glove and used to scan the area to locate the vessel. A local anesthetic (without epinephrine) is administered subcutaneously at the puncture site. After 2 to 3 minutes, a small incision is made at the site of the anesthetized area. Mosquito forceps are used to separate the tissue for needle entry. The middle and index fingers are placed above and below the incision, respectively, with the hand farthest from the patient, while the other hand is used to puncture the vessel. The needle is inserted medially at a 25- to 30-degree angle.

The Seldinger technique is used for catheterization of the vessel. The best entry level is at the apex of the femoral arch. Introducing the needle above the arch results in missing the artery (Fig. 19–3, *1*); this is most likely to occur in slim patients. Entering below the femoral arch may result in puncturing the deep femoral artery (Fig. 19–3, *2*); this is most likely to occur in obese patients.

The femoral approach is indicated in studies of pathologic conditions in the following areas:

1. lower extremities
2. pelvic area
3. abdominal aorta and its branches
4. thoracic aorta
5. brachiocephalic vessels
6. coronary arteries and the left ventricle of the heart

The femoral approach is contraindicated in the following cases:

1. occlusive disease of the iliac or common femoral arteries
2. marked tortuosity of the iliac artery
3. severe blood dyscrasia present
4. grafts of the femoral artery
5. aneurysm of the femoral artery

## Percutaneous Brachial

Brachial catheterization is the second most common approach for angiography. The brachial artery is slightly smaller than the femoral artery, and the complication rate is slightly higher than for the femoral approach. The brachial artery is superficial and lies on the anteromedial aspect of the humerus. The median nerve is medial to the artery, the radial nerve is posterior, and the ulnar nerve is posteromedial. The brachial artery is best palpated at the lower third of the arm. However, the arterial needle puncture is most successfully introduced just above the antecubital fossa (Fig. 19–4). The needle is inserted using the Seldinger technique. For a high pressure retrograde injection after catheter placement, a sphygmomanometer is placed just below the puncture site and inflated 50 mm Hg above the patient's systolic blood pressure. This helps force the contrast medium into the brachiocephalic vessels and alleviates the pain that may be caused by the contrast medium in the distal end of the extremity.

The brachial approach is indicated in, but not limited to, the following instances:

1. to assess pathology of upper extremities
2. to assess cerebral atherosclerosis
3. where the femoral approach is unfeasible or unsuccessful
4. where cardiac catheterization is required
5. to assess internal mammary artery grafts

The left brachial approach is primarily employed in the study of the left vertebral artery, the basilar artery, and the posterior fossa. The right brachial approach is most useful in examinations of the right vertebral artery, the basilar artery, and the posterior fossa. Puncture of either the right or left brachial artery has a low complication rate; however, occasionally the median or radial nerve may be damaged by the puncture. The most common complication of this approach is brachial arterial spasm.

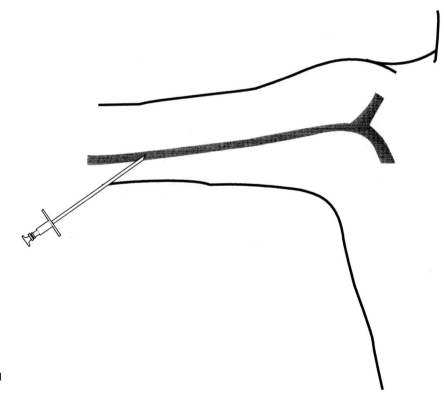

**Figure 19–4.** Location of needle for brachial approach.

## Percutaneous Axillary

Axillary catheterization is the least desirable approach to angiography. One reason the axillary approach is undesirable is that the brachial plexus (nerve complex), located near the axillary artery, can suffer permanent damage as a result of trauma or from compression by a hematoma on the nerves. The small diameter and mobility of the vessel are further reasons for discouraging the selection of the axillary artery as a puncture site. This approach should be employed only when the others are not feasible. If the axillary artery puncture is used, the side that is catheterized is determined by the vessel(s) to be studied. The left axillary artery is catheterized to evaluate the following:
1. descending thoracic aorta and abdominal aorta
2. pelvic area
3. lower extremities

The right axillary artery is most effective when assessing the following:
1. ascending aorta and left ventricle of the heart
2. selective coronary
3. four-vessel study of the cerebral vessels

The axillary approach is contraindicated in the following cases:
1. occlusive disease of the axillary artery
2. aneurysm of the axillary artery
3. graft of the subclavian artery

In the axillary approach, the patient's arm is abducted 90 degrees or is positioned using maximum arm abduction with the patient's hand under his or her head. The latter position is preferred because it places the vessel in a "fixed" position, making it less likely to move. The Seldinger technique is used to catheterize the artery. The needle is inserted at a 45-degree angle to the arm over the lateral axillary fold and the proximal area of the surgical neck of the humerus (Fig. 19–5). Care must be taken to avoid injecting the anesthetic into the brachial plexus, which might result in permanent damage.

## Cutdown

The cutdown approach is a minor surgical procedure to isolate a vessel for the introduction of a catheter (Fig. 19–6). Although a cutdown may be performed on almost any vessel, the brachial vein is usually the vessel of choice. In the brachial approach, the arm is placed in an anatomic position and the antecubital area is scrubbed and draped. A 1-inch, superficial, transverse incision is made medial to and just above the antecubital fossa. The tissues are separated with curved mosquito forceps in a direction parallel to the vessel until the vein is uncovered. When the vein is visualized, the walls of the vessel are freed and the vessel is isolated by placing closed forceps under the artery or vein and then opening the jaws of the forceps. Two sutures are placed around the vessel, one at the proximal end and one at the distal end. A transverse incision penetrating the intima is made on the anterior surface of the vein. To introduce the catheter, vessel dilators are inserted in the vessel. Small dilators are inserted first, and the size is gradually increased until the last dilator inserted is one size smaller than, or the same size as, the vascular catheter. After the vessel is dilated, the catheter is introduced into the vessel and the forceps are removed. The sutures are tightened around the catheter to prevent bleeding. The catheter is placed in the desired area with the aid of fluoroscopic visualization. After the procedure, the catheter is removed and the vessel and skin are sutured. A bandage is placed over the surgical site, and the sutures are removed in a few days.

## Translumbar

The translumbar approach is indicated when the femoral, axillary, or brachial methods cannot be performed. The translumbar approach is contraindicated in the following cases:
1. blood dyscrasia

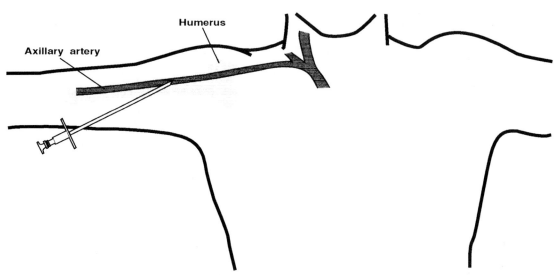

**Figure 19–5.** Location of needle for axillary approach.

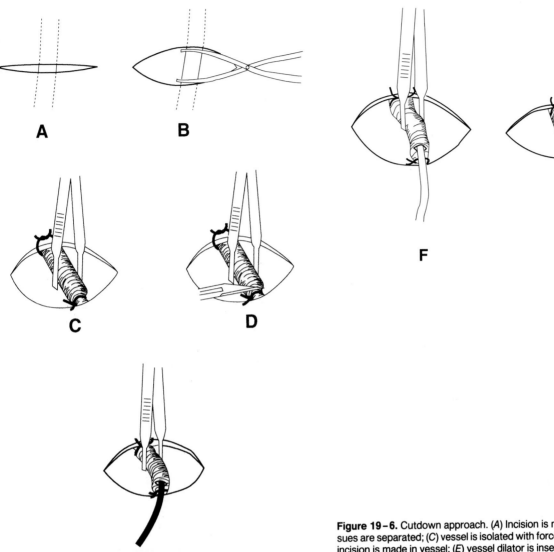

**Figure 19–6.** Cutdown approach. (*A*) Incision is made in skin; (*B*) tissues are separated; (*C*) vessel is isolated with forceps and sutures; (*D*) incision is made in vessel; (*E*) vessel dilator is inserted; (*F*) catheter inserted; (*G*) forceps removed and catheter secured with sutures.

2. abdominal or dissecting aneurysm
3. aortic graph
4. severe hypertension

The needle puncture for the translumbar technique may be performed at one of two levels. The puncture level may be at either the 12th thoracic (T-12) or second lumbar (L-2) vertebra (Fig. 19–7). The techniques for these methods are similar.

Translumbar puncture of the upper aorta is performed by placing the patient in a prone position with a positioning sponge or pillow under the abdomen to straighten out the lordotic curve of the lumbar spine. The 12th thoracic vertebra is located by palpating the 12th rib. A local anesthetic is administered 1 to 2 cm below T-12 and 8 to 10 cm left of the spine; a small nick is made in the skin. A puncture is made using a short bevel 8-inch 18-gauge Teflon-sheathed needle with a sharp obturator. The needle is inserted and directed ventrad and cephalad until the needle reaches the lateral border of T-12. The needle is then withdrawn about 5 cm and directed laterally and ventrally until the pulsations of the aorta are felt. When the needle strikes the aorta, resistance is felt; when the needle is advanced into the aorta, there is a sudden release of the tension. Only the wall of the aorta nearest the spine is punctured. The needle should be placed in the middle of the aortic lumen. Placement of the needle in the aorta is confirmed by a backflow of bright red blood. After the obturator is removed and the bloodflow is observed, a high torque guide wire is introduced through the Teflon sheath. If resistance is felt when the guide wire is introduced, the needle is probably too close to the opposite wall of the aorta and should be repositioned. When the needle is in the proper position, plastic tubing is connected to the hub. The tubing allows an injection to be made without moving the position of the needle; this is especially important during manual injections of the contrast medium.

To perform a lower translumbar puncture, L-2 is located either by fluoroscopy or by a preliminary abdom-

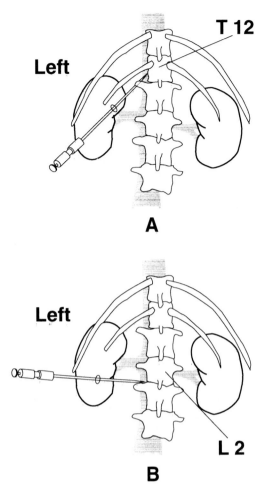

Left

**T 12**

**A**

Left

**L 2**

**B**

**Figure 19-7.** Translumbar approach (patient is prone). (A) Placement of needle for T-12 approach; (B) placement of needle for L-2 approach.

inal radiograph with a lead marker on the patient. The L-2 puncture requires the same size needle as the upper puncture. The patient is placed in the same position as the T-12 puncture, and the needle is introduced 8 to 10 cm lateral to L-2. The needle is directed at a 30- to 40-degree angle until it is lateral to L-2, after which the needle is withdrawn about 5 cm and advanced at a higher angle, until it enters the aorta. Care should be taken to avoid entering the renal or other visceral arterial branches. Ideally the needle should be placed just below the inferior mesenteric artery. By placing the needle at this level, the visceral arteries will not be opacified; this is important when attempting to demonstrate the femoral arteries. After the needle is properly positioned, plastic tubing is connected to the bulb.

Translumbar aortography is not without its hazards. Care should be taken to avoid puncturing the lung when performing a T-12 puncture. Misalignment of the needle may cause a hemothorax or pneumothorax. It is also recommended that aortic punctures be limited to three during the procedure to prevent retroperitoneal hemorrhage.

## ANTITHROMBIC METHODS

Regardless of the methodology of approach used, blood clot formations on the guide wire or in the catheter present one of the greatest risks to the patient. Should a clot form and be released in an artery, it can cause an embolism, which can be fatal, especially if the embolus is in the cerebral or the coronary artery. To reduce the possibility of blood clot formation, catheter and guide wire manufacturing companies have designed their products to be coated with heparin. Independent research has proved that this is effective for preventing blood clots. If the patient's condition does not contraindicate the injection of heparin into the vessels, then heparin should be administered during the examination.

There are two schools of thought regarding the best procedure to keep the blood vessels clot-free: one procedure is systemic heparinization, and the second method is use of the constant pressure pump. In the systemic heparinization method, an initial dose of 1000 to 5000 units of aqueous heparin is injected through the catheter. This is contraindicated in the translumbar approach or in patients with internal bleeding, severe hypertension, aortic insufficiency, or following needle aspiration. When systemic heparinization is to be used, the amount of the initial heparin injection is determined by the size and weight of the patient. A guideline for dosage is 45 units/kg of the patient's weight. After the initial injection, the catheter is flushed every 2 to 3 minutes with 5 to 10 ml of a solution of 1000 units of heparin in 500 ml of normal saline solution. The periodic flushing keeps the lumen of the catheter open and replaces some of the original heparin as it is metabolized. At the end of the procedure, the patient is given 10 mg of protamine sulfate for each 1000 units of the initial heparin injection; this counteracts the heparin to control bleeding after the catheter is removed.

The constant pressure pump method involves placing a plastic bag of saline-heparin solution in a pressure pouch. The pressure pouch is inflated to a pressure slightly greater than the systolic pressure of the patient. The saline solution flows through the catheter into the vessel by overcoming the resistance of the arterial pressure. As the saline bag empties, the pressure pouch must be reinflated to maintain the necessary pressure to keep the saline solution flowing into the vessel. The constant pressure pump is set up so that the saline pump is hung from an intravenous pole with tubing attached to the saline bag. A three-way stopcock connects the tubing to the catheter, allowing a syringe to be attached to one end of the stopcock. By adjusting the valve, an injection of contrast medium can be made through the stopcock.

After the desired injections are made, or blood samples are removed, the valves of the stopcock may be readjusted to permit the constant saline solution to flow through the catheter. The constant pressure pump is used between filming and catheter manipulation. The pressure pump is most commonly used with an end-hold catheter.

# POSTANGIOGRAPHIC CARE

After the catheter is removed, compression over the puncture site is applied until hemostasis is obtained. This may take from 5 to 45 minutes, depending on the patient's blood pressure status, anticoagulative status, and bleeding and clotting times. Care is taken to avoid undue pressure to the arterial site, which may impede blood flow distal to the point of stasis, inducing thrombosis. Thus, it is imperative to check peripheral pulses during the time that pressure is applied. There is controversy as to whether or not to use a dressing on the puncture site. Those opposed to compression say that it prohibits the visualization of the site. Proponents of compressing believe that it reduces the possibility of postprocedural bleeding.

Regardless of the approach or location of the puncture, it is important that the patient remain in bed. He or she may elevate the head 30 degrees. The patient is encouraged to drink fluids. The extremity where the puncture site is located should be immobilized for at least 12 hours. Vital signs are taken every 15 minutes for the first hour, then every 30 minutes for the next 2 hours, and hourly for an additional 4 hours. At the time the vital signs are taken, the distal pulses on the extremity of the puncture site are recorded. Additionally, a visualization of the puncture site for the femoral puncture and a sensory and motor check for the percutaneous brachial and axillary punctures should be performed when the vital signs are recorded.

When checking the peripheral pulses, the color and temperature of the punctured extremity are noted, as well as the neurologic status. These factors, combined with peripheral pulse data, comprise a fair assessment of the patient's circulatory status in the affected extremity. When a translumbar approach (TLA) is used, it is impossible to apply direct manual pressure to the site. Hemostasis is obtained by aortic tamponade, where blood is lost into the musculature surrounding the puncture site, thus providing an internal pressure. Often, the patient experiences epigastric or flank pain, relieved by narcotic analgesia. Evidence of the hematoma is obtained by an abdominal x ray, demonstrating a deviated left ureter.

Slight changes occur in the aftercare of angioplasty patients. Bed rest is maintained for 12 to 24 hours, longer than for routine angiography. Blood pressure readings are taken and trends noted, especially when renal angioplasty has been performed. Following an appropriate time interval, the patient may be placed on anticoagulant therapy.

Although the patient leaves the x-ray room after the filming, angiographic care is not completed until 12 hours after the examination. Table 19–2 summarizes the routine postangiographic care.

In addition to routine postangiographic care, after a femoral approach, an abdominal radiograph is sometimes taken to observe the contour of the urinary bladder. Displacement of the bladder may indicate hematoma formation.

Pressure dressings at the puncture site are discouraged because they hinder observation of the site. Research studies have shown that the local complication rate without pressure dressings compares favorably with those rated with pressure dressings. All complications should be recorded and the necessary follow-up procedures administered.

# COMMON ANGIOGRAPHIC COMPLICATIONS

The majority of angiographic complications usually occur at the puncture site during and after the procedure, during manipulation of the catheter or guide wire, and during injection of a contrast medium during the procedure.

Table 19–2. **Postcatheterization Care**

| Care | Catheterization Approach | | | |
| --- | --- | --- | --- | --- |
| | **Femoral** | **Brachial** | **Axillary** | **Translumbar** |
| Bed rest | Bed rest; patient may elevate head 30 degrees | Bed rest; patient may elevate head 30 degrees | Bed rest; patient may elevate head 30 degrees | Bed rest; patient may elevate head 30 degrees |
| Punctured extremity | Leg straight | Arm immobile in sling | Arm immobile in sling | N/A |
| Vital signs | 15 min × 4<br>30 min × 4<br>1 h × 4 | 15 min × 4<br>30 min × 4<br>1 h × 4 | 15 min × 4<br>30 min × 4<br>1 h × 4 | 15 min × 4<br>30 min × 4<br>1 h × 4 |
| Additional pulse check with vital signs check | Femoral, dorsalis pedis, and posterior tibia | Radial and ulnar | Radial and ulnar | N/A |
| Other checks at time of vital signs check | Groin for hematoma | Sensory and motor function | Sensory and motor function | N/A |
| Postangiography order | Resume care as physician ordered prior to angiography | Resume care as physician ordered prior to angiography | Resume care as physician ordered prior to angiography | Resume care as physician ordered prior to angiography |
| Fluids | Encourage unless patient is restricted by physician orders | Encourage unless patient is restricted by physician orders | Encourage unless patient is restricted by physician orders | Encourage unless patient is restricted by physician orders |

The more common complications at the puncture site include bleeding, hematoma, and thrombosis. Bleeding is usually a result of poor technique. Unnecessary bleeding may occur because of multiple vessel punctures, multiple catheter changes, prolonged catheterization time, catheters that are poorly constructed, or damaged vessels. Sometimes bleeding occurs around the catheter at the puncture site. This type of bleeding may be stopped by manual compression for a few moments. Hematomas at the puncture site are often a result of inadequate manual compression of the vessel after catheter withdrawal. Unless the hematoma is severe enough to require therapy, it is not considered a complication. Thrombosis may develop several hours after the procedure. Accurately recording the pulses prior to and after the procedure is a critical aspect of the proper diagnosis of the patient's condition. A cold, pale extremity in which the pulses are absent or diminished indicates a possible thrombosis. Severe femoral thrombosis and ischemia of the lower extremity may result in loss of the limb. Other complications include arteriovenous fistula, pseudoaneurysm, thrombophlebitis, and infection. These complications are extremely rare.

Complications resulting from catheter manipulation include embolization, dissection, impaction of the catheter, and breakage of the guide wire. Embolization may occur because of pressure injections, catheter manipulation, or catheter construction. Excessive pressure injections may dislodge loose thrombi attached to a vessel, causing emboli. Catheter construction itself facilitates the formation of emboli; this is especially true with side-hole catheters, in which it is difficult to keep the holes free from thrombi. In addition, different catheter materials have different clotting factors. Some materials actually promote clotting.

Vessel dissection resulting from catheter manipulation is often unavoidable. Most vessel dissections occur because the vessels are degenerated, tortuous, or fibrotic. In these instances, forceful manipulation of the catheter or a pressure injection may cause dissection. Some dissections are a result of placement of the catheter into the vessel wall. The location of the dissection is a major factor in determining the seriousness of the injury. Even the slightest dissection in the brain, heart, or kidneys is critical. Small dissections in large vessels may not have a serious effect.

Impaction of the catheter is a result of placing too large a catheter in a vessel. Because the catheter is too large for the vessel, the catheter can occlude the blood flow. Usually this situation is rapidly diagnosed by visual observation of a contrast medium test injection. If a test injection does not "wash out," then an obstructed blood flow is indicated. If the blood flow is disrupted, the catheter should be withdrawn immediately. Prolonged occlusion in the kidney, brain, or heart may result in ischemia, infection, or chemical damage to the organ.

Guide wires have been known to break inside the vessels. Modern guide wire construction has significantly decreased the incidence of guide wires breaking within the vessels. Many instances of guide wire breakage are a result of sharp, beveled needles.

Lastly, complications occur during the injection of a contrast medium. All contrast media marketed today have documented incidences of patient reactions. Some contrast media have a lower incidence of reaction than others. The proper use of contrast media is as important as the proper manufacturing of the product. The greatest areas of risk of contrast media reaction are in the coronary arteries and in cerebral and kidney circulation. The heart is sensitive to sodium ion contrast media. Thus, contrast media that use methylglucamine are safer than those containing sodium. Large doses of contrast media injected into the brain (150 ml or more) have been known to cause neurotoxic effects. The least damaging contrast media employed in cerebral circulation are those with a combination of methylglucamine and sodium salts. Injection of a contrast medium in the renal arteries results in vasoconstriction; this is the converse of what normally occurs in other vessels, namely, vasodilation. Nonionic contrast media have less reaction than ionic media. It is interesting to note that contrast media reactions in patients having general anesthesia are virtually nonexistent. However, the use of anesthesia introduces the possibility of complications resulting from the anesthetic. The types of reactions resulting from contrast media range from nausea and vomiting to cardiac arrest (see discussion of contrast media reactions and treatments in Chapter 3, Contrast Media).

## REVIEW QUESTIONS

1. Select the answer below that is *not* considered a high risk condition when performing angiography.
   A. Anuria
   B. Ulcers
   C. Heart failure
   D. Myocardial infarction

2. An intramuscular injection of 0.4 to 1.0 mg of _____ may be administered prior to angiography to protect against vasovagal reaction.
   A. atropine
   B. meperidine hydrochloride
   C. diazepam
   D. Versed

3. Patients with chronic renal disease may have _____ to reduce the possibility of renal failure.
   A. Valium
   B. Versed
   C. sodium secobarbital
   D. fluids

4. An advantage of including the patient advocate is _____.
   A. reduced patient costs
   B. freeing the scrub person from patient tasks
   C. reducing the number of lawsuits
   D. keeping the patient's family out of the room

5. _____ is a laboratory procedure performed to assess renal function.
   A. Hematocrit
   B. Hemoglobin
   C. Creatinine
   D. Partial thromboplastin

6. To determine which vessel to puncture, assessment of the _____ is performed.
   A. peripheral pulses
   B. heart
   C. neurologic system
   D. all of the above

7. _____ sedation is the administering of drugs producing a depressed level of consciousness while allowing retention of a patent airway and ability to respond to physical or verbal stimuli.
   A. Transient
   B. Conscious
   C. Superficial
   D. Neurologic

8. It is incumbent upon the _____ conscious sedation to be knowledgeable of the pharmacology of the medication.
   A. technologist observing
   B. scrub person witnessing
   C. family members witnessing
   D. professional administering

9. List two common adverse reactions to opioids.

10. _____ is an antagonist to benzodiazepines.
    A. Valium
    B. Flumazenil
    C. Versed
    D. Meperidine

11. The oxygen saturation level should be _____ during the procedure.
    A. 80%
    B. no less than 85%
    C. 75%
    D. above 90%

12. During the Seldinger technique of vessel puncture, an anesthetic is administered to help prevent _____.
    A. vasospasm
    B. cardiac arrest
    C. high blood pressure
    D. bronchospasm

13. In the Seldinger technique, after the needle punctures the vessel walls, it is angled _____ to the skin and is slowly withdrawn until there is a backflow of blood.
    A. perpendicularly
    B. 45 degrees
    C. parallel
    D. 30 degrees

14. A forceful, but irregular, backflow of blood through the needle may indicate _____.

A. hypotension
B. stenosis
C. needle is subintimally located
D. myocardiac infarction

15. The most desirable approach is the _____.
    A. translumbar
    B. cutdown brachial
    C. percutaneous axillary
    D. percutaneous femoral

16. For a percutaneous femoral puncture, the pulse is palpated 1 cm below the _____.
    A. iliac artery
    B. inguinal ligament
    C. pectineus muscle
    D. femoral arch

17. In the percutaneous brachial approach, needle placement is _____ the antecubital fossa.
    A. at
    B. 1 cm below
    C. medial to
    D. just above

18. To help force the contrast medium into the brachiocephalic vessel and alleviate pain in the distal extremity, a _____ may be employed.
    A. warm compress
    B. sphygmomanometer
    C. high pressure injection
    D. manual injection

19. The axillary approach is undesirable because the _____ may suffer permanent damage as a result of the trauma or hematoma.
    A. medial nerve
    B. humerus
    C. biceps
    D. brachial plexus

20. The most common location of a cutdown approach is the _____.
    A. femoral artery
    B. axillary artery
    C. brachial vein
    D. aorta

21. In a cutdown, _____ around the vessel to prevent bleeding.
    A. sutures are tied
    B. gauze is wrapped
    C. clamps are applied
    D. sterile bandages are placed

22. A translumbar approach may be performed at _____.
    A. T-10
    B. T-12
    C. L-1
    D. L-4

23. Select the answer below that is *not* a contraindication for systemic heparinization.
    A. Internal bleeding

B. Aortic insufficiency
C. Severe hypertension
D. Vessel stenosis

24. After heparinization as a part of the postprocedural care, the patient may be given _____ to counteract the heparin.
    A. Valium
    B. Benadryl
    C. protamine sulfate
    D. aspirin

25. After an angiogram, the patient's vital signs are monitored every _____ minutes for the first hour.
    A. 15
    B. 20
    C. 25
    D. 30

26. As part of postprocedural care, at the time the vital signs are taken, _____ also occurs.
    A. administration of Benadryl
    B. visual inspection of the puncture site
    C. deheparinization
    D. cleaning the puncture site

27. List three common complications that may occur at the puncture site.

28. List three common indications for the percutaneous brachial approach.

## BIBLIOGRAPHY

Abrams, H: Angiography, Vol 2, ed 3. Little, Brown & Co, Boston, 1983.

Altin, RS, Flicker, S, and Naidech, HJ: Pseudoaneurysm and arteriovenous fistula after femoral artery catheterization: Association with low femoral punctures. AJR 152:626, March 1989.

Anderson, JH, et al: Anticoagulation techniques for angiography: An experimental study. Radiology 111:573, June 1974.

Cook Guide Wire Catalog. Cook Incorporated, Bloomington, IN, 1974.

Ducor sterile disposable angiographic catheter instructions for use. Cordis Corp., Miami, FL, 1976.

Eisenberg, R and Mani, R: Pressure dressing and postangiographic care of the femoral puncture site. Radiology 122(3):677, March 1977.

Epstein, B: The use of a constant pressure pump for maintaining the patency of catheters and needles during angiography. AJR 113(3):572, November 1971.

Gaspare, M: Evaluation of trauma with angiography. JAMA 238(22): 2366, November 1977.

Grollman, JH and Marcus, R: Transbrachial arteriography: Techniques and complications. Cardiovasc Intervent Radiol 11(1):32, January 1988.

Hawkins, I and Melichar, F: Application of new torque wire in visceral, extremity and neuroangiography. Radiology 125(3):821, December 1977.

Johnsrude, I, Jackson, D, and Dunnick, NR: A Practical Approach to Angiography, ed 2. Little, Brown & Co, Boston, 1987.

Kadir, S: Diagnostic Angiography. WB Saunders, Philadelphia, 1986.

Kandarpa, K: Handbook of Cardiovascular and Interventional Radiologic Procedures. Little, Brown & Co, Boston, 1989.

Katzen, B: Interventional Diagnostic and Therapeutic Procedures. Springer-Verlag, New York, 1980.

Kohlberg, W: To stop post-angiography bleeding. Med Times 106(10):82, October 1978.

Lechner, G, et al: Technical notes: The relationship between the common femoral artery, the inguinal ligament: A guide to accurate angiographic puncture. Cardiovasc Intervent Radiol 11(3):165, June 1988.

Medi-tech: 1991 Angiography and Interventional Catalogue. Meditech, Watertown, MA.

Merrick, P: Nursing care for the patient undergoing intravenous conscious sedation for imaging studies. Images 12(1):1, Winter 1993.

Saxton, H and Strickland, B: Practical Procedures in Diagnostic Radiology, ed 2. Grune & Stratton, New York, 1972.

Schwartz, HW (ed) and Parks, GW (assoc. ed): Current Concepts in Radiology Management. American Healthcare Radiology Administrators, Sudbury, MA, 1992.

Sigstedt, B and Lunderquist, A: Complications of angiographic examinations. AJR 1305(3):455, March 1978.

Snopek, A: Fundamentals of Special Radiographic Procedures. WB Saunders, Philadelphia, 1992.

Torees, L: Basic Medical Techniques and Patient Care for Radiologic Technologists. JB Lippincott, Philadelphia, 1989.

Vitale, R. Pharmacology of conscious sedation. Images 12(1):7, Winter 1993.

Wallace, S, et al: Systemic heparinization for angiography. AJR 116(1):204, September 1972.

White, R: Fundamentals of Vascular Radiology. Lea & Febiger, Philadelphia, 1976.

Wojtowycz, M: Handbook in Radiology, Interventional Radiology, and Angiography. Year Book Medical Publishers, Chicago, 1990.

# PROCEDURES

## CHAPTER 20

# Cardiac Catheterization

*Dennis A. Bair, AS, AART(R)(CV)*
*Carol A. Mascioli, AS, ARRT(R)(CV)*

Cardiac catheterization is one of the most common angiographic procedures performed in the United States. The widespread use of cardiac catheterization is due in part because it is a relatively easy, safe, and accurate procedure. Cardiac catheterization may be divided into two autonomous diagnostic procedures: coronary arteriography and angiocardiography. Although these procedures are separate, they are often performed on a combined basis. Because many cardiac problems are not singular in nature but can be part of a larger picture, basic angiographic techniques, hemodynamic measurements, and calculations are all part of the cardiac catheterization process. Cardiac catheterization techniques and the information that may be obtained from the procedure vary greatly. This procedure is so complex that there are numerous publications on this subject. This chapter is designed to provide the reader with a basic understanding of cardiac catheterization. The reader is referred to the bibliography for more in-depth information on this procedure.

## ANATOMY

### Chambers of the Heart

The heart is the pump of the circulatory system and is divided into two halves: the right half or deoxygenated blood flow, and the left half or oxygenated blood flow. Each half is further divided into two chambers, the atrium and ventricle. The atria, or upper chambers, are separated by an intra-atrial septum, whereas the ventricles, or lower chambers, are divided by the intraventricular septum. The atria serve as receiving chambers for blood from the various parts of the body, and the ventricles serve as pumping chambers. The left atrium is smaller in size than the right atrium, but the wall of the left atrium is thicker. Because the left ventricle is responsible for pumping the blood to the majority of the circulatory system (i.e., systemic circulation) and for maintaining blood pressure, it is thicker than the right

193

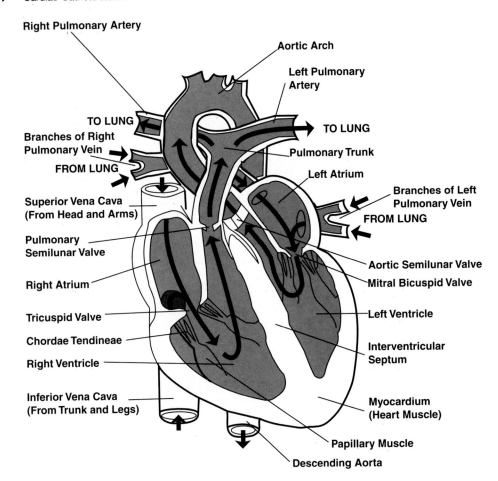

Right Pulmonary Artery

Aortic Arch

Left Pulmonary Artery

TO LUNG

Branches of Right Pulmonary Vein

FROM LUNG

Superior Vena Cava (From Head and Arms)

Pulmonary Semilunar Valve

Right Atrium

Tricuspid Valve

Chordae Tendineae

Right Ventricle

Inferior Vena Cava (From Trunk and Legs)

TO LUNG

Pulmonary Trunk

Left Atrium

Branches of Left Pulmonary Vein

FROM LUNG

Aortic Semilunar Valve

Mitral Bicuspid Valve

Left Ventricle

Interventricular Septum

Myocardium (Heart Muscle)

Papillary Muscle

Descending Aorta

**Figure 20–1.** Cross-section of the heart demonstrating the chambers, major vessels, and valves. (Modified from Thibodeau, GA: Anatomy and Physiology, St Louis, CV Mosby, 1987, with permission.)

ventricle. The left ventricle is where blood pressure is initiated. Figure 20–1 is a diagram of the heart and is useful in demonstrating the following descriptions of blood flow and heart valves.

The right atrium is the receiving chamber for blood from the superior vena cava, inferior vena cava, and coronary sinus. These veins bring blood from the upper extremity, the lower extremity, and the heart itself, respectively. From the right atrium, the blood is pumped through the atrioventricular (tricuspid) valve into the right ventricle. The blood is pumped from the right ventricle into the main pulmonary artery through the pulmonary (semilunar) valve to the lungs, where it is oxygenated. Blood leaves the lungs and enters the left atrium through the four pulmonary veins. The blood is pumped from the left atrium through the mitral (bicuspid) valve into the left ventricle. The left ventricle pumps the blood through the aortic (semilunar) valve into the aorta and to the rest of the body except the lungs.

## Valves of the Heart

Blood flow is directed, in part, by the valves of the heart, which prevent the backflow of blood into adjacent chambers or vessels. Valves are often referred to as inlet (blood moves into the heart) or outlet (blood moves out of the heart) valves. The right atrioventricular valve is an inlet valve between the right atrium and the right ventricle. It is tricuspid (three flaps, or cusps) in nature. The pulmonary valve is an outlet valve between the right ventricle and the pulmonary artery. It is semilunar (three half-moon-shaped segments) in nature.

The left atrioventricular valve, or mitral valve, is an inlet valve between the left atrium and the left ventricle. It is bicuspid (two flaps or cusps) in nature. The aortic valve is an outlet valve between the left ventricle and the aorta. It is semilunar (three half-moon-shaped portions) similar to the pulmonary valve in nature.

## Blood Supply to the Heart

Because the chambers of the heart are nonpermeable enclosures, the heart has a separate blood circulation (Fig. 20–2) that supplies the myocardial tissues (heart muscle) with oxygen. The coronary arteries are the first branches of the ascending aorta and provide the blood supply to the myocardial tissues. There are normally two coronary arteries: the left main and right main coronary. The left main coronary artery branches immediately into the left anterior descending artery (LAD) and the circumflex arteries. The LAD supplies the anterior portion of the left ventricle and a small part of the anterior and posterior portions of the right ven-

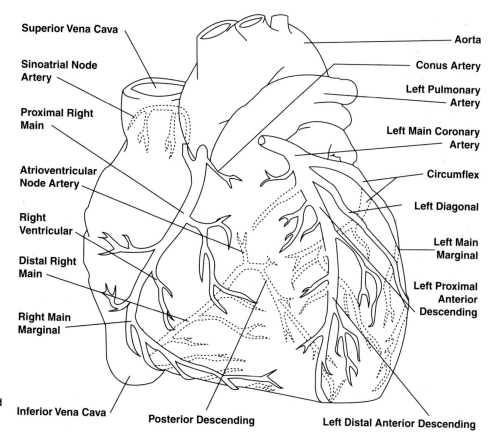

**Figure 20-2.** Coronary artery blood supply.

tricle. The proximal LAD divides into the diagonal branch and the distal LAD. Septal perforators branch off the LAD. The circumflex artery supplies the left atrium and the superior anterior and posterior areas of the left ventricle. The circumflex artery divides into the first and second obtuse marginals.

The right coronary artery supplies the blood to the right atrium, the right ventricle, and a portion of the left ventricle. Branches of the right coronary artery include the sinoatrial (SA) nodal artery, the atrioventricular (AV) nodal artery, the conus artery, the right ventricular artery, and the posterior descending artery. Blood leaves the heart muscle primarily by the coronary sinus, which empties directly into the right atrium. Other venous drainage occurs by deep channels emptying directly into the right ventricle. Figure 20-3 is a diagram of the venous circulation of the heart.

## INDICATIONS

Cardiac catheterization is performed for a wide scope of problems associated with the heart. The most common indication is coronary artery disease. The following represents a list of additional indications for cardiac catheterization:

1. angina: new onset, unstable angina unresponsive to medical therapy, or unstable angina postinfarction
2. highly positive exercise tolerance test
3. evaluation before major surgery
4. silent ischemia
5. atypical chest pain
6. coronary spasm
7. recurrent symptoms in patients with coronary artery bypass

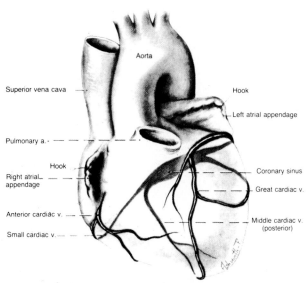

**Figure 20-3.** Venous drainage of the heart. (From Jacob, Francone, and Lossow: Structure and Function in Man, ed 3, WB Saunders, Philadelphia, 1982, p 373, with permission.)

8. unstable angina postinfarction
9. failed thrombolysis
10. major complication after acute myocardial infarction (shock, congestive heart failure [CHF], mitral regurgitation caused by ruptured papillary muscle, ventricular septal defect)
11. valvular heart disease
12. congenital heart disease
13. aortic dissection
14. pericardial constriction or tamponade
15. cardiomyopathy
16. initial or follow-up assessment for heart transplant

## CONTRAINDICATIONS

The presence of cardiac disease accounts for most contraindications to cardiac catheterization. The irony is that cardiac catheterization is used as a means to diagnose and assess heart disease. In these instances, the physician needs to determine if the information obtained from a cardiac catheterization outweighs the risk associated with the contraindications. Fortunately, many heart pathologies can be controlled or stabilized prior to performing the procedure. The following is a list of conditions that may be stabilized:
1. congestive heart failure
2. hypertension
3. arrhythmias, ventricular irritability
4. infection
5. electrolyte imbalance
6. anemia
7. medication intoxication, for example, digitalis

Other conditions that are contraindications for cardiac catheterization, but not correctable prior to the procedure, are:
1. recent myocardial infarction unless therapeutic intervention is contemplated
2. recent cerebral vascular accident (less than 1 month)
3. fever of unknown origin
4. poor left ventricular function

As with all ionizing radiation examinations, cardiac catheterization is contraindicated in women who are pregnant, especially during the first trimester.

## APPROACHES

Cardiac catheterization may be performed by using one of two approaches: brachial or femoral. Both approaches were developed by a pioneer in cardiac catheterization, and each bears the name of the respective individual who established the technique.

### Sones Technique

The brachial approach was first described by Mason Sones and involves a surgical cutdown at the antecubital area of the arm. The artery or vein is directly visualized, and the catheter is inserted by arteriotomy or venotomy. The catheters most often used are multipurpose and are noted in Fig. 20–4. When the procedure is completed, the artery or vein must be sutured and the cutdown incision on the arm repaired. The cutdown method has been modified so that most brachial approaches performed today utilize a percutaneous needle entry of the artery or vein. This is still referred to as the Sones technique. The catheters used in the percutaneous method are the same as those used in the cutdown method. Although the Sones technique is rarely used, it was the original approach to cardiac catheterization and it is indicated when femoral access is contraindicated because of iliac or femoral atherosclerotic disease, for example, occlusion, stenosis, vessel tortuosity, or previous femoral artery bypass surgery. Both left and right heart catheterizations can be performed by the brachial approach.

### Judkins Technique

The percutaneous femoral approach is the preferred catheterization method. It was described by Melvin Judkins and employs the Seldinger technique (refer to Chapter 19, Catheterization Methods and Patient Management, for a discussion of the Seldinger technique). In this method any one of three different sets of preshaped catheters may be used to visualize the left coronary artery, right coronary artery, and left ventricle, respectively (Fig. 20–5). While the Judkins technique is more frequently used for left heart catheteri-

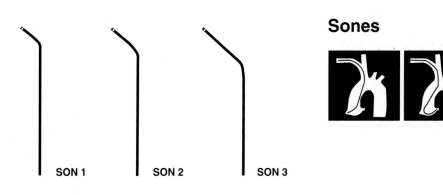

**Sones**

SON 1          SON 2          SON 3

**Figure 20–4.** Catheters commonly used for Sones approach. (Courtesy of Cordis Corporation, Miami, FL.)

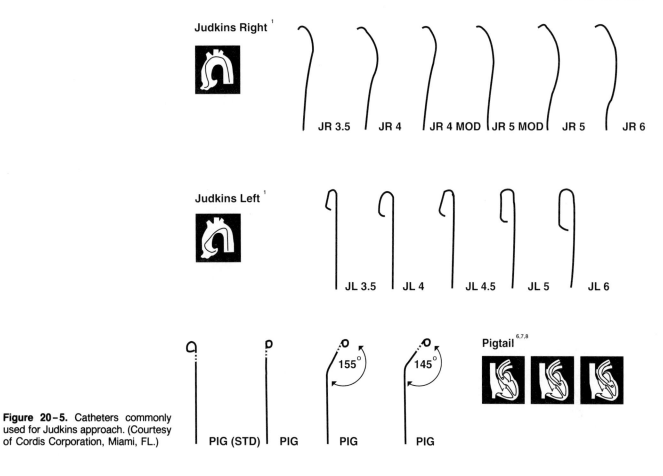

Judkins Right [1]

JR 3.5  JR 4  JR 4 MOD  JR 5 MOD  JR 5  JR 6

Judkins Left [1]

JL 3.5  JL 4  JL 4.5  JL 5  JL 6

155°  145°  Pigtail [6,7,8]

**Figure 20-5.** Catheters commonly used for Judkins approach. (Courtesy of Cordis Corporation, Miami, FL.)

PIG (STD)  PIG  PIG  PIG

zation, right heart catheterization can also be easily accomplished.

## PATIENT MANAGEMENT

### Preprocedural Care

Management of the cardiac catheterization patient begins with proper preprocedural education and securing an informed consent for the procedure. Proper patient education is useful in relieving anxiety, fear, and anticipation concerning the procedure. It is important to remember that the patient may be very anxious when confronted with the possibility of heart disease and the actual procedure itself. Cardiac catheterization is an invasive procedure and has risks associated with it. When patients are at ease and understand the procedure, they are generally more cooperative and fewer reactions may occur. Any premedication of the patient is the decision of the physician and varies relative to the patient's condition.

### Intraprocedural Care

Although Chapter 19 fully explains the preprocedural, intraprocedural, and postprocedural care, patient management during cardiac catheterization has many unique situations. Table 20-1 identifies some

Table 20-1. **Intraprocedural Patient Management for Cardiac Catheterization**

| Specific Problem | Type of Monitoring | Treatment |
|---|---|---|
| Bradycardia/ hypotension | ECG, intra-arterial blood pressure, pulse oximetry | 1. have patient cough<br>2. administer atropine or epinephrine<br>3. insert temporary pacemaker |
| Contrast medium reaction (the intensity of the reaction will dictate the exact treatment) | ECG, intra-arterial blood pressure, pulse oximetry | 1. administer diphen-hydramine<br>2. atropine or epinephrine<br>3. may use other drug or equipment on emergency cart |
| ST segment changes or chest pain | ECG | 1. administer sublingual nitroglycerin<br>2. administer sublingual nifedipine |
| Premature ventricular contraction, ventricular tachycardia, ventricular fibrillation | ECG | 1. reposition catheter<br>2. possible use of defibrillator or cardioverter<br>3. administer lidocaine<br>4. possible CPR |

monitoring procedures and suggested care that should be administered when these unique problems occur.

## Postprocedural Care

Postprocedural management is a continuation of earlier management. Much of the patient's discomfort often occurs when the catheter is removed and manual compression is used to maintain hemostasis. Vasovagal responses may occasionally occur at this time. It is important to observe for loss of pulse, hematoma formation, or excessive bleeding occurring at the catheter insertion site. The dermitotomy site should be dressed according to the preference of the physician, and postprocedural care should be explained to the patient. The following represent a list of care and instructions that should be followed after a cardiac catheterization:

1. Bed rest with leg extended for 8 hours; head may be slightly elevated; patient may be "log" rolled with assistance.
2. Check blood pressure and pulse every 30 minutes for the first 4 hours, then every hour for the next 4 hours.
3. Check groin for bleeding or hematoma every 15 minutes for the first 4 hours, then every 30 minutes for the next 4 hours, and finally every hour for the next 4 hours.
4. Resume diet and previous orders unless specified.
5. Drink plenty of fluids to flush contrast medium from kidneys or run intravenous fluids according to physician orders.
6. Void when necessary using bedpan or urinal; if unable to void, a urinary catheter may be placed in the patient's bladder.
7. Have patient observe for a "warm, wet sensation" at the puncture site, because this may be an indication of bleeding. If these symptoms appear, the patient should compress the bandage and call the nurse.

## EQUIPMENT

Much of the radiologic equipment in a cardiac catheterization laboratory is similar to that in most angiographic procedure rooms. The reader is referred to Chapters 11, 12, 13, 16, and 17 for more information on room design and equipment. In cardiac catheterization, the areas of greater emphasis are electrocardiogram (ECG) and hemodynamic or physiologic pressure monitoring. The physiologic recorder is an important piece of equipment in the cardiac catheterization laboratory. A multichannel unit is usually the equipment of choice because it displays the ECG and multiple pressure signals. Pressure transducers are used to obtain pressure signals. It is important to ensure that this equipment is calibrated daily as well as prior to each procedure according to the manufacturer's guidelines. This equipment is essential to assuring a safe diagnostic study and accurate cardiac measurements such as hemodynamic pressure measurements, cardiac output

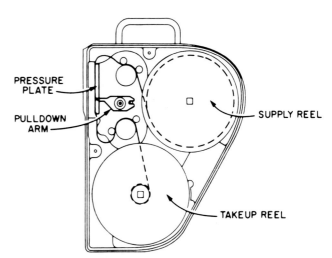

**Figure 20–6.** Cross-section of cine camera. (From Curry, Dowdy, and Murray: Christensen's Introduction to the Physics of Diagnostic Radiology, ed 3, Philadelphia, Lea & Febiger, 1984, with permission.)

measurements, and blood oximetry. Because ventricular tachycardia and fibrillation are risks associated with cardiac catheterization and present a life-threatening situation, electric defibrillation equipment is essential in case of an emergency.

Cineangiographic (cine) equipment is another item necessary for optimal cardiac catheterization. Thirty-five-millimeter single-emulsion continuous film is exposed at an average of 30 frames/sec. A cine is a relatively simple mechanism. It operates in a similar manner to a movie camera. The primary components of the camera are a supply reel, pressure plate, pulldown arm, shutter, aperture, take-up reel, and gears to move the film (Fig. 20–6). The supply reel contains the unexposed film, which is threaded past the pressure plate and connected to the pull arm, ending at the take-up reel. During exposure, the shutter moves (opens), revealing the aperture for film exposure (Fig. 20–7),

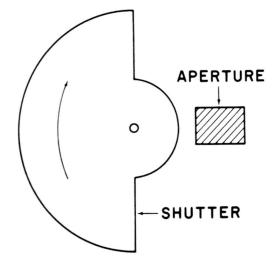

**Figure 20–7.** Frontal view of an opened shutter. (From Curry, Dowdy, and Murray: Christensen's Introduction to the Physics of Diagnostic Radiology, ed 3, Philadelphia, Lea & Febiger, 1984, with permission.)

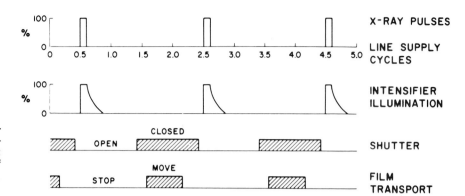

**Figure 20–8.** Correlation of x-ray pulse, intensifier illumination, shutter, and film transportation. (From Curry, Dowdy, and Murray: Christensen's Introduction to the Physics of Diagnostic Radiology, ed 3, Philadelphia, Lea & Febiger, 1984, with permission.)

and the pressure plate moves forward, pressing the film against the aperture. After exposure, the shutter moves backward (closes), covering the aperture, and allows the pull arm to move the film to the take-up reel.

The speed with which the heart beats requires an exact correlation among the x-ray pulse (exposure), intensifier illumination (cine exposure), closing-opening of the cine shutter, and cine film transportation (Fig. 20–8). Proper filming requires the intensifier illumination to occur simultaneously with the x-ray pulse. The cine shutter must be opened and the film must be stationary during this time. The shutter closes and film is transported between x-ray pulses.

Catheters used for cardiac catheterization are highly specialized. These catheters are available in a large variety of precurved shapes, each with its own application (Fig. 20–9).

## CONTRAST MEDIA

When choosing a contrast medium for cardiac catheterization, conditions specific to the heart must be taken into account. These include contrast medium–induced hypotension, bradycardia, changes in electrolytes, left ventricular depression, and whether the contrast agent promotes or retards thrombus formation.

The trend in coronary arteriography and left ventriculography is to employ nonionic, low osmolar contrast agents. Although these media are more expensive, they are safer and significantly reduce reactions.

Because the heart is a very dense organ, higher kilovoltage techniques (80 to 110 kV) are required to properly penetrate this structure. Therefore, the medium used for coronary arteriography and left ventriculography contains a high concentration of iodine. These concentrations range from 320 to 370 mg of iodine per milliliter.

## POSITIONING AND FILMING

Prior to discussing the views employed in cardiac catheterization, the reader is advised that in conventional radiography, the term "view" relates specifically to how the equipment "sees" the image and how a radiologist interprets a radiograph. However, in this section, the term is used generally, for example, to describe right anterior oblique (RAO) and left anterior oblique (LAO) positions. Although in conventional radiography, RAO and LAO are body positions, in cardiac catheterization, the patient remains supine while the equipment moves to simulate these positions.

To obtain optimal information from coronary arteriography, it is necessary to use various views. The use of multiple views provides a means of demonstrating a three-dimensional organ (the heart) on a two-dimensional recording medium (cine). These views are highly specific for each portion of the coronary anatomy and help to unravel superimposed vessels.

The left coronary artery is best demonstrated using the RAO and LAO views with various degrees of cranial or caudal angulation. These positions often use varying tube angulations to demonstrate different vessels. For example, a 30-degree RAO provides an anterior-posterior projection of the first marginal branch, the entire circumflex, the distal LAD artery, and the septal branches (Fig. 20–10A). A 30-degree RAO with cranial angulation highlights the distal two thirds of the LAD artery as well as the origin of the first diagonal artery. A 30-degree RAO with caudal angulation view straightens the circumflex artery and demonstrates the origins of the marginal arteries. An AP view best demonstrates the left main coronary artery. A 30- to 45-degree LAO cranial (Fig. 20–10B) is useful in visualizing the left main coronary artery and demonstrates the bifurcation of the LAD artery and diagonal branch as well as the circumflex and first marginal branch. A 30-degree LAO caudal visualizes the left main coronary artery and the origins of the LAD artery and circumflex artery. A 45-degree LAO can visualize the body of the circumflex artery. A lateral (90 degree) view visualizes the entire length of the LAD artery and septal branches.

The right coronary artery (RCA) is best demonstrated using the RAO and LAO views. The RCA, right ventricular branch, and posterior descending artery are visualized in the 30-degree RAO (Fig. 20–11A). A 30- to 45-degree LAO demonstrates the RCA, right ventricular branch, posterior descending artery,

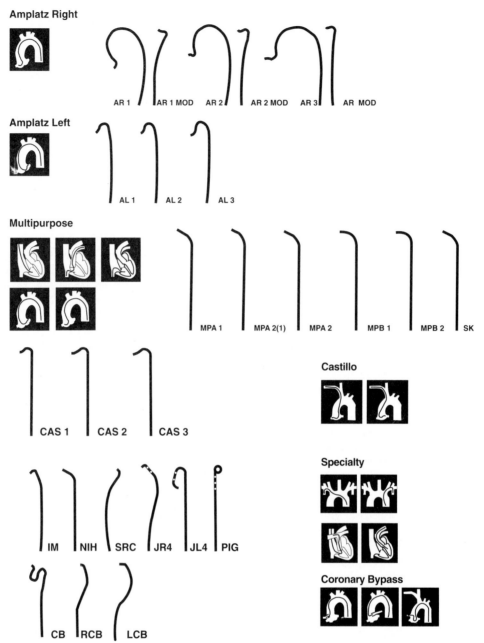

**Figure 20-9.** Commercial catheters that may be employed for cardiac catheterization. (Courtesy of Cordis Corporation, Miami, FL.)

and posterolateral branch (Fig. 20-11B). Caudal angulation may need to be added to separate the posterior descending artery and posterolateral artery.

Body habitus and coronary anatomy can vary from one patient to another. These variations make it important to "tailor" the views required to obtain a complete filming procedure needed for proper diagnosis.

## ANGIOCARDIOGRAPHY

As previously mentioned, cardiac catheterization is useful in evaluating several disorders. Besides coronary

filming, angiography (heart circulation) and hemodynamic monitoring are other diagnostic tools used in cardiac catheterization. Angiocardiography is the radiographic evaluation of the chambers of the heart and the various valves. Hemodynamic monitoring is the evaluation and recording of the function of the heart. These measurements include, but are not limited to, oxygen saturation, pressure tracings and measurements, and cardiac output. Computations and comparisons of these measurements establish the norms. Common intracardiac conditions are:

1. valvular gradients and stenoses
2. valvular regurgitation

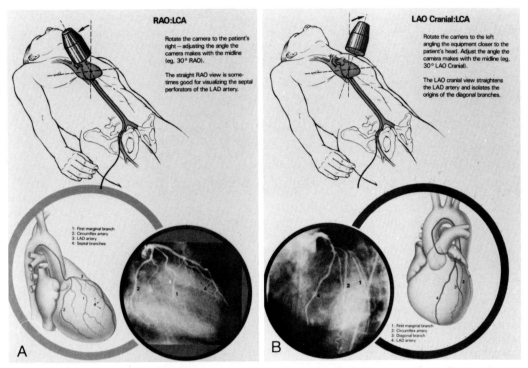

**Figure 20-10.** (*A*) RAO for left coronary artery; (*B*) LAO cranial for left coronary artery. (From Brogno and Kemp: Cardiovascular Angiography: Correlation to Normal Cardiac Anatomy. Sanofi Winthrop Pharmaceuticals, New York, NY, with permission.)

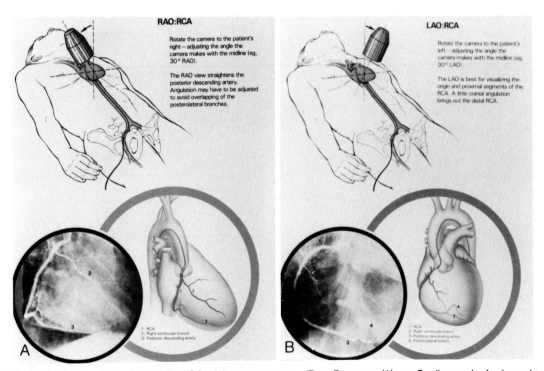

**Figure 20-11.** (*A*) RAO for right coronary artery; (*B*) LAO for right coronary artery. (From Brogno and Kemp: Cardiovascular Angiography: Correlation to Normal Cardiac Anatomy. Sanofi Winthrop Pharmaceuticals, New York, NY, with permission.)

3. intra-atrial shunts (atrial septal defects)
4. intraventricular shunts (ventricular septal defects)
5. patent ductus arteriosum
6. coarctation of the aorta
7. congestive heart failure

## COMPLICATIONS

Risks and complications are a part of any invasive procedure. These must be weighed against the benefits obtained by performing a cardiac catheterization. Because cardiac catheterization is an invasive procedure of the heart, the complications associated with it are more serious than other procedures. Therefore, the staff of the cardiac catheterization team must be prepared to handle all complications and emergencies in a quick and effective manner. Although rare, among the complications associated with cardiac catheterization are:

1. myocardial infarction
2. stroke or cerebrovascular accident (CVA)
3. life-threatening arrhythmia
4. vascular damage (dissection, embolus, thrombus)
5. cardiac perforation or tamponade
6. contrast reaction or renal failure
7. infection
8. vasovagal reaction
9. hemorrhage or hematoma
10. in rare cases, death

## REVIEW QUESTIONS

1. The pumping chambers of the heart are called _____.
   A. auricles
   B. atria
   C. ventricles
   D. septa

2. The first branch(es) of the ascending aorta is/are the _____ artery(ies).
   A. bracheocephalic
   B. left and right coronary
   C. left carotid
   D. left subclavian

3. The left main coronary artery divides to form the circumflex and the _____ arteries.
   A. left cardiac
   B. posterior descending
   C. left anterior descending
   D. first obtuse marginal

4. One indication for cardiac catheterization might be _____.
   A. heartburn and indigestion
   B. coronary artery disease
   C. hiatal hernia
   D. irregular heartbeat

5. Which of the following contraindications can be corrected?

A. poor left ventricular function
B. recent myocardial infarction
C. recent stroke
D. hypertension

6. The femoral approach for cardiac catheterization is called the _____ approach.
   A. Sones
   B. Judkins
   C. Seldinger
   D. Hartzler

7. The Judkins technique uses one of _____ catheter(s) available for cardiac catheterization.
   A. 1
   B. 2
   C. 3
   D. 4

8. Images obtained during cardiac catheterization are recorded with a _____ film.
   A. A 35-mm cine
   B. 8-mm movie
   C. 16-mm double emulsion
   D. cut

9. _____ iodine concentration contrast media are required for cardiac catheterization because the heart is an extremely dense organ.
   A. Lower
   B. Higher
   C. Midrange

10. Which of the following is *not* a complication of cardiac catheterization?
    A. myocardial infarction
    B. infection
    C. hematoma
    D. reaction to general anesthesia

## BIBLIOGRAPHY

Abrams, HL: Angiography, Vol 3, ed 3. Little, Brown & Co, Boston, 1983.

Cordis Diagnostic Cardiology and Biopsy Forceps. Cordis Corporation, Miami, 1992.

Curry, TS, Dowdy, JE, and Murray, RC: Christensen's Introduction to the Physics of Diagnostic Radiology, ed 3. Lea & Febiger, Philadelphia, 1984.

Grossman, W and Baim, DS: Cardiac Catheterization, Angiography, and Intervention, ed 4. Lea & Febiger, Philadelphia, 1991.

Hole, JW: Human Anatomy and Physiology. Wm C Brown Group, Dubuque, IA, 1980.

Jacob, SW, Francone, C, and Lossow, WJ: Structure and Function in Man, ed 5. WB Saunders, Philadelphia, 1982.

Kandarpa, K: Handbook of Cardiovascular and Interventional Radiologic Procedures. Little, Brown & Co, Boston, 1989.

Kerns, MJ: The Cardiac Catheterization Handbook. Mosby-Year Book, St Louis, 1991.

Mallett, M: Handbook of Anatomy and Physiology for Students of Medical Technology, ed 3. Burnell Company/Publishers, Mankato, MN, 1981.

Soto, B, Kassner, EG, and Baxley, WA: Imaging of Cardiac Disorders, Vol 2: Acquired Disorders. JB Lippincott, Philadelphia, 1992.

Spindola-Franco, H and Fish, BG: Radiology of the Heart. Springer-Verlag, New York, 1985.

Thibodeau, GA: Anatomy and Physiology. CV Mosby Company, St Louis, 1987.

# CHAPTER 21

# Thoracic Aortography

*Marianne R. Tortorici, EdD, ARRT(R)*

Thoracic aortography is not a frequently performed angiographic procedure, although it can be of great diagnostic value. Often a pathologic condition, especially one involving the aortic valve, can be demonstrated by an angiocardiogram (cardiac catheterization) or a thoracic aortogram. Where angiocardiography is mentioned in this chapter as an alternate diagnostic method, no attempt is made to explain the specifics of the angiocardiographic procedure. Rather, the reader is referred to Chapter 20, Cardiac Catheterization, for more specific information on angiocardiography. Thoracic aortography is usually reserved for those patients whose clinical data are inconclusive and for patients who are seriously ill.

This chapter presents the anatomy of the aorta and techniques of thoracic aortography. There is a brief discussion of related complications and angiographic findings.

## ANATOMY

The aorta is the largest artery in the body. It originates at the aortic valve of the heart and extends to approximately the fourth lumbar vertebra, where it bifurcates into the right and left common iliac arteries. The aorta is divided into three parts, or segments (Fig. 21–1):

1. ascending, which extends upward from T-3 to T-2 (5 cm in length)
2. aortic arch, which begins at the second sternocostal joint to T-4
3. descending, which consists of the thoracic and abdominal portions. The thoracic portion extends from T-4 to T-12, and the abdominal aorta runs from T-12 to L-4.

This chapter concentrates on the aortic arch and the thoracic aspect of the descending aorta.

The most proximal aspect of the aorta is the aortic bulb, or root, located at the left ventricle of the heart. The bulb consists of the three sinuses of Valsalva: the left, right, and posterior sinus (Fig. 21–2). It is important to note that the left sinus contains the left coronary artery, and the right sinus contains the right coronary

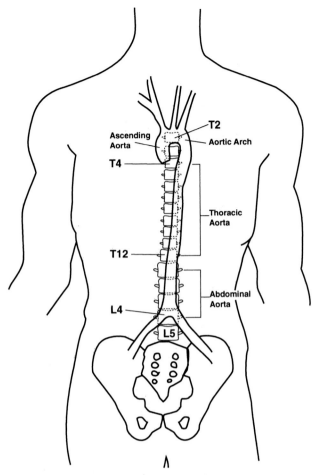

**Figure 21–1.** Segments of the aorta.

artery. During filming, the aortic bulb is best demonstrated with the patient in a 10- to 15-degree left posterior oblique position.

The ascending aorta measures approximately 5 cm in length. It extends superiorly from the aortic bulb, then anteriorly and to the right, and ends at the level of the second sternocostal joint, where it continues as the aortic arch.

The arch begins at the level of the second sternocostal joint and runs superiorly, posteriorly, and to the left, and then extends inferiorly, terminating at about T-4 (the isthmus). The most superior aspect of the arch is at the level of the manubrium of the sternum. The arch measures 5 to 6 cm in length and has a diameter of 2 to 3 cm, narrowing to 1.7 to 2.5 cm distally. Extending from the arch are the three great vessels, or branches. The most proximal great vessel is the brachiocephalic (innominate), followed by the left common carotid and left subclavian vessels (Fig. 21–3A). The right common carotid and right subclavian arteries originate from the brachiocephalic. The ductus arteriosus (isthmus area in the adult), which connects the left pulmonary artery to the aorta in a fetus, is located anteriorly 1 to 1.5 cm distal to the left subclavian artery.

There are several variations of the branches of the arch and the arch itself, which include:

1. Only two arteries originating from the arch — the innominate and left subclavian (Fig. 21–3B). In this case, the left common carotid originates from the innominate instead of the aortic arch (a common branch variation that occurs in approximately one in four people).
2. The left vertebral artery originates from the arch

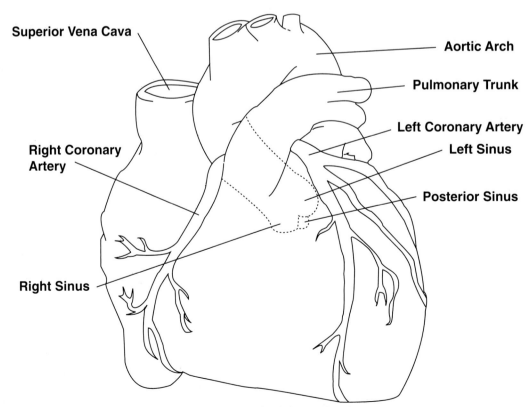

**Figure 21–2.** Aortic bulb, demonstrating sinuses.

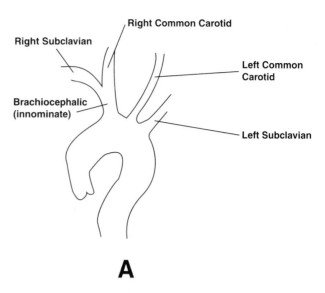

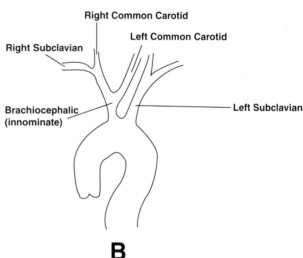

**Figure 21–3.** Branches of aortic arch: (A) normal branch; (B) one type of branch variation.

(instead of the left subclavian) between the left common and left subclavian (occurs in about 3 percent of the population).

3. The innominate, left vertebral artery, and left subclavian originate from the arch, while the left common carotid originates from the innominate (seen in about 1 percent of the population). In this case, the left vertebral artery is located between the innominate and left subclavian arteries.

There are numerous other branch variations and to mention them all is beyond the scope of this text. Generally, branch variations can be seen in the form of alternate origins of branches and an increase or decrease in the number of branches.

There are several variations of the arch itself including:

1. The left circumflex aorta, which has a normal arch with the descending aorta extending inferiorly and to the right (Fig. 21–4A).

2. The inverse aorta, which is characterized by the aorta arching to the right (reverse of a normal arch). The branches may be normal or abnormal (Fig. 21–4B).

3. Pseudocoarctation, characterized by an arched descending aorta (Fig. 21–4C).

As with branch variations, there are numerous abnormalities of the arch itself. To discuss them all is beyond the scope of this text. Readers interested in other variations are referred to an anatomy text.

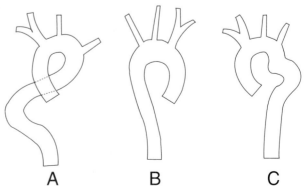

**Figure 21–4.** Some variations of aortic arch. (A) Left circumflex; (B) inverse aorta; and (C) pseudocoarctation.

The descending aorta is a continuation of the arch, extending inferiorly, medially, and ending at the level of the 12th thoracic vertebra, where it continues as the abdominal aorta. At this level, the aorta has numerous intercostal arterial branches that are rarely of diagnostic value.

## INDICATIONS

Thoracic aortography is indicated when abnormalities or pathologies of the aorta, or the great branches, cannot be determined by other diagnostic means. The more common indications for the procedure are disorders of the great branches of the arch, patent ductus arteriosus, aortic aneurysm, coarctation, aortic arch anomalies, aortic insufficiency, aortic stenosis, arteriovenous malformations or fistulae, and aortic valve disease. The accuracy of thoracic aortography diagnosis varies. In the case of aneurysms, a large percentage of studies are performed with false-negative results. A common cause of this phenomenon is the simultaneous and equal opacification of the true and false lumina during injection of the contrast medium. This presents a false appearance of a dilated aortic lumen. The accuracy rate for diagnosis of all other aortic disorders is much better than it is for aneurysms.

Another clinical symptom indicating the need for a thoracic aortogram is a variation of blood pressure of 30 mm Hg or more in the upper extremities; this variation may indicate a pathologic condition in the thoracic aorta. Other indications include deceleration injury (auto accident) and aortic dissection.

## EQUIPMENT

The major equipment for thoracic aortography includes an electromechanical injector, an electrocardiograph unit, emergency cardiac equipment, and a system for recording the image. For pathologic conditions involving the aortic valve or left ventricle, the best recording system is a cineradiograph. The optimal filming rate is in the range of 30 to 60 frames/sec. Discussion of this type of filming is presented in Chapter 20, Cardiac Catherization. Satisfactory images of pathologic conditions involving the other sections of the aorta can be produced by a rapid film changer.

## PREPROCEDURAL CARE AND CAUTIONS

Premedicating a patient for thoracic aortography adheres to the normal procedure for any angiographic examination. It is suggested that atropine in combination with diazepam be administered as a premedication to prevent bradycardia. Angiographers may also elect to order a specific premedication protocol to decrease the possibility of contrast media reaction (refer to Chapter 3, Contrast Media). In addition to administering the normal preprocedural medications and

completing consent forms, the patient should have a preangiographic clinical examination. The clinical examination should include overpenetrated chest radiographs to assess the condition of the aorta. It is desirable to compare the patient's previous chest radiographs with the current ones.

## APPROACHES

In general there are two approaches for thoracic aortography: the forward and the retrograde. The forward approach is rarely used and involves the catheterization of the femoral vein to puncture the septum of the heart. In this approach, the catheter enters the heart through the inferior vena cava. The most common retrograde approaches include the introduction of the catheter via the brachial, carotid, femoral, or axillary arteries. In these approaches, the catheter is manipulated through an artery to a predetermined location of the aorta. In both approaches, it is important to avoid placing the catheter in a coronary artery.

Introduction of the catheter in the retrograde method is usually performed using the Seldinger technique. The brachial method is useful for assessing coarctation and patent ductus arteriosus. The left brachial artery approach is preferred because introduction of a catheter into the right brachial artery can produce problems in catheter manipulation. This can occur when attempting to introduce the catheter through the brachiocephalic artery. An alternate method using a Robb needle placed in the brachial artery can be used when the contrast medium injection is made directly through the needle.

A general anesthetic is usually employed in the retrograde carotid approach. This approach demonstrates coarctation and patent ductus arteriosus. Catheterization of the left carotid artery is easiest and most desirable because it arises directly from the aorta. The distal carotid artery should be temporarily occluded during injection to prevent the contrast medium from entering the brain. Cerebral damage is one of the most common complications of thoracic aortography. Both the brachial and carotid approaches are rarely used for assessment of the aortic arch because these procedures are risky and the arch is not well visualized.

The most desirable approach for thoracic aortography is the femoral artery puncture. Unlike the brachial or carotid methods, the femoral approach permits placement of the catheter in any part of the aorta. If for some reason the femoral artery cannot be catheterized, an alternative is the left axillary approach.

The forward thoracic aortographic approach is limited to cases in which there is severe aortic stenosis and when the retrograde method cannot be used. One type of forward approach is the transseptal catheterization method. This method requires a Brockenbrough catheter (Fig. 21–5). The catheter has a distal curve and a proximal end that can accommodate various fittings. One fitting accommodates a long stainless steel transseptal needle with a metallic arrow on the hub to indi-

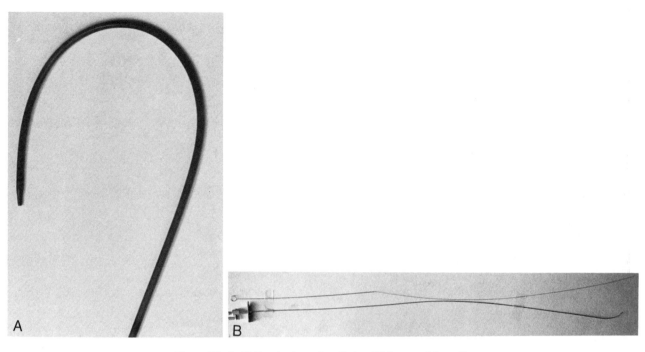

**Figure 21–5.** (*A*) Brockenbrough catheter; (*B*) transseptal needle.

cate the direction in which the needle is pointed. The following is a summary of the transseptal method:

1. A Brockenbrough catheter is introduced into the femoral vein and placed in the right atrium of the heart.
2. The transseptal needle is placed in the Brockenbrough catheter 1 to 2 cm distal to the catheter opening.
3. The catheter is placed at the fossa ovalis (small depression in septum wall).
4. The needle is advanced through the catheter to puncture the septum.
5. After oxygenated blood is returned, confirming proper needle placement, the needle is removed and the catheter is positioned in the left ventricle.

During the puncture of the septum, the patient tends to experience a transient sensation of fullness in the mediastinum or a sharp sensation under the sternum. The pain should not persist. If it does, the angiographer should reassess the location of the transseptal needle. Transseptal puncture is not without its hazards and should be performed only in cases in which no other method of approach is available. Complications that may result from transseptal puncture include placement of the needle in the aorta, perforation of the heart into the pericardium, perforation of the free atrial wall, and pericardial tamponade caused by blood accumulation.

## CATHETERS

The pigtail catheter with an end hole and multiple side holes provides the greatest amount of contrast medium delivery for thoracic aortography. A closed-end catheter may be employed to reduce the chances of the catheter's recoiling and injecting contrast medium into the carotid arteries.

## CONTRAST MEDIA

The amount of contrast medium employed depends on the area and the pathology to be visualized. When it is necessary to see the entire aortic arch, a minimum of 60 ml is required. If the aorta is obviously dilated, a larger dose is necessary; for a smaller aorta, a lesser dose is used. The injection rate is usually 30 ml/sec for a total of 60 ml. The optimal concentration of the contrast medium is 70 percent. However, a 70 percent concentration has been known to cause cerebral damage if it reaches the brain in its highly concentrated form. Lower concentrations of a medium have been employed, but they produce a lower quality radiograph.

## POSITIONING AND FILMING

The patient position employed for thoracic aortography depends on the area of interest. If the suspected pathology is patent ductus arteriosus or coarctation, a 45-degree left posterior oblique position should be employed. A 45-degree right posterior oblique position demonstrates ventricular septal defect. However, in cases of ventricular septal defect, it is recommended that angiocardiography be performed. The aortic arch and its great branches are demonstrated in a right posterior oblique position. All images should include the heart, the aortic arch, and the great vessels to demonstrate possible valvular insufficiency.

Regardless of the area under investigation, the catheter should be positioned in the midascending aorta. Catheterization of the coronary arteries should be avoided. Placing the catheter too close to the aortic valve may result in the pressure from the injection forcing a backflow of contrast medium into the left ventricle.

The patient's size, age, and sex affect the location of the aorta. Individuals with a high diaphragm tend to have the aortic arch displaced superiorly and the ascending and descending aorta shifted laterally. The ascending and descending aorta tend to be more elongated with lower diaphragms. Older individuals usually have a low diaphragm; female patients usually have a high diaphragm.

For rapid-sequence filming, the first 1.5 seconds after injection provides radiographs with the most information; therefore, the filming rate should be at least 4 frames/sec for the first 2 seconds. The rate can then be reduced to a minimum of 2 frames/sec for the subsequent 3 to 5 seconds. The latter films are of value to determine if there is collateralization of the vessels. As indicated previously, if the area of interest is the aortic or mitral valve, then cineradiography should be employed. The rate of filming for cineradiography should be 30 to 60 frames/sec (refer to Chapter 20, Cardiac Catheterization).

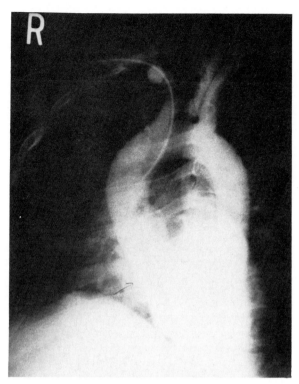

**Figure 21–6.** Aortic insufficiency.

## COMPLICATIONS

Thoracic aortography is not without complications. Of all types of angiographic procedures, thoracic aortography has the recorded death rate at 1.7 percent. There is a higher rate of deaths when a high concentration of contrast medium is employed and when the injection is made directly into the carotid artery. There appears also to be an increase in complication rate for patients on anticoagulants, patients with hypertension, and individuals with arteriosclerosis or aortic insufficiency. The largest percentage of deaths is attributed to brain damage. Many respiratory complications are a result of damage to the medullary respiratory centers. Other recorded severe reactions that have occurred, but did not result in death, are hemiplegia, convulsions, cardiac arrhythmias, pulmonary edema, bradycardia, tachycardia, and mental confusion. Complications resulting from catheter manipulation and procedural problems include perforation of the myocardium, intramural injections, kinking or looping of the catheter and the guide wire, and inadvertent entry into, and occlusion of, the coronary artery (usually the left coronary artery).

## SOME ANGIOGRAPHIC FINDINGS

Thoracic aortography can demonstrate a variety of anomalies and pathologic conditions. Some of the more common ones are aortic insufficiency, aortic positional

abnormalities, aneurysms, patent ductus arteriosus, and coarctation. Injuries resulting from blunt trauma can also be diagnosed by thoracic angiography. To demonstrate the pathologic condition or injury in question, it is vital to employ proper patient positioning and filming. This chapter presents some examples of radiographic findings that are demonstrated by serial filming. Angiographic findings demonstrated by cineradiography are illustrated in Chapter 20.

Figure 21–6 is an example of aortic insufficiency. Injection of a contrast medium into the aorta of a patient with a normal aortic valve will not show opacification of the left ventricle. Note that in Figure 21–6 the left ventricle is demonstrated. It is important to position the catheter in the midsection of the ascending aorta to prevent accidental filling of the left ventricle by the force of the injection. A second technique to reduce accidental filling of the ventricle is to use a closed-end catheter. One method of determining whether the opacification is a result of the injection or of aortic insufficiency is to observe the rate of opacification. In aortic insufficiency the left ventricle has a progressive opacification of the chamber that lasts for more than one heartbeat. If the filling of the chamber is a result of the pressure injection, opacification occurs during the injection of contrast medium and is ejected by the heart fairly rapidly.

As mentioned previously, there are a variety of aortic positional anomalies. For example, the right common carotid artery may originate directly from the arch instead of the right subclavian artery. These anomalies can exist in individuals without causing any problems.

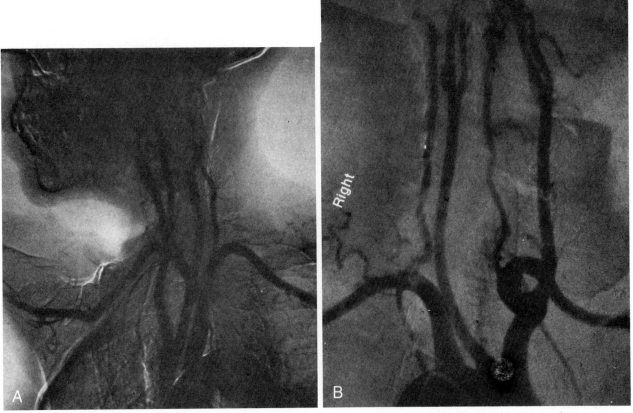

**Figure 21-7.** (*A*) Two brachiocephalic vessels, common left and right carotid and common left and right subclavian; (*B*) common origin of innominate artery and left carotid.

The positions of the great branches become important when the patient experiences complications caused by the vessel's (or vessels') abnormal location. Furthermore, prior to performing any surgical procedure in the area, it is also important to identify any anomalies that may exist. Variations of the arch or its branches may result in the need for alternate surgical techniques. Figure 21–7 illustrates examples of great-vessel anomalies.

It is important to diagnose aneurysms as soon as possible because undetected, untreated aneurysms often result in death. Of all aneurysms, 22 percent occur in the ascending aorta, 12 percent in the arch, and 7 percent in the descending aorta. There are a variety of aneurysms. The most common type is the atherosclerotic aneurysm. This aneurysm usually occurs in the ascending aorta and can rupture at any time.

A second type of aneurysm is the dissecting aneurysm. A dissecting aneurysm results in the separation of the vessel wall, causing blood to flow through both the split (false) lumen and true vessel lumen. This type of aneurysm is difficult to diagnose on radiographs because of the simultaneous and equal opacification of the false and true lumina. The reported diagnostic accuracy is 40 percent. The common sites for dissecting aneurysms are the mobile portions of the aorta near fixed parts of the aorta, including the aortic bulb and the brachiocephalic and supradiaphragmatic regions.

There are three types of dissecting aneurysms: the first type (50 percent) arises distal to, or at, the level of the left subclavian artery and extends peripherally; the second type (41 percent) involves the aortic bulb or root, to the descending thoracic aorta; and the third type (9 percent) involves the ascending aorta and sometimes the brachiocephalic artery.

A third type of aneurysm is the traumatic aneurysm (Fig. 21–8), which is usually a result of blunt trauma. These aneurysms often go undetected because the symptoms are frequently obscured by other injuries. A common site of injury is near the origin of the left subclavian artery. Sharp trauma aneurysms usually result in immediate death.

Other types of aneurysms that are not common are luetic, the result of an untreated syphilis infection; mycotic, caused by a fungal infection; nonsyphilitic infection; and congenital.

Thoracic aortography is usually performed in atypical cases of patent ductus arteriosus to determine whether the clinical findings are caused by a patent ductus arteriosus, an aortic septal defect, or a ruptured sinus of Valsalva. Figure 21–9 represents a patent ductus arteriosus.

It is important to perform thoracic aortography in cases of coarctation (Fig. 21–10), where surgery is indicated, to determine the type of surgery to be performed, for example, end-to-end anastomosis or a

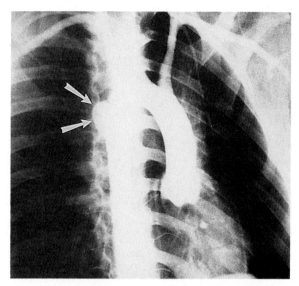

**Figure 21–8.** Small traumatic aortic aneurysm.

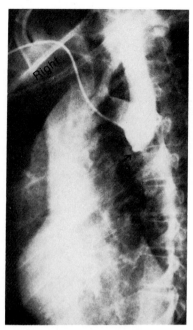

**Figure 21–10.** Coarctation.

graft. The radiographs determine the length and severity of stenosis, the degree of forward displacement of the stenotic area at the level of the ligamentum arteriosum, the appearance of the middle segment of the arch, associated malformations, the distance of the stenosis to the origin of the left subclavian artery, the width of the prestenotic segment, and information regarding collateral vessels.

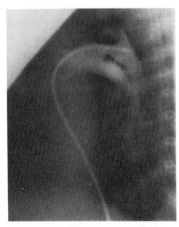

**Figure 21–9.** Patent ductus arteriosus.

## REVIEW QUESTIONS

1. The aortic arch begins at the second sternocostal joint and extends to _____.
   A. T-2
   B. T-3
   C. T-4
   D. T-5

2. The most proximal aspect of the aorta _____.
   A. is where the coronary arteries originate
   B. is located in the right ventricle
   C. terminates at T-4
   D. contains deoxygenated blood

3. The most proximal (first) branch of the aortic arch is the _____ artery.
   A. brachiocephalic
   B. right common carotid
   C. left common carotid
   D. right subclavian

4. The lowest diagnostic accuracy rate for thoracic aortography is when assessing _____.
   A. aortic stenosis
   B. aneurysms
   C. patent ductus arteriosus
   D. aortic insufficiency

5. A _____ is most useful in diagnosing aortic valve pathology.
   A. rapid film changer
   B. video tape
   C. digital subtraction angiography
   D. cineradiograph

6. A(n) _____ chest x-ray is recommended as a preangiographic clinical examination for thoracic aortography.
   A. overpenetrated
   B. decubitus
   C. underexposed
   D. expiration

7. The _____ artery is the most desirable approach for thoracic aortography.
   A. carotid
   B. axillary

C. brachial

D. femoral

8. Employing a pigtail multiside-hole catheter with _____ reduces catheter recoil.

A. four turns

B. parallel holes

C. no more than 10 holes

D. closed end hole

9. A minimum of _____ ml of contrast medium is recommended to visualize the aortic arch.

A. 20

B. 40

C. 60

D. 80

10. For contrast medium injection during a thoracic aortogram, the catheter should be positioned at the level of _____.

A. the aortic bulb

B. the midascending aorta

C. T-4

D. the proximal thoracic aorta

11. The filming rate for thoracic aortography is fastest during the _____.

A. last 2 seconds

B. 3- to 4-second interval

C. venous phase

D. first 2 seconds

12. The recorded death rate for thoracic aortography is about _____ percent.

A. 0.5

B. 1.7

C. 2.3

D. 2.6

13. The largest percentage of deaths for thoracic aortography is attributed to _____.

A. cardiac arrest

B. pulmonary emboli

C. aneurysms

D. brain damage

14. A(n) _____ is employed to demonstrate patent ductus arteriosus.

A. RPO

B. lateral

C. AP

D. LPO

15. Most aortic aneurysms occur in the _____.

A. ascending aorta

B. aortic arch

C. descending aorta

D. thoracic aorta

## BIBLIOGRAPHY

Abrams, H: Angiography, Vol 1, ed 3. Little, Brown & Co, Boston, 1983.

Anthony, C and Thibodeau, G: Textbook of Anatomy and Physiology, ed 10. CV Mosby, St Louis, 1979.

Johnsrude, I, Jackson, D, and Dunnick, NR: A Practical Approach to Angiography, ed 2. Little, Brown & Co, Boston, 1987.

Gray, H and Gross, CM: Anatomy of the Human Body. Lea & Febiger, Philadelphia, 1976.

Kandarpa, K: Handbook of Cardiovascular and Interventional Radiologic Procedures. Little, Brown & Co, Boston, 1989.

Katzen, B: Interventional Diagnostic and Therapeutic Procedures. Springer-Verlag, New York, 1980.

Luzsa, G: X-ray Anatomy of the Vascular System. JB Lippincott, Philadelphia, 1974.

Meschan, I: An Atlas of Anatomy Basic to Radiology. WB Saunders, Philadelphia, 1975.

Sagel, S: Special Procedures in Chest Radiology. WB Saunders, Philadelphia, 1976.

Snopek, A: Fundamentals of Special Radiographic Procedures. WB Saunders, Philadelphia, 1992.

White, R: Fundamentals of Vascular Radiology. Lea & Febiger, Philadelphia, 1976.

# CHAPTER 22

# Cerebral Angiography

*Joseph R. Bittengle, MEd, (ARRT)(R)*
*Donna C. Davis, MEd, (ARRT)(R)(CV)*

In 1927 Moniz* radiographically demonstrated a surgically exposed carotid artery following an injection of sodium iodide into the artery. Since that time, there have been substantial developments in cerebral angiography, including the design of catheters, the composition of contrast media, and the characteristics of the imaging equipment. The advent of computed tomography (CT), digital subtraction angiography (DSA), magnetic resonance angiography (MRA), and interventional techniques has contributed to the development of the subspecialty of neuroradiography.

Magnetic resonance angiography is gaining popularity as a screening technique for carotid and cerebral arterial occlusions. While it lacks the specificity of cerebral angiography, MRA is noninvasive and therefore a safer procedure. Used in conjunction with CT and prior to cerebral angiography, MRA is proving its diagnostic value.

This chapter presents the anatomy of cerebral circulations and the indications for and technique of performing cerebral angiography. A discussion of complications and angiographic findings is also included.

## ANATOMY

The cerebrovascular circulatory system arises from the aortic arch. The right and left carotid arteries supply blood to the anterior and middle portions of the brain. The right common carotid artery originates from the innominate artery, and the left common carotid artery originates directly from the arch of the aorta (Fig. 22–1). The cerebrovascular system also consists of the right and left vertebral arteries, which supply blood to the posterior portion of the brain. Venous drainage of the brain is achieved by the jugular veins.

---

*Antonio Caetano de Abreu Freire Egas Moniz (1874–1955) was a Portuguese neurologist, diplomat, and 1949 Nobel prize winner in physiology and medicine.

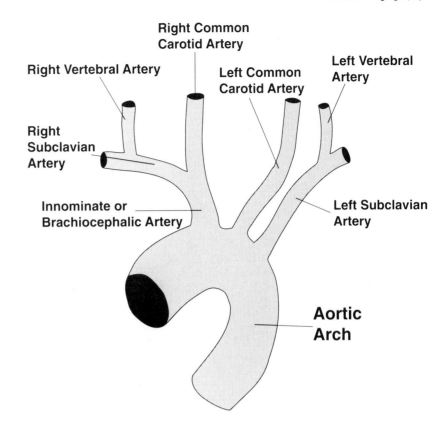

**Figure 22-1.** Branches of the aortic arch.

## Carotid Arteries

Each common carotid artery bifurcates into external and internal carotid arteries. The carotid bifurcation is usually located at the level of the fourth cervical vertebra, which corresponds to the superior surface of the thyroid cartilage. The thyroid cartilage is an important landmark during the percutaneous puncture technique of the carotid artery. To ensure proper placement of the percutaneous needle in the common carotid artery, the puncture site should be located approximately 1 inch inferior to the upper border thyroid cartilage.

The internal carotid artery, which is located laterally at the bifurcation, supplies blood to the anterior portion of the brain, the orbits, the anterior portion of the nasal cavity, and the forehead. The external carotid artery, which is located medially at the bifurcation, supplies blood to the anterior portion of the neck, the face, most of the scalp, and the temporal regions. Generally, the internal carotid arteries and their branches are examined more frequently through cerebral angiography than are the external carotid arteries.

Near its bifurcation point, the inferior portion of the internal carotid artery is dilated. This dilated region of each carotid artery is known as the carotid sinus and assists in the regulation of blood pressure. When viewed from the side, the superior portions of the internal carotid artery appear S-shaped within the cranium and are known as the carotid siphon (Fig. 22-2A). Any abnormality in the appearance of the carotid siphon, such as elongation or compression (Fig. 22-2B), may indicate the presence of a pathologic condition.

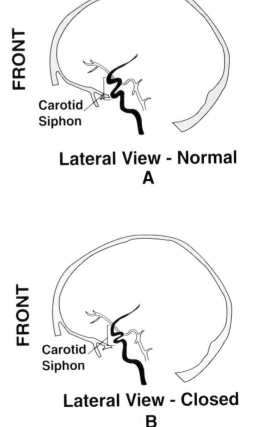

**Figure 22-2.** (A) Normal carotid siphon; (B) closed carotid siphon.

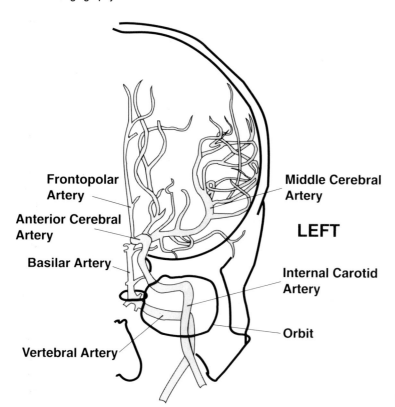

**Figure 22-3.** T shape of internal carotid artery.

The terminal portion of the internal carotid artery is T-shaped when viewed from the front (Fig. 22–3). The anterior cerebral artery and the middle cerebral artery originate from this T-shaped portion of the internal carotid artery. Any alterations in the shape of these T-shaped segments may also indicate the presence of a pathologic condition.

The sylvian triangle is another important diagnostic landmark sometimes used during cerebral angiography. It is best demonstrated with a lateral projection. The sylvian triangle is outlined by drawing a line connecting the tops of the insular loops (branches of the middle cerebral arteries) with the base of the first insular branch (Fig. 22–4). Identification of the sylvian triangle during cerebral angiography may be significant in the diagnosis of intracranial lesions because space-occupying lesions may cause a shift in the normal appearance of the sylvian triangle.

## Vertebral Arteries

The right and left vertebral arteries also form part of the cerebrovascular circulation. The right vertebral artery originates from the right subclavian artery, and the left vertebral artery originates from the left subclavian artery (Fig. 22–1). The vertebral arteries extend up the neck, passing through the transverse foramina of the cervical vertebrae, and supply blood to the posterior portion of the brain (Fig. 22–5).

The largest branch of the vertebral artery is the posterior inferior cerebellar artery (PICA). The PICA extends laterally just inferior to the union of the two ver-

tebral arteries. Branch arteries of the PICA include the anterior medullary, lateral medullary, supratonsillar, superior retrotonsillary, and vermian segments.

The single basilar artery is formed from the union of the right and left vertebral arteries. Branch arteries of the basilar artery include the pontine, internal auditory, anterior inferior cerebellar, and superior cerebellar arteries. The terminal portion of the basilar artery bifurcates into the right and left posterior cerebral arteries. The posterior cerebral arteries connect to the internal carotid arteries by the posterior communicating arteries. An important anastomosis is formed by the anterior communicating and the posterior communicating arteries. This anastomosis is known as the circle of Willis (Fig. 22–6).

## Veins

Venous drainage of deoxygenated blood from the intracranial area is accomplished through the jugular veins. The internal jugular veins receive blood from the dural sinuses, which include the sigmoid sinus, transverse sinus, straight sinus, and superior and inferior sagittal sinuses. Cerebral veins, which drain into the dural sinuses, include the superior cerebral, middle cerebral, inferior cerebral, and basal veins. The external jugular veins receive blood from the outer cranial vault and the inner structures of the face. Both the right and left internal and external jugular veins drain into the right and left brachiocephalic veins, respectively (Fig. 22–7). The brachiocephalic veins join to form the superior vena cava.

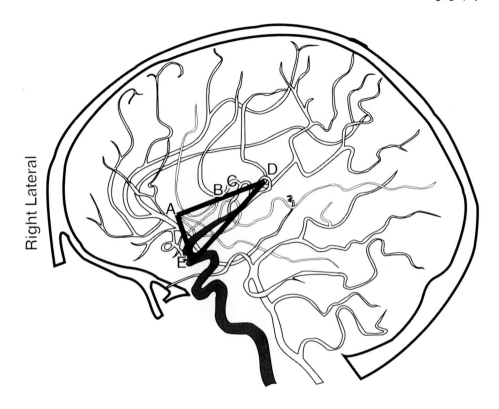

**Figure 22–4.** Sylvian triangle.

A.B.C.D = Insular Loops

E = Base of First Insular Branch

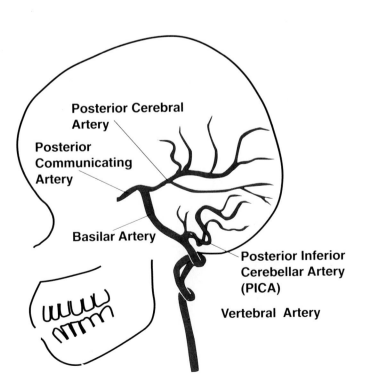

Posterior Cerebral
Artery

Posterior
Communicating
Artery

Basilar Artery

Posterior Inferior
Cerebellar Artery
(PICA)

Vertebral Artery

**Figure 22–5.** Vertebral blood supply to the brain.

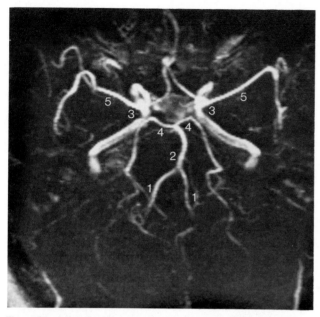

**Figure 22–6.** MRA of the circle of Willis. *1,* Vertebral arteries; *2,* basilar artery; *3,* internal carotid arteries; *4,* superior cerebellar arteries; *5,* middle cerebellar artery.

## INDICATIONS

Although cerebral angiography is no longer considered the primary means of diagnosing pathologic conditions of the cerebrovascular circulatory system, its use in conjunction with neurovascular interventional studies has not diminished. Cerebral angiography is still an effective tool in the diagnosis of occlusive diseases (atherosclerosis, thrombosis, emboli), aneurysms, arteriovenous malformations, and fistulae. Cerebral angiography performed following a positive CT or MRA scan is useful in determining the extent of vascular involvement.

## EQUIPMENT

A variety of equipment is used for cerebral angiography. Certain equipment, however, is common to most cerebral angiographic approaches, namely, rapid-sequence film changers, x-ray tubes equipped with small focal spots, image-intensified fluoroscopy with digital subtraction capabilities (Fig. 22–8), floating-

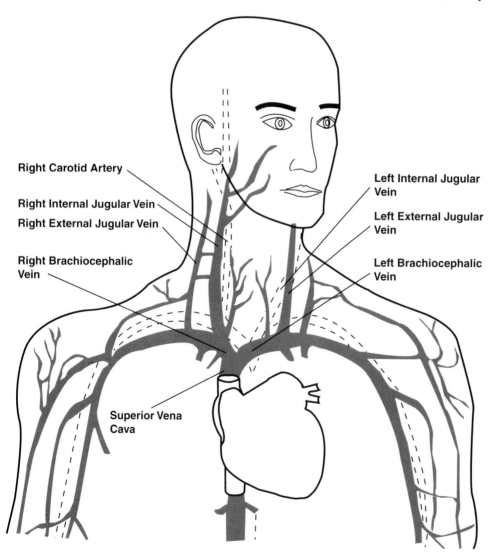

Right Carotid Artery

Right Internal Jugular Vein

Right External Jugular Vein

Right Brachiocephalic Vein

Left Internal Jugular Vein

Left External Jugular Vein

Left Brachiocephalic Vein

Superior Vena Cava

**Figure 22–7.** Jugular veins.

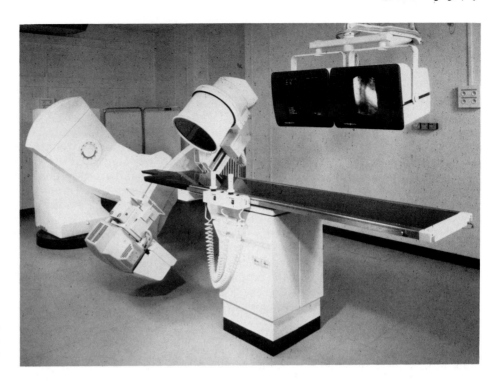

**Figure 22-8.** Advantx AFM—
Angiography Imaging System.
(Courtesy of GE Medical Systems,
Milwaukee, WI.)

top x-ray tables, and automatic electromechanical injectors.

Rapid filming is required during cerebral angiography because of the rapid flow of blood through the vessels. The use of rapid serial film changers capable of performing either single-plane or biplane imaging is required. Biplane imaging has the advantage of simultaneously performing two right-angle radiographic projections, thereby reducing the amount of radiographic contrast medium used and radiation exposure to the patient. However, because of the excessive scattered radiation emitted during the procedure, biplane angiography does have the disadvantage of producing images of reduced quality. One method of decreasing the quantity of scattered radiation produced is to alternate the exposures.

An x-ray tube with a focal spot of 0.3 mm or less is necessary to perform magnification studies of the cerebral vessels. By magnifying the vessels, small pathologic conditions may be better visualized. To maintain optimum recorded detail during the macroradiographic technique, the smallest focal spot available should be used.

Image-intensified fluoroscopy equipped with digital subtraction capabilities offers several advantages over rapid serial imaging. The advantages include the use of considerably less contrast medium per injection, instant playback of computerized images, instant availability of subtracted images, and greater imaging speed. A detailed discussion of digital imaging is presented in Chapter 15, Digital Subtraction Angiography.

A floating x-ray table top is needed to move the patient into position for the floor-mounted rapid serial filming sequence and a C-arm imaging system. The table top, therefore, must be mobile enough to accommodate both intensified fluoroscopy and serial filming.

An automated electromechanical injector is routinely used with all catheterization approaches except the direct puncture method. The direct puncture technique uses a manual syringe injection.

## PREPROCEDURAL CARE AND CAUTIONS

Preprocedural patient care for cerebral angiography adheres to the normal procedure for any angiographic examination. For scheduled patients, on the day prior to the angiogram, a review of the patient's medical history is conducted before medications are prescribed. In emergency cases, the patient's medical history may not be as comprehensive. Therefore, the prescription of any premedication is based on the data available at the time of the procedure.

Relative to the patient's condition, the following items in the patient's medical history should be assessed: prothombin time (PT), partial thromboplastin time (PTT), blood urea nitrogen (BUN), creatinine, allergic history, cardiac arrhythmias, and blood pressure instability (hypertension or hypotension).

It is important to review the patient's laboratory results prior to the procedure. The PT and PTT will assess the patient's coagulation ability. High values will result in an increased bleeding risk for the patient. BUN and creatinine will assess the patient's renal function. Contrast media can be detrimental to the patient with decreased renal function, indicated by high BUN and creatinine values.

It is also important to palpate and record the patient's pulse rate, pulse characteristics, and blood pressure prior to the procedure. If the femoral approach is to be used for catheterization, the pedal pulses should also be recorded. The angiographer must be aware of any differences in blood pressure, pulse strength, or delay in pulses between the right and left upper extremities. Decreased carotid pulse and bruits should be identified because they may be an indication of a pathologic condition of the vessel.

## APPROACHES

Cerebral angiography may be performed by using the direct percutaneous method of the common carotid artery or catheterization method via a femoral or transaxillary puncture. All methods have their advantages and disadvantages.

Although the direct percutaneous method was one of the first methods developed for performing cerebral angiography, it is rarely used today. In this method, the patient is placed in a supine position on the x-ray table. The head is positioned in moderate extension to permit easier palpation of the vessel and to facilitate puncturing the artery. A local anesthetic is typically used. The patient must be fully informed and instructed on the particulars of the procedure to reduce the possibility of needle displacement caused by patient motion. A support should be placed under the patient's head and shoulders to help maintain the patient's position.

The direct percutaneous method was commonly used on the carotid artery. The needle is placed in the common carotid artery below the level of its bifurcation. The puncture site is about 2.5 cm below the upper border of the thyroid cartilage. Needle position is verified by a test injection of contrast medium under image-intensified fluoroscopy. Often the injection of contrast medium is performed directly through the needle. Alternately, after needle placement, a small sheath catheter may be placed in the carotid artery for the injection. The use of a catheter reduces the possibility of accidental displacement of the needle and facilitates patient positioning.

Direct percutaneous punctures do have disadvantages and hazards. The major disadvantage is that to study more than one vessel, more than one puncture must be performed. For example, to demonstrate the anatomy of both carotid arteries, the angiographer must puncture both the right and left common carotid arteries. Complications associated with the direct percutaneous method include the development of a hematoma at the puncture site, which can result in deviation of the trachea and possible respiratory impairment; the formation of thrombi; the production of emboli; vessel occlusion; and puncturing the wrong vessel.

Using the Seldinger technique, the femoral puncture method is the preferred approach for cerebral angiography. This method proves to be the safest and least traumatic to the patient. For this approach, the femoral artery is punctured just below the inguinal ligament, and a catheter is manipulated into the cerebral vessel of choice. By guiding the catheter and appropriate positioning of the patient's head, any of the cerebral vessels may be catheterized. The most common complication associated with the femoral puncture method is hematoma formation at the puncture site, which is usually transient. Hemiparesis, loss of vision, and gangrene of the lower extremity are also complications of the femoral approach but rarely occur. Complications can be minimized by proper flushing of the catheter, good postprocedural compression, limiting catheterization time, and limiting the quantity of contrast medium injected. While the femoral puncture approach is the preferred method, it may be contraindicated in patients with aortic occlusion or vessel tortuosity. If the vessels are tortuous and prohibit manipulation and advancement of the catheter, a transaxillary approach should be attempted.

The transaxillary approach to catheterization of the cerebral vessels is used with the patient in the supine position and the right upper extremity in abduction. The needle is inserted into the axillary artery. Because of the anatomic alignment, the right axillary artery is used because it facilitates examination of all the cerebral vessels. A complication associated with the transaxillary approach is damage to the brachial plexus, caused by repeated punctures or hematoma formation and compression of the brachial plexus.

## CEREBRAL CATHETERS

Knowledge of the patient's anatomy, understanding of the various types of catheters available, and the skill of the angiographer contribute to the successful placement of a catheter into the correct cerebral vessel. The choice of cerebral catheter used by the angiographer is usually based on personal preference. All cerebral catheters have a single end hole and no side holes. The various catheters available differ in their materials and types of tip configurations (Fig. 22–9).

A selection of catheters used for cerebral angiography may include the Berenstein, Headhunter (H1H), Simmons (Sidewinder), Newton, Mani, Bentson, and Vinuela. With the exception of the Vinuela, each of these catheter types offers more than one catheter curve. The curve is usually identified by a number, such as Simmons 1. The Vinuela is a 5.5 French catheter that tapers to a 4 French and is typically used for neuroembolizations. Most manufacturers produce separate catheters for normal and tortuous vessels. Some manufacturers produce special catheters for pediatric patients. Table 22–1 is a summary of the various types of catheters and their suggested uses.

## CONTRAST MEDIA

Many research studies have been performed to determine the best contrast media for use in cerebral angiography. These studies compare the relationship be-

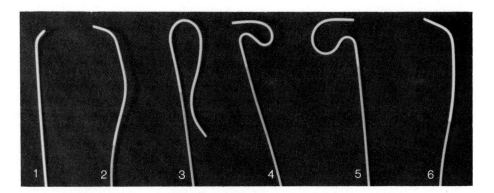

**Figure 22-9.** Common catheter curves for cerebral angiography: *1,* Berenstein; *2,* Headhunter; *3,* Simmons; *4,* Newton; *5,* Mani; *6,* Bentson.

tween contrast medium chemical composition to patient pain response, radiographic image quality, and patient complications.

While some institutions use organic ionic iodinated contrast media for cerebral angiography, today many use the nonionic contrast agents. Examples of the nonionic contrast media used for cerebral angiography include iohexol (Omnipaque), iopamidol (Isovue), and ioversol (Optiray).

When used for cerebral angiography, the nonionic contrast media tend to produce fewer adverse reactions in patients. Nonionic contrast agents will not disassociate in solution and have a lower neurotoxicity. These characteristics are thought to contribute to their greater safety. An additional beneficial characteristic of nonionic contrast media is lower osmolality, which is believed to be responsible for their inability to cross the blood-brain barrier.

The amount of contrast medium injected is dependent on such factors as patient condition, age, and weight; pathologic condition of the vessel; and the specific vessel to be imaged. Table 22-2 lists the common ranges for doses of contrast medium used for cerebral angiography.

The volume of contrast medium injected can affect the rate of complications because higher complication rates are associated with larger volumes of contrast medium. Cerebral angiography often involves the investigation of both carotid and vertebral arteries. Occasionally the angiographic study may be limited to one or two vessels. Because of the probability of multiple injections, care should be taken to record the amount of

contrast medium used for each injection. The total amount of ionic contrast medium injected for any one session should not exceed 150 ml. The total amount of nonionic contrast medium injected for any one session should not exceed 2 ml/kg of patient weight per hour, an amount that is especially useful in pediatric angiography. However, the patient's pancreatic and renal functions should be considered when calculating the maximum safe contrast medium load of the patient.

## POSITIONING AND FILMING

To ensure immobilization of the patient during the cerebral angiographic procedure, a specially designed head-positioning sponge is used. Velcro straps may also be placed across the forehead and chin of patients who are unable to cooperate (Fig. 22-10). Because of the intricacy of the vessels to be demonstrated, patient motion must be minimized.

After the catheter has been placed in the desired vessel, a sterile covering is placed over the catheter to maintain the sterile field as the film changer is rotated into position.

### Carotid Arteries

Filming for most carotid angiograms consists of anteroposterior axial, lateral, and anteroposterior oblique transorbital projections with the patient in the supine position. In the anteroposterior axial projec-

Table 22-1. **Summary of Catheters and Their Suggested Uses**

| Catheter | Vessel Characteristics |
|---|---|
| Berenstein | Young patients, normal aortic arch, normal vessel origins |
| Headhunter (H1H) | Normal aortic arch, normal vessel origins |
| Simmons (Sidewinder) | Tortuous aorta, tortuous vessel origins |
| Newton | Tortuous aorta, tortuous vessel origins |
| Mani | Tortuous aorta, tortuous and atypical vessel origins |
| Bentson | Normal vessel origins |

Table 22-2. **Common Ranges for Doses of Contrast Medium for Cerebral Angiography**

| Vessel | Volume for Single Dose of Contrast Medium |
|---|---|
| Common carotid artery | 8-12 ml |
| Internal carotid artery | 5-9 ml |
| External carotid artery | 4-8 ml |
| Vertebral artery | 6-10 ml |

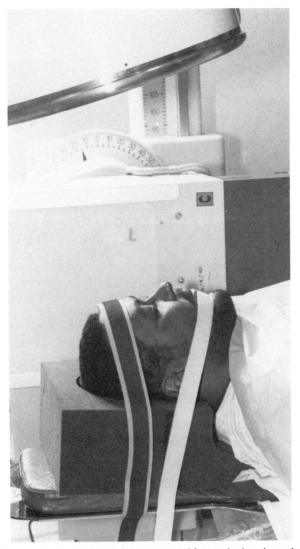

**Figure 22–10.** Angiographic sponge used for cerebral angiography.

tion, the patient is positioned with the midsagittal plane and the orbitomeatal line adjusted perpendicularly to the plane of the film (Fig. 22–11). The central ray is directed 15 to 20 degrees caudad to exit the foramen magnum. The lateral projection is performed with the patient's interpupillary line adjusted perpendicularly to the plane of the film and the midsagittal plane adjusted parallel to the plane of the film. The central ray is directed horizontally to be perpendicular to the film plane and centered to enter approximately 1 to 1.5 inches superior to the external auditory meatus (Fig. 22–12). For the anteroposterior oblique transorbital projection, the head is rotated away from the injected side and adjusted so that the midsagittal plane forms a 60-degree angle with the plane of the film. The central ray is directed 20 degrees cephalad and centered at the midpoint of the orbit.

These views demonstrate various cerebral vascular anatomy. The anteroposterior axial projection demonstrates a frontal view of the anterior and middle cerebral arteries. The lateral projection is used to demonstrate a lateral view of the anterior and middle cerebral arteries and the carotid siphon (Fig. 22–13). The anteroposterior oblique transorbital projection demonstrates the internal carotid bifurcation, the anterior communicating artery, and the middle cerebral artery projected in the orbital shadow.

Filming sequence varies from institution to institution. In general it is important to obtain at least one radiograph without contrast medium. The noncontrast image may be used for manual subtraction. All phases of circulation should be demonstrated, including the arterial, the capillary, and the venous phases. An example of a filming sequence for carotid angiography might be 2 frames/sec for 4 seconds and 1 frame/sec for 6 seconds for a total of 14 radiographs.

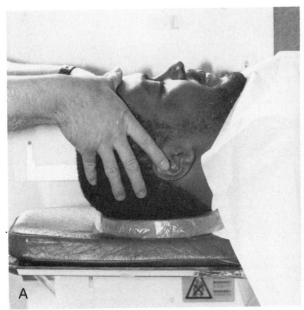
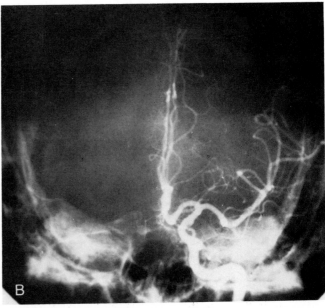

**Figure 22–11.** (A) Anteroposterior axial position; (B) anteroposterior axial projection of the internal carotid artery.

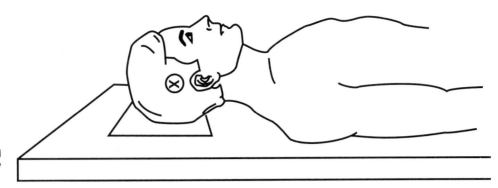

**Figure 22-12.** Location of central ray for lateral carotid angiography position.

## Vertebral Arteries

The radiographic positioning for vertebral angiography usually consists of the anteroposterior axial and lateral projections with the patient supine. In the anteroposterior axial projection, the midsagittal plane and the orbitomeatal line are adjusted perpendicular to the plane of the film. The central ray is directed 30 to 35 degrees caudad to exit the foramen magnum (Fig. 22-14). For the lateral projection, the patient's midsagittal plane is adjusted parallel to the plane of the film and the interpupillary line is adjusted perpendicular to the film plane. The central ray is directed horizontally to be perpendicular to the film plane and centered approximately 1 inch posterior and 1 inch superior to the external auditory meatus (Fig. 22-15).

The anatomy demonstrated during vertebral angiography also varies according to the position used. The anteroposterior axial projection demonstrates the basilar artery, the right and left posterior cerebral arteries, and the superior cerebellar artery. The lateral projection will demonstrate the basilar artery and the posterior cerebral artery.

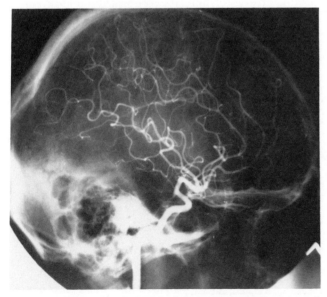

**Figure 22-13.** Lateral projection of the internal carotid artery and branches.

The filming sequence for vertebral angiography is similar to that used for carotid angiography. An example of a filming sequence for vertebral angiography might be 2 frames/sec for 4 seconds, 1 frame/sec for 3 seconds, and 1 frame every other second for 6 seconds for a total of 14 radiographs. Again, it is important to image all phases of the circulation.

## COMPLICATIONS

Complications associated with cerebral angiography may be classified as local, neurologic, or systemic. Local complications occur at the puncture site. Neurologic complications are adverse reactions affecting the nervous system. Systemic complications are related to the patient's hypersensitivity to the iodinated contrast medium and affect organs or areas of the body other than the central nervous system. Most complications associated with cerebral angiography are minor and transient.

The most common local complications include hematoma and extravasation of the contrast medium at the puncture site. Usually these local complications last only a few days. Some hematomas, however, may be large enough to cause difficulties. These local complications can be avoided by limiting the time of the procedure, limiting the amount of catheter manipulation, and checking for proper needle placement.

Neurologic complications are associated with the tendency of ionic contrast media to pass across the blood-brain barrier, resulting in a toxic chemical effect. This effect is usually manifested by seizures. The use of nonionic contrast media reduces the likelihood of neurologic complications.

Systemic complications may include hypotension, pain and heat, vasospasm or vasodilation, shock, and laryngospasm. These systemic reactions tend to be idiopathic, and the use of nonionic contrast media reduces the likelihood of systemic complications. Other complications that may occur are embolization, cerebral infarction, and the formation of arteriovenous fistulas.

## SOME ANGIOGRAPHIC FINDINGS

The most common angiographic findings are pathologic conditions associated with atherosclerosis, aneu-

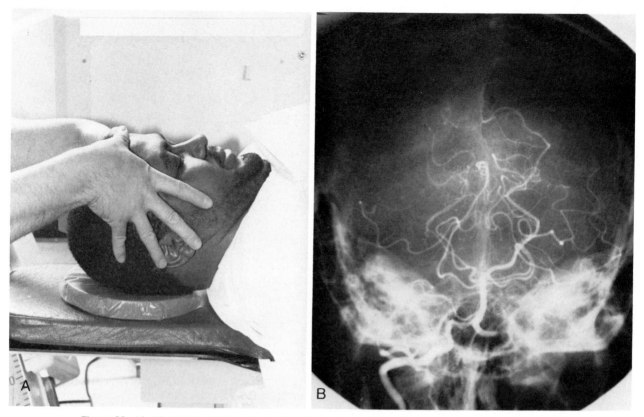

**Figure 22-14.** (A) Anteroposterior axial position; (B) anteroposterior axial projection of the vertebral artery.

rysms, arteriovenous malformations, traumatic intracranial hemorrhage, and tumors.

Atherosclerosis, a form of arteriosclerosis, affects the vessel by dilating and elongating the vessel, resulting in tortuosity. Intimal thickening and plaque formation result in a narrowing of the vessel and a reduction in the size of the vessel lumen. If the narrowing is severe, occlusion of the vessel may result. Often the plaque will contain calcium, making diagnosis easier. Common sites for atherosclerosis are at the bifurcation of the common carotid artery (Fig. 22-16), at the carotid siphon, at the origin of the vertebral arteries, and in the basilar artery.

Collateral circulation often develops in younger pa-

tients exhibiting slow development of atherosclerotic disease. It is important to examine all the brachiocephalic vessels to determine the true extent of collateralization in patients demonstrating occlusive disease.

Most aneurysms are found in the circle of Willis. Common sites include the origin of the posterior communicating artery, the junction of the anterior communicating artery, the anterior cerebral and middle cerebral branches, and the supraclinoid region of the internal carotid artery (Fig. 22-17). For anticipated surgical intervention, it is important to demonstrate the size of the aneurysm, the relationship of the aneurysm to other vessels, and the presence of hemorrhage.

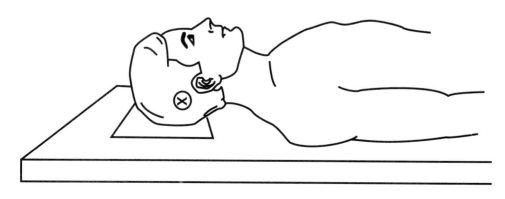

**Figure 22-15.** Location of central ray for lateral vertebral angiography position.

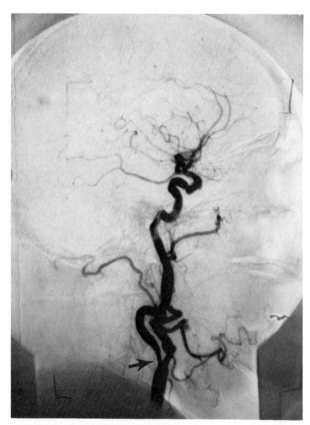

**Figure 22–16.** Lateral carotid projection demonstrating narrowing of the internal carotid artery at the bifurcation.

Arteriovenous malformations (AVMs) are characterized by many tortuous irregular vessels, dilated arteries feeding the malformation (Fig. 22–18), and dilated veins draining blood. The rapid shunting of blood because of the high arterial pressure causes greater dilation of the involved veins. An early venous phase will be evident on the radiograph. This rapid flow of blood and dilated vessels may require the use of larger doses of contrast medium and an increased filming rate. A rate of 6 frames/sec may be required to adequately image AVMs.

Traumatic intracranial hemorrhage may be demonstrated as a subdural hematoma, extradural hematoma, or intracerebral hematoma. Displacement of adjacent arteries is common with each type of hematoma. Most subdural hematomas are located in the midparietal region near the sylvian fissure. Extradural hematomas are usually located in the temporal area. Intracranial hematomas are usually located in the frontal or temporal regions. Cerebral angiography performed to assess tumors may be used to determine the development of vessels near the tumor and to evaluate the vascularity of the tumor.

Cerebral angiography is used to determine the location of the tumor, the direction of any displaced vessels, and tumor vascularity. The characteristics of the vessels feeding the tumor can assist in determining the pathologic condition. The most frequent hypervascular tumors are glioblastomas, meningiomas (Fig. 22–19), and metastases.

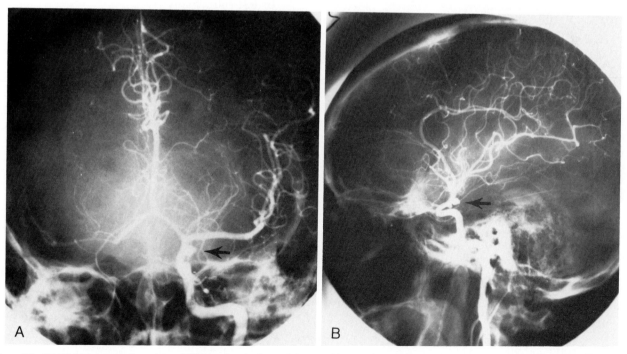

**Figure 22–17.** (*A*) Anteroposterior axial and (*B*) lateral projections of the carotid artery demonstrating two aneurysms on the supraclinoid region of the internal carotid artery.

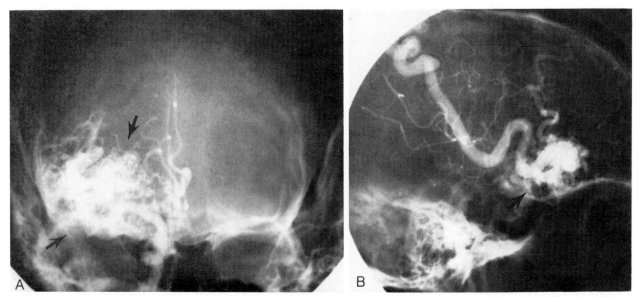

**Figure 22–18.** (A) Anteroposterior axial and (B) lateral projections of internal carotid artery demonstrating a gross arteriovenous malformation.

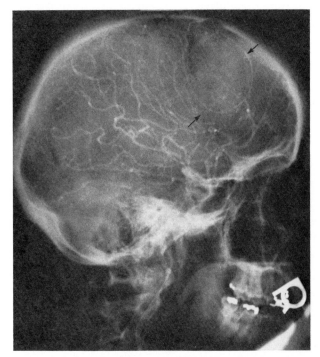

**Figure 22–19.** Meningioma.

## REVIEW QUESTIONS

1. The dilated regions on each internal carotid artery near the bifurcation are known as the _____.
   A. insular loops
   B. carotid siphon
   C. carotid sinus
   D. sylvian triangle

2. The largest branches of the vertebral arteries are the _____.
   A. AICA
   B. lateral medullary
   C. middle cerebral
   D. PICA

3. The left common carotid artery originates from the _____.
   A. aortic arch
   B. left subclavian
   C. left vertebral
   D. right subclavian

4. Cerebral veins include all of the following *except* the _____.
   A. basal
   B. dural sinus
   C. middle cerebral
   D. superior cerebral

5. One method for reducing scatter radiation during biplane cerebral angiography is to _____.
   A. alternate the exposures
   B. magnify the images
   C. use a focal spot less than 0.3 mm
   D. use low-speed intensifying screens

6. Which of the following items should be assessed prior to performing a cerebral angiogram?
   I. patient's allergic history
   II. BUN, creatinine
   III. CBC
   IV. PT, PTT
   A. I, II only
   B. II and IV only
   C. I, II, IV only
   D. I, II, III, IV

7. For the direct percutaneous method of the common carotid artery, the puncture site should be localized _____.
   A. 2.5 cm below the upper border of the thyroid cartilage
   B. 2.5 cm above the upper border of the thyroid cartilage
   C. at the level of C-3
   D. at the level of C-5

8. The preferred access method for cerebral angiography is the _____ artery.
   A. brachial
   B. direct puncture of the carotid
   C. femoral
   D. axillary

9. The most common complication of femoral artery catheterization is _____.
   A. embolism
   B. hematoma
   C. intimal tear
   D. stroke

10. Catheters used for cerebral angiography are typically _____.
    A. single end hole
    B. single end hole with multiple side holes
    C. side holes only
    D. single end hole with two alternating side holes

11. Nonionic contrast media have all of the following characteristics *except* _____.
    A. ability to cross the blood-brain barrier
    B. low osmolality
    C. low neurotoxicity
    D. will not disassociate in solution

12. The anteroposterior oblique transorbital projection using a 60-degree head angle and a 20-degree cephalic central ray will demonstrate the _____.
    I. anterior communicating artery
    II. basilar artery
    III. internal carotid bifurcation
    IV. middle cerebral artery
    A. II only
    B. II and IV only
    C. I, III, IV only
    D. I, II, III, IV

13. The average, single-dose contrast medium injection for the internal carotid artery is _____.
    A. 4–8 ml
    B. 5–9 ml

C. 8–12 ml
D. 10–15 ml

14. An early venous phase evident on a cerebral angiogram could be an indication of _____.
    A. aneurysm
    B. atherosclerosis
    C. AVM
    D. glioblastoma

15. A common filming sequence for the carotid artery is _____.
    A. two frames for 4 seconds followed by one frame for 6 seconds
    B. two frames for 3 seconds, one frame for 4 seconds, and two frames for 6 seconds
    C. two frames for first 4 seconds, one frame for next 2 seconds, and two frames for 4 seconds
    D. two frames for 4 seconds, one frame for next 2 seconds, and one frame for 6 seconds

## BIBLIOGRAPHY

Bontrager, KL: Textbook of Radiographic Positioning and Related Anatomy, ed 3. Mosby-Year Book, St Louis, 1993.

Borgstein, RL, et al: Digital subtraction angiography (DSA) of the extracranial cerebral vessels: A direct comparison between intravenous and intra-arterial DSA. Clin Radiol 44:402, 1991.

Ehrlich, RA and McCloskey, ED: Patient Care in Radiography, ed 4. Mosby-Year Book, St Louis, 1993.

Eisenberg, RL and Dennis, CA: Comprehensive Radiographic Pathology. CV Mosby, St Louis, 1990.

Hutson, J, et al: Prospective blinded comparison of two-dimensional time-of-flight MR angiography with conventional angiography and duplex US. Radiology 186:339, 1993.

Meschan, I: An Atlas of Anatomy Basic to Radiology. WB Saunders, Philadelphia, 1975.

Nussel, F, Wegmuller, H, and Huber, P: Comparison of magnetic resonance angiography, MRI and conventional angiography in cerebral arteriovenous malformation. Neuroradiology 33:56, 1991.

Rose, JS: Invasive Radiology Risks and Patient Care. Year Book Medical Publishers, Chicago, 1983.

Snopek, AM: Fundamentals of Special Radiographic Procedures, ed 3. WB Saunders, Philadelphia, 1992.

Squire, LF and Novelline, RA: Fundamentals of Radiology, ed 4. Harvard University Press, Cambridge, MA, 1988.

Stimac, GK: Introduction to Diagnostic Imaging. WB Saunders, Philadelphia, 1992.

Tsuruda, JS: Magnetic Resonance Angiography. Sanofi Winthrop Pharmaceuticals, New York, 1991.

Whitley, JE and Whitley, NO: Angiography Techniques and Procedures. Warren H Green, St Louis, 1971.

Wolper, SM: Current role of cerebral angiography in the diagnosis of cerebrovascular disease. AJR 159:191, 1992.

# CHAPTER 23

# Pulmonary Angiography

*Marianne R. Tortorici, EdD, ARRT(R)*

Pulmonary angiography is a study of the blood circulation leading from the right ventricle of the heart to the lungs and returning to the left atrium of the heart. Frequently, the pathologic condition demonstrated on the radiographs is secondary to another condition. For example, gross dilation of the main pulmonary artery with normal hilar branches and small peripheral branches suggests pulmonary valvular stenosis.

Recording the pressures in various parts of the heart and pulmonary artery aids in diagnosis. By comparing the recorded pressures to the normal pressures, it is possible to successfully predict the type of pathologic condition that may be found. This is important because often it can dictate the best approach for the angiogram.

This chapter outlines the anatomy, techniques, and complications of pulmonary angiography with a brief summary of some pathologic findings. The reader is referred to other texts for a discussion of interventional pulmonary procedures.

## ANATOMY

The trunk of the pulmonary artery rises from the right ventricle of the heart at the pulmonary semilunar valves. It ascends medially and posteriorly (just to the left side of the aorta) and gives rise to the left and right branches at a level just below the aortic arch. The left pulmonary artery is about 1 cm higher than the right pulmonary artery.

### Left Lung Circulation

In the fetus, the left pulmonary artery is connected by an opening to the aortic arch (ductus arteriosus). Upon birth, the blood flow between the left pulmonary artery and aorta ceases. The ductus arteriosus closes with the formation of fibrous tissue called the ligamentum arteriosum.

The left pulmonary artery enters the hilum of the left lung. It is anterior to the descending aorta and is connected to the inferior aspect of the aortic arch by the

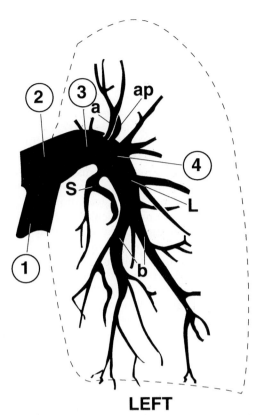

**Figure 23–1.** Pulmonary circulation: *1*, Trunk of the pulmonary artery; *2*, left pulmonary artery; *3*, ascending artery—*a*, anterior artery, and *ap*, apical posterior artery; *4*, descending artery—*L*, lingular artery, *b*, basal artery, and *S*, superior artery.

ligamentum arteriosum. The left pulmonary artery has two main branches, the ascending and descending, which feed the upper and lower lobes, respectively. The ascending branch gives rise to the apical posterior segmental artery and anterior segmental artery. These branches have numerous extensions, which are responsible for delivering blood to the various areas of the upper lobe. The descending branch of the left pulmonary artery is divided into the lingular artery, the superior segmental artery, and the arteries supplying the basal areas. Similarly, as in the case of the ascending branches, these divisions have numerous extensions that bring blood to the lower lobe. Figure 23–1 is a diagram of the major divisions of the left pulmonary circulation.

## Right Lung Circulation

The right pulmonary artery divides into an ascending branch, which feeds the right upper lobe, and the descending branches, which feed the right middle and right lower lobes. The ascending artery has three branches, the apical, posterior, and anterior segmental arteries. The apical segmental artery divides into the apical and posterior rami, which feed the apical and posterior portions of the apical segment of the right

upper lobe, respectively. The posterior segmental artery supplies the posterior portion of the right upper lobe. The anterior segment feeds the anterior aspect of the right upper lobe. The descending artery has the following branches: the middle lobe artery (which feeds the right middle lobe); the superior segmental artery (supplies the right lower lobe); the medial basal segmental artery (which feeds the right lower lobe); the anterior basal segmental artery (supplies the right lower lobe); the posterior basal segmental artery (which feeds the right lower lobe); and the lateral basal segmental artery (which feeds the right lower lobe). The branches of both the ascending and descending arteries have numerous divisions that feed the specific lobular areas. Figure 23–2 is a diagram of the right pulmonary circulation.

## THEORIES OF BLOOD FLOW

When discussing pulmonary circulation, the lungs can be divided or classified into three zones (Fig. 23–3). The amount of blood flowing in each zone depends on the gravity and the vascular pressures of the pulmo-

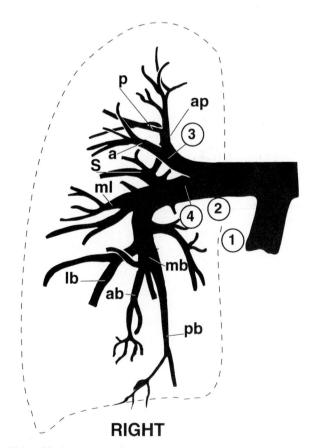

**Figure 23–2.** Right pulmonary circulation: *1*, Pulmonary artery; *2*, right main pulmonary artery; *3*, ascending artery—*ap*, apical, *p*, posterior, and *a*, anterior; *4*, descending artery—*ml*, middle lobe artery, *S*, superior, *mb*, medial basal, *ab*, anterior basal, and *pb*, posterior basal, and *lb*, lateral basal.

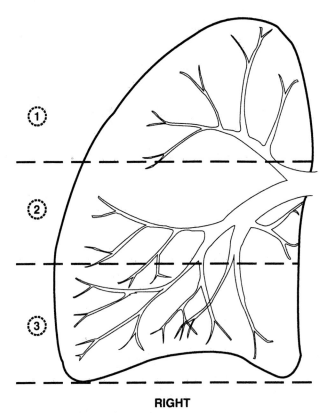

**RIGHT**

**Figure 23-3.** Lung zones 1, 2, and 3.

nary artery, the pulmonary veins, the alveoli, and interstitial pressures.

Pulmonary vascular pressures are relatively low. Also, the weight of the blood in the lung is considerable. Thus, the direction of blood flow is influenced by the cumulative weight of the blood (the blood throughout the lung), low vascular pressures, and gravity. For example, when a patient is supine, gravity helps create a greater flow of blood to the posterior areas of the lung. This is important to remember because it is possible to increase the amount of contrast medium in a specific lung area by altering the patient's position.

Pressures also influence blood flow. Alveolar pressure is responsible for the flow of blood from the capillaries to the veins. When the alveolar pressure exceeds the pulmonary arterial and venous pressures (i.e., zone one in an erect position), blood flow in the capillaries is diminished, reducing the vascular blood flow. If the pulmonary arterial pressure is greater than the alveolar pressure, and both pressures exceed the pulmonary venous pressure, then the flow of blood on the venous side of the capillary is decreased (i.e., zone two in an erect position). In this case, the blood flow is determined by the difference between the arterial and alveolar pressures, which can vary within the zone. It is possible to have an area in which the pulmonary arterial pressure is the greatest (i.e., zone three) and the pulmonary venous pressure is greater than the alveolar pressure. In this case, the blood flow is determined by the difference between the pulmonary arterial and pulmonary venous pressures, which can vary within the zone.

In summary, in the erect position, the greatest blood flow is in zone three, zone two has the second greatest blood flow, and zone one has the least amount of blood flow.

Another factor affecting blood flow is the pressure within the interstitial space. Located in this space are the pulmonary vessels. As the pressure of the interstitial space increases, the vessels are constricted and blood flow reduced. When the interstitial pressure is decreased, the diameter of the vessel and subsequent blood flow increases. Thus, if edema, air, or fluid is in the plural space, the interstitial pressure increases, which substantially decreases blood flow.

Interstitial pressure and alveolar pressure are the primary factors affecting blood flow. Secondary factors include blood gas concentration, hydrogen ion concentration, lung volumes, pulmonary blood flow rate, bronchial arterial flow rate, and neurogenic reflexes. A description of these factors is beyond the scope of this text. For further explanation regarding these factors, the reader is advised to consult the bibliography at the end of this chapter.

## INDICATIONS

Pulmonary angiography demonstrates pulmonary vessel status and anatomy. The procedure is indicated in vascular anomalies, for example, arteriovenous malformations, to demonstrate reverse shunting across patent ductus arteriosus and, most commonly, in cases of pulmonary embolization. Pulmonary embolization is very difficult to diagnose. It is not uncommon for the symptoms of aortic dissections or thoracic aneurysms to mimic pulmonary emboli. Therefore, in pulmonary angiography, it is important to examine the venous phase of the circulation. When performing pulmonary angiography for pulmonary embolization, it is important to determine whether an embolus or other pathologic condition exists; to assess the status of the venae cavae; and to evaluate the size, location, and extent (number) of the emboli.

## CONTRAINDICATIONS

Pulmonary angiography is contraindicated in patients who have had a recent myocardial infarction. Performing a pulmonary angiogram on these patients may cause cardiac arrhythmias. Pulmonary hypertension (mean arterial pressure above 60 mm Hg) can be a contraindication for performing pulmonary angiography, which may warrant selective or superselective injection.

As with all contrast studies, pulmonary angiography is also contraindicated in patients with a known allergy to contrast media. If the procedure must be performed on these patients, proper steroid and antihistamine premedication protocols should be followed. Also, the appropriate emergency equipment should be readily available in case of a contrast medium reaction.

## PREPROCEDURAL CARE AND CAUTIONS

Preangiographic care includes an in-depth clinical evaluation of the patient to determine if the procedure should be performed. The clinical examinations should include blood gas determinations, an electrocardiogram, a chest x-ray examination, and a perfusion and inhalation lung scan. Of these examinations, it is important to correlate the findings of the chest x-ray examination with the lung scan. The results of these examinations and comparison with the results of the angiogram are vital in assessing the pathologic condition. The clinical examinations should determine which branches of the pulmonary system are to be studied. Unfortunately, this does not always occur, and several injections are performed to properly evaluate the status of the pulmonary system. After it has been determined that a pulmonary angiogram is indicated, the routine preangiographic medication and preparation are implemented.

## EQUIPMENT

The equipment employed for pulmonary angiography varies with the diagnosis. In general, a rapid film changer, automatic injector, electrocardiograph, and some form of manometer to measure pressures should be employed. When digital subtraction angiography (DSA) is being performed, a digital subtraction unit is needed. In cases concerning problems with the pulmonary valve or the right side of the heart, a cineradiograph is usually more valuable than filming with a rapid film changer. Although it is common practice to employ automatic injectors, pulmonary angiography has been performed with excellent results by manual injection.

## APPROACHES

There are several approaches for pulmonary angiography, including a percutaneous venous puncture of the upper extremity, a cutdown of the antecubital vein, a transjugular, and a percutaneous puncture of the femoral vein. Catheterization of the femoral vein is a common route. However, in cases of suspected pulmonary embolization, the upper extremity puncture is preferred. This is because most emboli occur in the pelvis or the lower extremity; therefore, employing the femoral vein approach may further complicate the matter. It is also easier to manipulate the catheter from the upper extremity than from the femoral vein.

When performing a percutaneous upper extremity puncture, it is best to employ the right arm, which facilitates catheter placement. Once the catheter has been introduced into the vein, the arm should be abducted (Fig. 23–4) to straighten out the vein and assist in catheter positioning. To further facilitate catheter placement, the Valsalva technique can be employed in conjunction with the abduction of the arm.

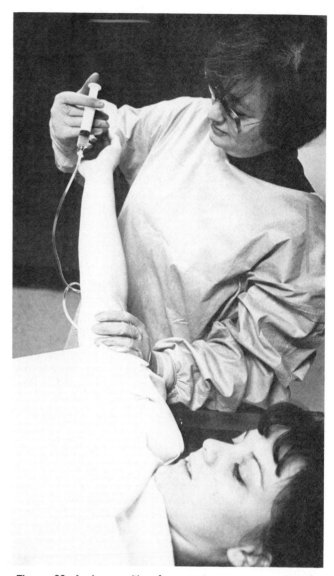

**Figure 23–4.** Arm position for percutaneous upper extremity puncture.

In the venous approach, a large gauge needle (12 to 16 gauge) is inserted in the vein after the area has been anesthetized and a 1- to 2-mm nick has been made slightly below the entrance of the needle in the vein. Injection may be made directly through the needle, or a catheter may be inserted in the vessel and advanced to the desired position. However, it should be noted that the closer the injection is to the area being filmed, the better the filling of the part and the film quality.

Some angiographers prefer to use the cutdown antecubital approach. An explanation of the cutdown approach is found in Chapter 19, Catheterization Methods and Patient Management.

The transjugular approach is performed by puncturing the jugular vein. A catheter is inserted in the vein and advanced to the right or left pulmonary artery.

The femoral vein approach may be used for pulmonary angiography. If the femoral approach is used, a catheter is inserted into the femoral vein using the Seldinger technique. The catheter is manipulated into the right atrium or pulmonary artery via the inferior vena cava. Because emboli often occur in the lower extremity or pelvis, there is the risk that catheter manipulation may cause complications.

## CATHETERS

The two most common catheters employed for pulmonary angiography are the closed-end, multiple-side-hole catheter and the pigtail. The closed-end, multiple-side-hole catheter has the advantage of preventing recoil in the right ventricle while delivering a large bolus of contrast medium. When a closed-end catheter is employed, a guide wire cannot be used to position the catheter; rather, catheter positioning is accomplished by inserting a sheath over the catheter. The sheath is used in much the same manner as the guide wire.

The pigtail catheter contains multiple side holes and an end hole. It is angled about 15 to 20 cm prior to the "pigtail." The most common pigtail employed is the Grollman (Fig. 23–5).

Steerable catheters are also useful in pulmonary angiography. These catheters require the attachment of a special handle (refer to Chapter 17, Supplementary Catheterization Equipment) for manipulation. The advantage of a steerable catheter is that no guide wire is needed.

## CONTRAST MEDIA

Research indicates that the iso-osmolar contrast media have a significantly decreased effect on pulmonary arterial pressure, patient discomfort, blood pressure, and heart rate than the ionic media. Thus, nonionic contrast media are preferred over ionic media.

Besides being safer, some angiographers believe that nonionic media demonstrate better radiographic quality in the venous phase.

The amount of contrast medium employed depends on the injection site. In general, 50 to 60 ml is used when the injection is in the trunk of the pulmonary artery; 30 to 40 ml is employed for a right or left pulmonary artery injection. If the lobes are the injection site, 15 to 20 ml of contrast medium is used.

The rate of injection depends on the amount of contrast medium employed. It is desirable to introduce the total amount of contrast medium within 1 to 2 seconds. Thus, if the injection site is the trunk of the pulmonary artery, then the rate is 25 to 30 ml/sec, resulting in delivery of all the contrast medium within 2 seconds. When a 30- to 40-ml/sec rate is employed for selective injection in the right or left pulmonary artery, a 2-second delivery of 15 ml/sec is recommended. For a superselective injection of the lobes, a 1-second total contrast medium delivery is suggested.

The primary site of injection is the trunk of the pulmonary artery. The location of the catheter in this area is confirmed by recording right atrium, right ventricle, and pulmonary artery pressures. When systolic pressure of the pulmonary artery is close to the systemic arterial pressure, the injection should not occur in the pulmonary main artery. The average pressure of the pulmonary artery in the adult is 15 mm Hg. If hypertension is present (60 mm Hg or higher), the injection should be made into the right atrium. Injection into the trunk of the pulmonary artery with severe pulmonary hypertension may cause an arrhythmia or pulmonary edema. A right atrium or selective injection is employed as an alternative rather than a primary injection site. Injection of the contrast medium into the right atrium creates loss of radiographic quality, caused by dilution of contrast medium. Also, the contrast in the right atrium may superimpose the pulmonary artery. If no pathologic condition is observed with an injection of the trunk of the pulmonary artery, the selective injection into the right or left pulmonary artery and superselective injection of the segments or lobes may be performed.

## POSITIONING AND FILMING

Regardless of the filming method used, the supine position is the first position employed during pulmonary angiography. This position is used to assess the symmetric flow of the arteries and the size of the vessels. Other positions used during the procedure are the left and right posterior obliques. A 10- to 15-degree left posterior oblique position is used to demonstrate the right pulmonary artery, while a 30- to 45-degree right posterior oblique demonstrates the left main pulmonary artery.

Filming may be accomplished by using either serial film changers or digital subtraction technique (DSA). DSA is advantageous because it has high density (contrast) resolution and real time capability. DSA has been

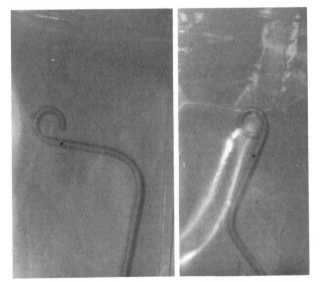

**Figure 23–5.** Grollman catheter.

known to record emboli as small as 2 to 3 mm. However, DSA is susceptible to motion artifacts, has poor spatial resolution, and often can visualize only a small field size. Motion artifacts are usually caused by patient respiration or the natural beating of the heart. Thus, DSA is often restricted to very cooperative patients who can hold their breath to reduce motion artifacts. It should be noted that motion artifacts can be reduced by providing the patient with explicit breathing instructions and by employing an ECG-initiated injection. Because of the small field size, multiple injections are often required to visualize all involved areas. Some success has been recorded in reducing the number of injections by increasing the area visualized using a 14" field size.

In DSA, the injection may be made into the peripheral antecubital vein using a 16-gauge needle or by catheterizing the right atrium (a right atrium injection is not recommended for patients with renal failure). The peripheral injection uses 45 ml of contrast medium injected at a rate of 15 ml/sec. A suggested filming rate is 27 frames/sec for 20 seconds. This method is becoming attractive because it costs significantly less than the catheterization method using a film changer.

The rapid filming method has the disadvantage of requiring patient catheterization. However, it demonstrates a larger field than DSA filming. Since a larger area is visualized, the number of injections is often fewer with film changer technique than with DSA. The radiographic image quality with film changers is excellent. When filming is performed using a film changer, the filming rate should be 2 to 3 frames/sec (for a total of 8 to 10 frames) for the main pulmonary artery, and 1 to 1½ frames/sec (for a total of 8 to 10 frames) for the right or left pulmonary artery and segmental filming. If the injection is performed manually through a needle in a vein, the filming rate should be 2 to 4 frames/sec.

## COMPLICATIONS

Because pulmonary angiography often involves placement of a catheter in the heart, some complications that occur during pulmonary angiography are cardiac-related. Among these are premature ventricular contractions, perforation of the heart, arrhythmia, a twisted catheter in the heart, and severe bradycardia. All of these complications are primarily the result of catheter manipulation. Other complications that may or may not be a result of catheter manipulation include dislodgement of a blood clot, air emboli, and thrombi in the catheter.

## SOME ANGIOGRAPHIC FINDINGS

By far the most common finding of pulmonary angiography is pulmonary embolization. Radiographically, pulmonary emboli may appear as a filling defect of the vessel or as a complete occlusion of the vessel. In the latter case, the cause of the occlusion may be something

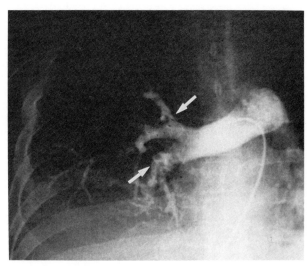

**Figure 23–6.** Pulmonary embolism.

other than pulmonary emboli. Therefore, to determine the cause, the angiogram should be correlated with other diagnostic procedures, especially lung scans. Figure 23–6 illustrates an example of pulmonary emboli.

Although the presence of pulmonary emboli is the major pathology demonstrated by pulmonary angiography, other findings include pulmonary stenosis, pulmonary vascular changes, coarctation of the pulmonary artery, patent ductus arteriosus, and tumors.

## REVIEW QUESTIONS

1. At birth, the ductus arteriosus closes with the formation of a fibrous tissue called _____.
   A. lingular ligament
   B. ligamentum arteriosum
   C. patent ductus
   D. segmental cartilage

2. The ascending and _____ arteries are the two main branches of the left pulmonary artery.
   A. descending
   B. posterior
   C. superior
   D. inferior

3. The ascending branch of the right pulmonary artery feeds the right _____ lobe.
   A. lower
   B. upper
   C. middle
   D. posterior

4. Alveolar pressure is responsible for the flow of blood from the _____ to the _____.
   A. veins, arteries
   B. capillaries, veins
   C. arteries, veins
   D. veins, capillaries

5. In cases of suspected pulmonary embolization, the _____ puncture is performed.
   A. transjugular
   B. femoral
   C. upper extremity
   D. translumbar

6. To facilitate catheter placement during a percutaneous upper extremity puncture, _____ may be employed.
   A. the adduction of the right arm
   B. having the patient pant
   C. hand elevation
   D. the Valsalva technique

7. Approximately _____ ml of contrast medium is employed for injection of the lobes.
   A. 5 to 10
   B. 10 to 15
   C. 15 to 20
   D. 20 to 25

8. If hypertension is present in the main pulmonary artery, the injection should be made in the _____.
   A. left ventricle
   B. right ventricle
   C. right atrium
   D. left atrium

9. In DSA of the lungs, it is common to have _____.
   A. multiple injections
   B. poor image quality
   C. a large field size
   D. low contrast

10. Recommended DSA filming rate is _____ frames/sec.
    A. 27
    B. 33
    C. 42
    D. 60

11. List two complications associated with pulmonary angiography that may occur in the heart.

12. List three pathologies that may be demonstrated on pulmonary angiography.

## BIBLIOGRAPHY

Abrams, H: Angiography, Vol 1, ed 3. Little, Brown & Co, Boston, 1983.

Baltaxe, H and Levin, D: A modified technique of pulmonary arteriography. Radiology 100:425, August 1971.

Beachley, M, et al: Alternate technique for pulmonary arteriography. AJR 134(1):195, June 1980.

Bjork, L: Digital angiography in pulmonary embolism. Acta Radiol Diagn 27(2):179, March–April 1986.

Courey, W, de Villasante, JM, and Waltman, AC: A quick, simple method of percutaneous transfemoral pulmonary arteriography. Radiology 113(2):475, November 1974.

Glenn, J and Ranniger, K: A variation of the technique of transfemoral pulmonary arteriography. Radiology 117(2):473, November 1975.

Gray, H: Anatomy of the Human Body, ed 29. Lea & Febiger, Philadelphia, 1976.

Johnsrude, I, Jackson, D, and Dunnick, NR: A Practical Approach to Angiography, ed 2. Little, Brown & Co, Boston, 1987.

Kozak, BE and Rosch, J: Curved guide wire for percutaneous pulmonary angiography. Radiology 167(3):864, June 1988.

Kumazaki, T: Ioxaglate versus diatrizoate in selective pulmonary angiography: II. Cardiovascular responses. Acta Radiol Diagn 26(5):635, September–October 1985.

Kumazaki, T: Ioxaglate versus diatrizoate in selective pulmonary angiography: I. Subjective reactions. Acta Radiol Diagn 26(5):635, July–August 1985.

Lach, RD: Technique for transfemoral percutaneous pulmonary angiography. Cardiovasc Intervent Radiol 10(2):114, 1987.

Lopez, A, et al: Pulmonary artery versus pulmonary angiography catheters (letter). Crit Care Med 18(4):459, April 1990.

Luzsa, G: X-ray Anatomy of the Vascular System. JB Lippincott, Philadelphia, 1974.

Meschan, I: An Atlas of Anatomy Basic to Radiology. WB Saunders, Philadelphia, 1975.

Meyerovitz, MF: How to maximize the safety of coronary and pulmonary angiography in patients receiving thrombolytic therapy. Chest 97(4)(suppl):132S, April 1990.

Mills, CS and Van Aman, ME: Modified technique for percutaneous transfemoral pulmonary angiography. Cardiovasc Intervent Radiol 9(1):52, 1986.

Musset, D, et al: Acute pulmonary embolism: Diagnostic value of digital subtraction angiography. Radiology 166(2):455, February 1988.

Pinet, F and Forment, J: Angiography of the thoracic systemic arteries. Radiol Clin North Am 16(3):441, December 1978.

Rees, CR, et al: The hemodynamic effects of the administration of ionic and nonionic contrast materials into the pulmonary arteries of a canine model of acute pulmonary hypertension. Invest Radiol 23(3):184, March 1988.

Saeed, M, et al: Pulmonary angiography with iopamidol: Patient comfort, image quality and hemodynamics. Radiology 165(2):345, November 1987.

Sagel, S: Special Procedures in Chest Radiology. WB Saunders, Philadelphia, 1976.

Tajima, H, et al: Effect of an iso-osmolar contrast medium on pulmonary arterial pressure at pulmonary angiography. Acta Radiol 32(2):134, March 1991.

White, R: Fundamentals of Vascular Radiology. Lea & Febiger, Philadelphia, 1976.

# CHAPTER 24

# Angiography of Liver and Spleen

*Marianne R. Tortorici, EdD, ARRT(R)*

The spleen and liver may be demonstrated through a variety of imaging modalities. Institutions with more advanced imaging equipment like a computed tomography (CT) scanner may perform a limited number of angiograms of the spleen or the liver. Conversely, institutions without CT scanners must rely on the older angiographic method of assessing the liver and spleen.

This chapter concentrates on the angiographic demonstration of the arterial phases of the liver and the spleen and of the portal system. The focus is on the diagnostic versus therapeutic aspect of the procedure.

## ANATOMY

### Arterial System

The celiac axis is the major branch of the abdominal aorta that supplies oxygenated blood to the liver and spleen. It arises from the anterior aspect of the aorta at the level of T-12. The celiac axis has three branches: the common hepatic, the splenic, and the left gastric arteries (Fig. 24–1). The common hepatic artery gives rise to the gastroduodenal, right hepatic, left hepatic, and middle hepatic arteries. The splenic artery feeds the pancreatic branch and the left gastroepiploic arteries. The superior mesenteric artery rises 1 to 20 mm below the celiac and supplies blood to the pancreas and drains into the portal vein.

### Portal System

The afferent tributaries of the portal vein are the splenic, the superior mesenteric, the inferior mesenteric, and the left gastric veins. Thus, injection of contrast medium into the celiac or superior mesenteric artery flows to the portal vein and provides a means to demonstrate the portal system. The efferent divisions of the portal vein are the right and left main branches. The portal vein is 6 cm long and is formed by the union of the superior mesenteric and splenic veins (Fig. 24–2).

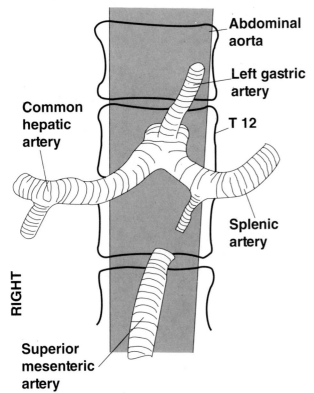

**RIGHT**

Figure 24-1. Celiac axis branches.

## INDICATIONS

Angiography of the portal system is indicated when portal hypertension or a possible retroperitoneal tumor exists. It is also useful in determining the existence of an aneurysm, cirrhosis of the liver, hepatitis,

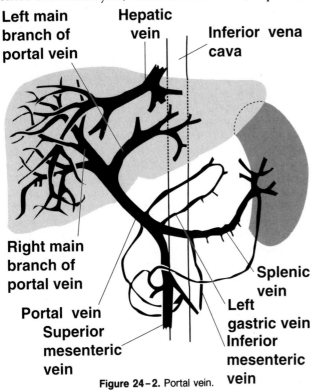

Figure 24-2. Portal vein.

vascular narrowing (common causes of vascular stenosis are atherosclerosis, trauma to the spleen, congenital malformation, and tumors), or bleeding.

## CONTRAINDICATIONS

Evaluation of the portal system by the direct percutaneous method is contraindicated for patients with blood dyscrasia, an absent spleen, or severe ascites. Other contraindications include a platelet count less than 50,000 per cubic millimeter of blood and a prothrombin time greater than 5 seconds. The primary contraindication for an indirect approach is a history of contrast media reaction.

## PREPROCEDURAL CARE AND CAUTIONS

Preprocedural patient care for the arterial assessment of the liver and spleen follows the normal routine of preprocedural care for any catheterization examination. Preprocedural patient care for portal assessment follows the general preprocedural care for any percutaneous procedure, with the added precautions of prothrombin time assessment and removal of ascitic fluid, if present. Also, because many patients with portal hypertension tend to be anemic, tests for hemoglobin and hematocrit levels should be performed. Normal hemoglobin (protein in erythrocytes that transports oxygen) levels are 13.5 to 18.0 g/dl in men and 12.0 to 16.0 g/dl in women. Normal hematocrit (the volume percentage of erythrocytes in whole blood) levels are 40 to 54 volumes/dl in men and 37 to 47 volumes/dl in women. Since percutaneous punctures for splenoportography have been known to cause hemorrhages, it is strongly advised that a surgical suite be available, if needed.

## EQUIPMENT

The major equipment employed for angiography of the liver or spleen is similar to that used for other angiographic procedures and includes a rapid serial film changer and an automatic injector. Accessory equipment for the indirect approach includes catheters, guide wires, and other supplementary equipment normally employed. For a percutaneous puncture, a Teflon sheath needle with an inner sharp stylet is used. A manometer may be used to measure arterial pressures.

## APPROACHES

There are two basic approaches for liver and spleen angiography—the direct and the indirect. The direct approach involves percutaneous puncture of the splenic vein or percutaneous trans-hepatic puncture of the intrahepatic vein radicals. The percutaneous trans-hepatic is rarely performed for diagnostic purposes and is not discussed in this text. The indirect approach via the femoral artery is the most common and often the preferred method.

The indirect approach for demonstrating the portal system may be performed by separate or simultaneous injections into the celiac axis and the superior mesenteric arteries. In the separate injection method, the catheter is introduced into the femoral artery via the Seldinger method and guided through the vessels until it reaches the celiac axis. After catheter placement, a contrast medium is injected and the vessels are radiographed. On completion of the filming, the catheter is repositioned into the superior mesenteric artery, and a second contrast medium injection is made with appropriate filming.

In the separate celiac axis catheterization, it may be necessary to perform a superselective catheterization. This involves the catheterization of the hepatic artery or splenic artery, which are branches of the celiac axis. Superselective catheterization provides a better demonstration of the splenic and hepatic arterial system. This is particularly true when the hepatic artery is catheterized, because there is no superimposition by the left gastric, gastroepiploic, or splenic arteries. Catheterization of the celiac axis or its branches provides visualization of the arterial, capillary, and portal phases.

The same results may be obtained by simultaneously catheterizing the celiac axis and superior mesenteric arteries. This is accomplished by catheterizing both femoral arteries, with one catheter positioned in the celiac axis and the other in the mesenteric artery. The injections into the arteries should be simultaneous. The demonstration of the venous system may be improved by injecting a vasodilator about 30 seconds before the contrast medium is injected. Typical vasodilators are tolazoline (Priscoline) and papaverine. Vasodilators should not be used in patients with arteriovenous malformations or with acute bleeding.

The direct approach to portal vein evaluations is not as popular as the indirect method. In the direct approach, the patient is placed in a supine position on the angiographic table with the left arm raised over the head. This position exposes the puncture site. The angiographer palpates the spleen to determine its size, shape, and location. A preliminary radiograph of the splenic area is taken to locate the spleen. Often, prior to exposing the preliminary radiograph, a lead marker is placed on the patient to assist in locating the spleen during the puncture. After the location of the spleen has been determined and the injection site prepared, a 20-gauge, 4″ needle with a sharp inner stylet and Teflon sheath is introduced into the appropriate intercostal space (generally, this is the 10th intercostal space). In patients with a small spleen, the puncture is made at a more posterior and superior location; in patients with a large spleen, the puncture is made at a more anterior and inferior site. To avoid puncturing the colon, the needle is introduced first transversely, then in a superior direction (Fig. 24–3). During the introduction of the needle, the patient suspends respiration on inspiration. After the needle is in the appropriate vessel, 1 to 3 ml of saline solution is injected to clear the needle. A venous backflow of blood confirms the proper location

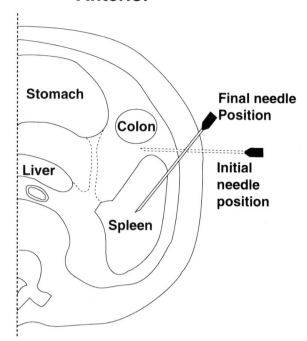

**Anterior**

Stomach

Colon

Liver

Spleen

**Final needle Position**

**Initial needle position**

**Posterior**

# Left side of patient

**Figure 24–3.** Needle placement for percutaneous splenic approach (transverse section).

of the needle. With the needle in the proper place, contrast medium is injected and filming is completed. A small amount of Gelfoam may be injected to reduce the possibility of hemorrhage before removing the needle.

If good opacification of the vessels or arterial pressure recordings are of primary importance, then it is best to employ the direct approach. The direct approach cannot be performed if the spleen has been removed or if there is severe bleeding. This approach can cause splenic or hepatic trauma or hemorrhage. The indirect approach is advantageous because it does not injure the spleen or liver, can be performed in the presence of bleeding, can demonstrate the portal vein when the spleen has been removed, and can assess underlying pathology. Disadvantages of the indirect approach are that there is poor venous opacification and arterial pressures cannot be recorded. Table 24–1 is a summary of the advantages and disadvantages of each approach.

## CATHETERS

When the indirect approach is employed for selective catheterization of the celiac axis or the superior mesenteric artery, a catheter with two side holes should be used to prevent catheter recoil during the injection. The cobra catheter (Fig. 24–4) is most often used for the femoral approach to these arteries. Other catheters

Table 24-1. **Direct Versus Indirect Approach**

| Approach | Advantage | Disadvantage |
|----------|-----------|--------------|
| Direct | Better opacification | Cannot be done if spleen has been removed |
| | Can record pressures | Cannot do if severe bleeding is present |
| Indirect | No injury to liver or spleen | Poorer opacification |
| | Can do if bleeding diathesis is present | Cannot record pressures |
| | Can do if spleen is absent | |
| | Can assess underlying pathology | |

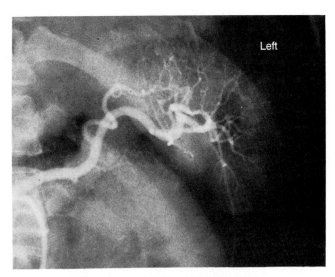

**Figure 24-5.** Normal splenoportography.

used are the Rosch curve, RC1 and RC2, or the shepherd's hook. A deflector wire can be employed to adjust the curve of the catheter to facilitate catheter placement. An end-hole catheter should be employed for superselective catheterization. As previously mentioned, the direct punctures for assessing the portal system require the use of Teflon sheath needles.

## CONTRAST MEDIA

Injections into the celiac or the superior mesenteric arteries require 35 to 50 ml of a high concentration contrast medium, injected at a rate of 8 to 12 ml/sec. A superselective injection into the hepatic artery requires 35 to 45 ml of contrast medium injected at a rate of 6 to 8 ml/sec.

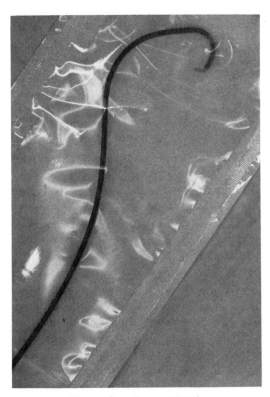

**Figure 24-4.** Cobra catheter.

## POSITIONING AND FILMING

The radiographic position that best demonstrates the liver and spleen is the supine position. Care should be taken to include the lower thoracic region and upper abdomen at midinspiration. The upper thoracic region is included if esophageal varices are suspected. A right posterior oblique position may be used for superior mesenteric injections to demonstrate the junction of the superior mesenteric and portal vein. This position is also useful for celiac injections to visualize esophagogastric varices.

Filming should last for a minimum of 20 seconds at a suggested rate of 2 frames/sec for 4 seconds (arterial phase) and 1 frame/sec for 16 to 20 seconds (capillary and venous phases). A postprocedural film is taken to assess extrasplenic contrast medium extravasation.

## COMPLICATIONS

The femoral approach is characterized by complications that are normally associated with angiographic punctures, for example, hematoma at puncture site. The direct percutaneous approach has been known to cause intra-abdominal hemorrhaging and extrasplenic deposits of contrast medium.

## SOME ANGIOGRAPHIC FINDINGS

During direct percutaneous splenoportography, the normal spleen is imaged as a small pool of contrast medium. The spleen is divided into several compartments; therefore, the entire spleen does not opacify (Fig. 24-5). The contrast medium drains from the spleen into the splenic vein and then into the portal vein. The portal vein forms a 40- to 55-degree angle with the vertebral column. If the angle is less than 40 degrees, liver atrophy may be indicated.

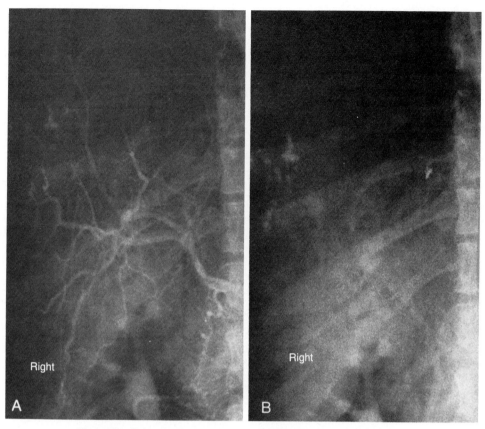

**Figure 24-6.** Hemangioma of liver: (*A*) arterial phase; (*B*) postinjection.

Other angiographic findings of splenoportography include obstruction of the portal vein, cirrhosis of the liver, ruptured spleen, and tumors (Figs. 24-6, 24-7). Arteriography has demonstrated aneurysms, tumors, vascular narrowing, and arteriovenous malformations.

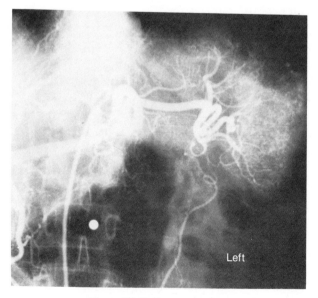

**Figure 24-7.** Ruptured spleen.

## REVIEW QUESTIONS

1. The celiac axis arises at the level of _____.
   A. T-10
   B. T-12
   C. L-2
   D. L-4

2. The afferent tributaries of the portal vein are formed by the union of the _____, inferior mesenteric, left gastric, and splenic veins.
   A. superior mesenteric
   B. inferior vena cava
   C. hepatic vein
   D. celiac axis

3. _____ is recommended as part of preprocedural care for angiography of the portal system.
   A. Prothrombin time assessment
   B. Chest x ray
   C. CBC
   D. Cardiac assessment

4. A normal hemoglobin level of a man or woman is _____ g/dl.
   A. 8
   B. 10
   C. 12
   D. 14

5. Superselective catheterization provides better visualization of the hepatic artery because _____.
   A. it requires less contrast medium
   B. the filming rate is faster
   C. it prevents catheter recoil
   D. there is no superimposition of other arteries

6. Demonstration of the venous system may be improved by injecting (a) _____ about 30 seconds before contrast medium injection.
   A. muscle relaxant
   B. vasoconstrictor
   C. vasodilator
   D. epinephrine

7. Indirect approach is advantageous because _____.
   A. it has good venous opacification
   B. it can be performed in the presence of bleeding
   C. arterial pressures can be recorded
   D. no catheter recoil occurs

8. A(n) _____ may be used for superior mesenteric injection to demonstrate the junction of the superior mesenteric and portal vein.
   A. LPO
   B. supine
   C. RAO
   D. RPO

9. List three branches of the celiac axis.

10. List three indications for angiography of the portal system.

## BIBLIOGRAPHY

Abrams, H: Angiography, Vol 2, ed 3. Little, Brown & Co, Boston, 1983.

Johnsrude, I, Jackson, D, and Dunnick, NR: A Practical Approach to Angiography. Little, Brown & Co, Boston, 1979.

Katzen, B: Interventional Diagnostic and Therapeutic Procedures. Springer-Verlag, New York, 1980.

Leger, L: Splenoportography. Charles C Thomas, Springfield, IL, 1966.

Luzsa, G: X-ray Anatomy of the Vascular System. JB Lippincott, Philadelphia, 1974.

McNulty, J: Radiology of the Liver. WB Saunders, Philadelphia, 1977.

Meschan, I: An Atlas of Anatomy Basic to Radiology. WB Saunders, Philadelphia, 1975.

White, R: Fundamentals of Vascular Radiology. Lea & Febiger, Philadelphia, 1976.

# CHAPTER 25

# Renal Angiography

*Jeanne L. Neuman, ARRT(R)(CV)*
*Marianne R. Tortorici, EdD, ARRT(R)*

There are several imaging modalities employed to image the kidneys. Computed tomography (CT), ultrasound, magnetic resonance imaging (MRI), nuclear medicine, and intravenous pyelography (IVP) may be used to demonstrate kidney pathology. However, renal angiography is the modality of choice for visualization of the renal blood circulation. Often, a renin study is performed in conjunction with a renal angiogram. This study is useful in assessing kidney function by analyzing the renin level in blood withdrawn from the kidney and inferior vena cava (IVC).

This chapter focuses on the technique and filming for renal angiography. Also presented is a summary of some angiographic pathologies, a brief description of a renin study, and interventional procedures.

## ANATOMY

The kidneys are bean-shaped, paired organs that remove waste products from the blood through the process of glomerular filtration. This process involves a tiny branch of the renal artery that divides into a net of capillaries inside a membranous sac called Bowman's capsule. This capillary net is called the glomerulus. Here filtration takes place by allowing water and finely dissolved particles to pass out of the capillary wall into the sac. The fluid filtered out of the blood is transformed into urine and passes through a system of tubules, finally emptying into the renal pelvis. The capillaries inside Bowman's capsule reunite to form another tiny arteriole that leaves the capsule and communicates with the renal venous system through another series of capillary beds.

The renal artery rises from the aorta between the inferior and superior mesenteric arteries (at approximately the level of L1-2) and enters the hilum of the kidney (Fig. 25–1). Approximately 70 to 75 percent of the population have a single main renal artery feeding each kidney. The right renal artery branches from the abdominal aorta, is directed downward, and is usually positioned a little more anterior and superior than the left renal artery. The renal arteries give rise to the anterior and posterior arterial branches, which in turn

**239**

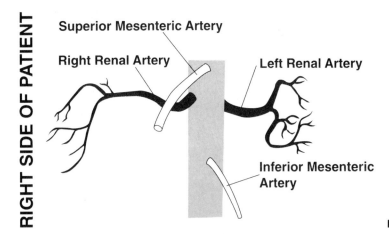

Figure 25–1. Location of the mesenteric and renal arteries.

branch into segmental arteries (Fig. 25–2). The anterior branch supplies the renal lobes of the lower pole and, as the name indicates, the anterior aspect of the kidney. The posterior branch supplies the renal lobes of the upper pole and the posterior aspect of the kidney. The segmental arteries feed the various parts of the kidney, including the apical, upper, middle, lower, and posterior segments. The segmental arteries divide into the interlobar arteries, which transport the blood to the glomeruli, tubules, and capillaries, where waste is filtered from the blood. The filtered blood is then returned to the heart via the renal veins and inferior vena cava.

In those individuals who have more than one renal artery entering one kidney, the additional arteries usually arise either superiorly or inferiorly to the main renal artery and provide blood to the area of the kidney they enter. For example, an accessory renal artery arising superiorly to the main renal artery would serve as the primary source of blood for the upper pole of the kidney. Multiple arteries are usually associated with such anomalies as horseshoe kidney and kidney dupli-

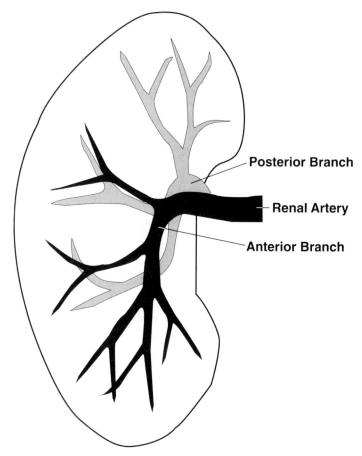

Figure 25–2. Renal circulation.

cation. It is important to identify multiple arteries, since all arteries must be catheterized and opacified to complete the angiogram. In general, multiple arteries only supply small portions of the kidney; therefore, nonopacification of these arteries may lead to a false diagnosis.

Often when the main renal artery is occluded, one or more other vessels collateralize to supply the kidney. The three primary vessel networks that collateralize are the pericapsular, perihilar, and periureteric arteries.

Blood return from the kidneys is through the renal veins. These vessels arise from the IVC at the level of L1-2. The right renal vein enters the inferior vena cava (IVC) posteriorly and is often noted for leaving a slight indentation in the wall of the IVC. The left renal vein is longer than the right, making the left kidney the organ of choice for kidney transplant.

## INDICATIONS

Renal arteriography is often performed after a mass or other pathology has been identified on an IVP, CT, nuclear medicine scan, or ultrasound scan. The renal arteriogram is helpful in identifying tumors and cysts. It is especially useful in distinguishing renal neoplasms in the perirenal area since this condition cannot be visualized by CT or ultrasonography. Renal angiography is also used to evaluate the condition of the kidneys in potential kidney donors and in recipients of kidney transplants (this helps determine if there is any rejection). Other indications for renal angiography include renal trauma, acute tubular necrosis and vascular occlusion, hypertension, and aneurysms.

Renal venography is performed to assess the patency of the renal veins, which may be occluded by a blood clot or tumor. Since it is not unusual for a tumor to extend into the IVC, renal venograms are often performed in conjunction with an IVC angiogram.

## PREPROCEDURAL CARE AND CAUTIONS

Renal angiography is contraindicated in cases where the patient's condition is too poor to undergo the procedure, for example, where there is kidney failure. Elevated creatinine and blood urea nitrogen (BUN) are indications of kidney failure. In these patients an injection of contrast medium may further worsen the condition of the kidney, especially if the patient is dehydrated.

Hydrating the patient is helpful in preventing renal failure and is recommended in patients with renal failure, multiple myeloma, sickle cell anemia, or pheochromocytoma. Hydration is especially important in pheochromocytoma because introduction of contrast medium in these patients may initiate uncontrollable paroxysmal hypertension. Premedicating these patients with a drug such as phentolamine (Regitine) often helps decrease the possibility of inducing hypertension.

The hypertensive patient has an increased risk of hematoma or postprocedural bleeding. To decrease the risk, these patients should be hydrated and premedicated with a drug such as nifedipine.

A history of adverse reaction to contrast media is also a contraindication to renal angiography. These patients may be premedicated with diphenhydramine (Benadryl) or corticosteroids, which will enable them to have the procedure. Where there has been a previous adverse contrast medium reaction, the radiologist, in consultation with the attending physician, should make the decision as to whether or not to proceed with the procedure.

Care should be taken to postpone renal angiography for 24 hours after retrograde pyelography. This will allow the kidney(s) to recover from any irritation or minor trauma that may have occurred during the retrograde procedure.

As with all angiographic procedures, it is important that the angiographer discuss the procedure and possible complications with the patient and obtain an informed consent.

## EQUIPMENT

The equipment employed for renal angiography is similar to that used for any standard angiographic procedure and includes a rapid serial film changer, an electromechanical injector, an electrocardiograph, and the normal supplementary equipment needed for catheterization. (Refer to Chapter 19, Catheterization Methods and Patient Management, and Chapter 17, Supplementary Catheterization Equipment, for more information.) Only a frontal film changer is needed since biplane filming is not performed. An alternate filming method is cine loop digital imaging with the ability to freeze frame images for transfer to a multiformat camera or laser imager. A cine loop captures, in real time, contrast medium on a video disk. The image may be viewed continuously, that is, as a movie, or by freezing the frame. The freeze-frame setting allows for transference of the image onto film.

## APPROACHES

The percutaneous femoral approach is the preferred method of catheterization, except for patients with advanced aortoileal atheromatous disease. In these instances a translumbar or transaxillary approach may be performed. If the translumbar approach is employed, the needle should be inserted into the abdominal aorta above the renal arteries. The translumbar approach is not conducive to selective renal angiography because intralobar tumors may not be demonstrated via the translumbar technique. The axillary method allows for selective catheterization of the renal arteries. Regardless of the approach employed, an abdominal aortogram should be performed to assess the number and status of the renal arteries. To properly assess the renal arteries, the injection should occur above the location of the renal branches.

After an abdominal aortogram has been completed, it may be necessary to perform a selective renal angiogram. In this approach, a catheter is placed in the renal artery. Care should be taken to avoid placing the catheter in a segmental artery because this may cause renal damage during the injection of contrast medium. Selective renal angiography is advantageous in assessing intralobar tumors and eliminates the superimposition of the superior mesenteric artery over the kidney as so often occurs in abdominal aortography.

## CATHETERS

The catheter most commonly employed for the abdominal aortogram is a pigtail catheter with multiple side holes. It should have a high pressure limit for rapid, high volume contrast medium injection. Selective renal angiography catheters are the visceral, the cobra, or a double- or single-curve catheter, with only one end hole. The catheter employed for renal transplants has a very sharp curve with one end hole (Fig. 25–3). The catheter is placed in the contralateral femoral artery to avoid injury to the transplanted kidney (Fig. 25–4). For an axillary approach, a single-curve catheter is most effective.

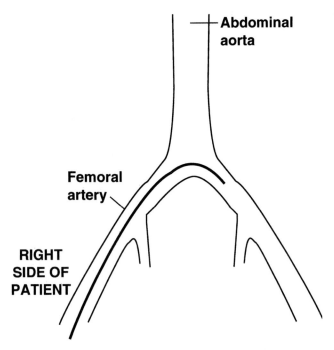

**Figure 25–4.** Catheter placement for left renal transplant.

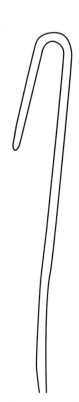

**Figure 25–3.** Renal transplant catheter.

## CONTRAST MEDIA

Either an ionic or a nonionic contrast medium is used for renal angiography. The nonionic medium reduces the risk and intensity of reaction and is more comfortable for the patient. The quantity of medium used depends on the area to be injected. Abdominal aortography employs 40 to 50 ml of a fairly high concentration contrast medium with a recommended rate of injection of 20 to 25 ml/sec. Thus, the total time of injection is 1½ to 2 seconds. Selective renal angiography requires a smaller volume of contrast medium. The suggested volume is 6 to 10 ml at a rate of 5 to 6 ml/sec. Selecting a rate rise of 0.1 second helps prevent catheter whipping, which in turn helps avoid dislodging the catheter. An inferior vena cavagram requires 30 to 40 ml of contrast medium delivered at a rate of 15 to 20 ml/sec. Selective renal venography employs a contrast medium volume of 18 to 24 ml delivered at a rate of 8 to 10 ml/sec.

Typical vessels in neoplastic tumors are dilated and are often obscured during renal angiography by the superimposition of the normal renal arteries. Administering epinephrine into the renal arteries just prior to introducing contrast medium helps delineate the tumor by constricting the renal artery and its branches. This causes the normal vessels to constrict and not opacify, while the dilated tumor vessels collect the contrast medium, thereby outlining the pathology (Fig. 25–5).

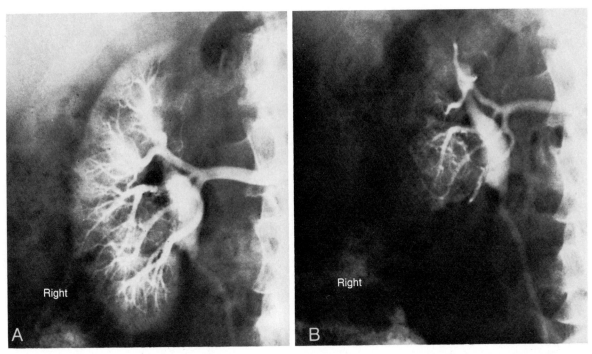

**Figure 25-5.** (*A*) Renal arteries before epinephrine administration and (*B*) after epinephrine administration.

A typical epinephrine dose is 5 to 10 micrograms ($\mu$g) (to obtain 10 $\mu$g of epinephrine/ml, dilute 1 ml of 1 : 1000 epinephrine in 100 ml of glucose and water or saline). Modern research indicates that the use of epinephrine is not without complications. It is important to perform a postepinephrine contrast injection to confirm that the vessels have returned to their normal size.

## POSITIONING AND FILMING

Recall that prior to selective renal angiography filming, an aortogram is performed using a high volume catheter. A rapid filming sequence for aortography requires the patient to be supine with the central ray directed at L2-3. The filming must include both kidneys and the iliac bifurcation. A common filming sequence is 2 films/sec for 3 seconds and 1 film/sec for 6 to 8 seconds for a total of 12 to 14 films.

In selective renal angiography, the high volume catheter is exchanged for a visceral catheter and placed in the selected renal artery. The patient is positioned supine and the central ray is directed to the kidney of interest. The angiogram should include the entire kidney and the abdominal aorta. Sometimes oblique positions (RPO and LPO) are used to demonstrate alternate views of the kidney. For example, a 30- to 45-degree posterior oblique position demonstrates the kidney of the side up "en face" or parallel to the image plane. Some institutions also perform magnification studies. However, there seems to be some controversy as to the necessity of performing magnification renal angiography routinely. The filming rate is usually 2 to

3 frames/sec during injection (1½ to 2 seconds), followed by 1 frame/sec for 2 seconds and 1 frame every other second for 6 seconds. If epinephrine is employed, the filming should begin 30 seconds after the injection of epinephrine and should be slower than the nonepinephrine filming rate because of vasoconstriction.

The filming rate should be set to demonstrate the arterial, nephron, and venous phases of the kidney. The arterial phase is useful in demonstrating the lumen size and the number and length of the renal arteries (the number of renal arteries can be evaluated only in abdominal aortography). The nephron phase represents the contrast medium in the glomeruli, tubules, capillaries, and small veins. This phase demonstrates filling defects, an abnormal silhouette of the kidney, and the extent of renal tissue patency. Since the kidney has filtered out most of the contrast medium prior to the venous phase, this phase is best demonstrated by renal venography. Arterial injection demonstrates the renal vein and the IVC, but care should be taken not to formulate an opinion regarding the condition of the venous circulation without further examination.

The filming for renal venography is very similar to that for renal arteriography. Filming of the IVC occurs prior to any selective catheterization. For the inferior vena cavagram, the patient is positioned in the same manner as for an aortogram. Since blood flow is cephalad, the catheter is positioned inferior to the renal veins. To opacify the renal veins, a selective catheterization is performed. The filming sequence is slower than for renal arteriography and occurs while the patient performs the Valsalva technique. A recommended renal venography filming rate is 1 frame/sec for 10 to 15 seconds.

After filming, the normal postprocedural care is provided. Refer to Chapter 19, Catheterization Methods and Patient Management, for specifics.

## RENIN STUDY

A renin study may be performed in conjunction with a renal angiogram. Renin is a chemical secreted by the kidneys to assist in the maintenance of blood pressure. To maintain homeostasis, when there is a decrease in blood pressure there is a corresponding increase in the secretion of renin from the kidneys. Each kidney manufactures renin separately corresponding to the amount of blood each kidney is receiving. If a kidney is subjected to decreased blood flow, renin is secreted to raise the blood pressure sufficiently to adequately perfuse that kidney. According to SmithKline Beecham Clinical Laboratories, normal renin levels depend upon the patient's diet and posture (supine or upright). For a patient on a normal sodium diet in the supine position, the renin level range is 0.2 to 2.3 ng/ml/h, which increases to 1.3 to 4.0 ng/ml/h in the upright position. An abnormal increase in renin secretion can result in hypertension. For assessment of renin levels, blood samples are taken from each kidney, the IVC, and peripheral sites. For example, if blood drawn from the right kidney has an elevated renin level while levels in other blood drawing sites are normal, then this may indicate the presence of a right renal artery stenosis. A similar conclusion may be made when the left renal vein renin level is elevated while other sites are normal; that is, there may be a left renal artery stenosis.

## INTERVENTIONAL PROCEDURES

Unlike many interventional procedures, renal interventional techniques are often performed along with the renal angiogram (based on the findings of the renal angiogram). An interventional procedure is performed by introducing the appropriate catheter following angiographic filming. Three common interventional procedures are angioplasty, embolization, and thrombolysis. The following is a brief summary of these procedures. The reader is referred to Chapter 29, Vascular Interventional Angiography, for an in-depth discussion of these examinations.

Renal angioplasty employs a balloon catheter to dilate a stenotic renal artery. Balloon length is 4 to 5 cm, and balloon width ranges from 2 to 3 mm. A vascular access introducer that can accommodate an angioplasty balloon enables catheter exchanges without difficulty. This procedure has a good success rate, especially in cases involving atheromatous plaques or fibromuscular disease.

Renal embolization is often performed as a preoperative procedure to stop the blood flow to a malignant part of the kidney or arteriovenous malformation. This may be achieved by using either a device, such as a balloon catheter, or pharmaceuticals, such as polyvinyl alcohol.

Thrombolysis employs a thrombolytic agent to dis-

solve clots within the renal artery. This procedure may be used in conjunction with angioplasty to restore renal artery patency.

## COMPLICATIONS

Besides the common angiographic complications, renal angiography has been known to cause fibrin intrarenal emboli, which are usually small and cause partial obstruction. Usually the emboli do not cause permanent damage and dissipate within an hour.

A more severe complication occurs when contrast medium is injected into a segmental artery, obstructing the flow of blood and causing the contrast medium to remain in the vessels. This complication may cause tissue necrosis and permanent kidney damage. A less traumatic complication is renal spasm, occurring during selective angiographic injection. Overfilling of a vessel should be avoided because it can simulate a vascular tumor.

## SOME ANGIOGRAPHIC FINDINGS

Most pathologies of the kidney are tumors or cysts and vascular abnormalities. Tumors may be malignant or benign. Approximately 65 to 75 percent of malignant tumors are hypervascular with large vessels, neovascularity, and irregular margins. Renal stenosis may be caused by either atheromatous disease or fibromuscular disease, resulting in hypertension that is poorly controlled by antihypertensive medication.

In children, the most common malignancy is Wilms' tumor. Benign tumors, such as angiomyolipoma or hamartoma, are composed of smooth muscle and fatty tis-

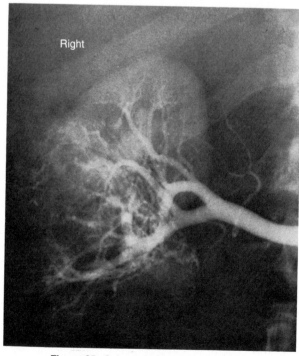

Right

**Figure 25-6.** Large right renal carcinoma.

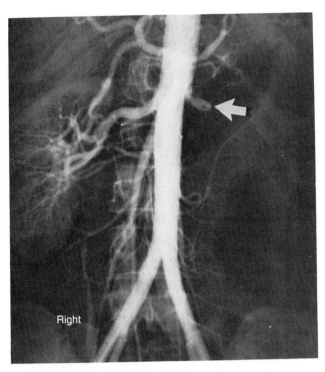

**Figure 25-7.** Traumatic dissection of left renal artery.

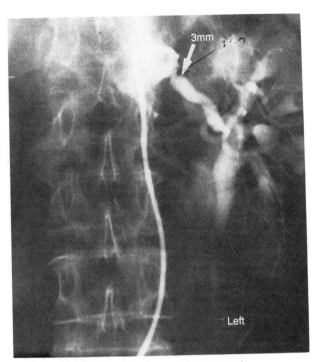

**Figure 25-9.** Left renal artery stenosis.

sue. Often the increased fatty tissue can be demonstrated on CT, which helps differentiate these tumors from malignancies. Adenomas vary in the degree of vascularity demonstrated radiographically and often require a biopsy for proper diagnosis.

Pathologies associated with hypertension may be caused by lesions near the kidney and include aortic atheroma at the origin of the renal artery, aortic dissection, aortic occlusion, and neurofibromatosis. Hypertensive lesions within the renal arteries, veins, and kidneys include renal artery stenosis caused by atherosclerosis; renal artery stenosis originating from fibromuscular dysplasia; trauma to the vessel; and renal vein thrombosis. Figures 25-6 through 25-15 demonstrate some common pathologies.

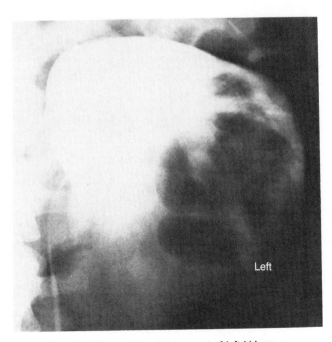

**Figure 25-8.** Large benign cyst of left kidney.

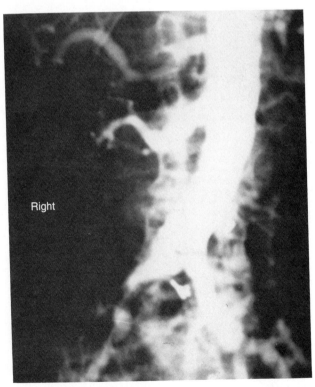

**Figure 25-10.** Abdominal aortogram on a 74-year-old woman with poorly controlled hypertension. Note absence of left renal artery. Her kidney had "autonephrectomized."

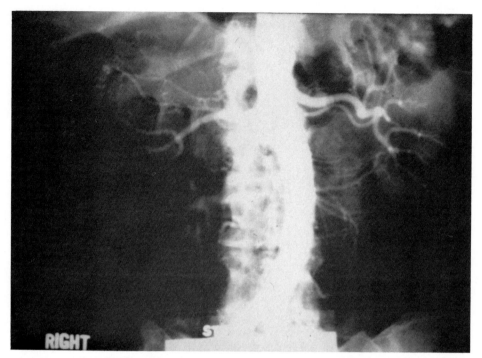

**Figure 25-11.** Abdominal aortogram on a 63-year-old woman with mass in the upper pole of the right kidney seen on an IVP, renal ultrasound, and CT scan. Arteriography performed for preoperative vascular map.

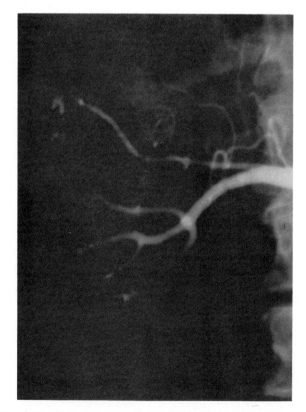

**Figure 25-12.** Selective catheterization of right renal artery of the 63-year-old woman depicted in Figure 25-11, showing hypervascular lesion in the right upper pole, as suspected.

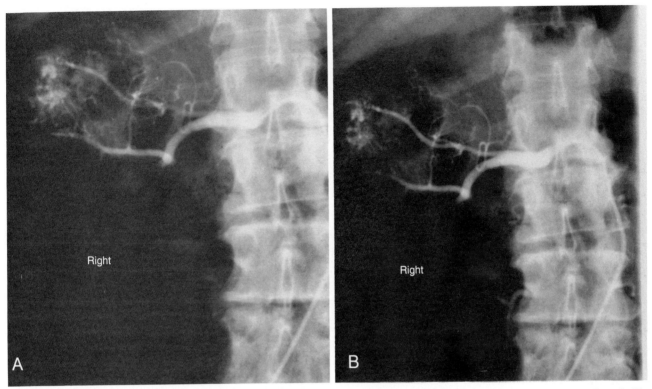

**Figure 25–13.** (*A*) Right renal arteriogram following injection of epinephrine, constricting normal vessels (tumor vessels remain unaffected); (*B*) post–epinephrine injection, 1 second later. Notice "puddling" of contrast in aberrant tumor vessels.

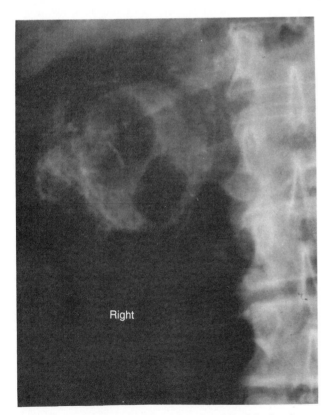

**Figure 25–14.** Venous phase following epinephrine injection demonstrates enhanced right renal arteriogram with remarkable tumor staining of right upper pole.

## REVIEW QUESTIONS

1. _____ examination(s) of the kidney is (are) often performed prior to a renal angiogram.
   A. CT
   B. Ultrasound
   C. IVP
   D. Nuclear medicine
   E. All of the above

2. The _____ approach is the preferred method of catheterization for a renal angiogram.
   A. axillary
   B. femoral
   C. translumbar
   D. brachial

3. _____ is often a result of renal artery stenosis.
   A. Hypertension
   B. Hamartoma
   C. Angiomyolipoma
   D. Neurofibromatosis

4. _____ percent of the population have multiple renal arteries.
   A. Ten
   B. Twenty-five
   C. Forty-five
   D. Sixty
   E. Seventy-five

5. Abdominal aortography requires ____ ml of contrast medium injection.
   A. 6 to 8
   B. 10 to 20
   C. 40 to 50
   D. 60 to 70

6. ____ is injected prior to contrast medium to help evaluate tumors.
   A. Valium
   B. Benadryl
   C. Saline
   D. Epinephrine

7. A balloon catheter may be employed as an interventional technique for ____.
   A. renal stenosis
   B. tumors
   C. cysts
   D. hypotension

8. List two lesions often demonstrated on a renal venogram.

9. ____ is a useful precaution for patients who have sickle cell anemia, myeloma, or kidney failure.
   A. Epinephrine
   B. Valium
   C. Hydration
   D. Fasting

10. Epinephrine is used to ____ the vessels.
    A. dilate
    B. flush
    C. constrict
    D. thin the blood in

11. Thrombolysis is used to ____.
    A. dissolve clots
    B. occlude the renal artery
    C. distend the vessel
    D. coagulate the blood

## BIBLIOGRAPHY

Abrams, H: Angiography, Vol 2, ed 3. Little, Brown & Co, Boston, 1983.

Blackwell, H and Lock, H: The role of angiography in renal trauma. Radiography 43(513):203, September 1977.

Bosniak, M, et al: Epinephrine-enhanced renal angiography in renal mass lesions: Is it worth performing? AJR 129(4):647, October 1977.

Bunnell, I: Selective Renal Arteriography. Charles C Thomas, Springfield, IL, 1968.

Gerlock, L and Goncharenko, V: The epinephrine effect in renal angiography revisited. Clin Radiol 29(4):387, July 1978.

Hudson, E: Renal Arteriography: X-ray Focus, Vol 12(2). Ilford, Limited, London, 1973.

Jander, H and Tonkin, I: Epinephrine enhanced renal angiography in diagnosis of hamartoma (angiomyolipoma): A reevaluation. Radiology 132(1):61, July 1979.

Johnsrude, I, Jackson, D, and Dunnick, NR: A Practical Approach to Angiography, ed 2. Little, Brown & Co, Boston, 1987.

Kandarpa, K: Handbook of Cardiovascular and Interventional Radiologic Procedures. Little, Brown & Co, Boston, 1989.

Katzberg, R, et al: Renal renin and hemodynamic responses to selective renal artery catheterization and angiography. Invest Radiol 12(5):381, September–October 1977.

Katzen, B: Interventional diagnostic and therapeutic procedures. Springer-Verlag, New York, 1980.

Kincaid, O and Davis, G: Renal Angiography. Year Book Medical Publishers, Chicago, 1966.

Lee, W, Pillari, G, and Wind, E: Lateral view in selective renal angiography. Radiology 123(1):227, April 1977.

Luzsa, G: X-ray Anatomy of the Vascular System. JB Lippincott, Philadelphia, 1974.

Meschan, I: An Atlas of Anatomy Basic to Radiology. WB Saunders, Philadelphia, 1975.

Moss, D and Freeman, R: Renal angiography and the management of severe closed renal trauma. Aust NZ J Surg 47(4):462, August 1977.

Rosenfield, A, Glickman, M, and Hodson, J: Diagnostic Imaging in Renal Disease. Appleton-Century-Crofts, New York, 1979.

Snopek, A: Fundamentals of Special Radiographic Procedures. WB Saunders, Philadelphia, 1992.

Spriggs, D and Brantley, R: Recognition of renal artery spasm during renal angiography. Radiology 127(2):363, May 1978.

White, R: Fundamentals of Vascular Radiology. Lea & Febiger, Philadelphia, 1976.

Wojtowycz, M: Handbook in Radiology: Interventional Radiology and Angiography. Year Book Medical Publishers, Chicago, 1990.

# CHAPTER 26

# Abdomen and Lower Extremity Angiography

*Marianne R. Tortorici, EdD, ARRT(R)*

Angiography of the abdominal aorta and its distal branches is a significant examination in the assessment of vascular disease of the abdomen and lower extremities. In addition to the diagnostic aspect, abdominal angiography is also employed for vascular interventional therapy. This chapter discusses the diagnostic aspect of abdominal angiography with lower extremity runoffs. The therapeutic aspect of this procedure is located in Chapter 29, Vascular Interventional Radiology.

## ANATOMY

The abdominal aorta is a continuation of the thoracic aorta. This vessel is located approximately midline (it rests slightly to the left of the spine) in the body and anterior to the vertebral column. The major branches of the abdominal aorta of radiographic interest, from the proximal to the distal end, are the celiac axis, superior mesenteric, renal, and inferior mesenteric arteries (Fig. 26–1).

The abdominal aorta bifurcates at about the level of L-4 into the right and left common iliac arteries, which then divide into external and internal iliac arteries. The internal iliac artery supplies blood to the pelvis and pelvic organs. The external iliac artery forms the common femoral arteries, which supply blood to the lower extremities.

The common femoral artery branches into the deep femoral and femoral (superficial femoral) arteries (Fig. 26–2). The deep femoral artery divides into the medial and lateral femoral circumflex and perforating arteries. The femoral artery continues down the leg to become the popliteal artery at the level of the knee. The popliteal artery branches into the anterior tibial, posterior tibial, and peroneal (fibular) arteries. The anterior tibial artery continues, becoming the malleolar vessels, the tarsal vessels, and the dorsal plantar and dorsal metatarsal arteries of the foot. The posterior tibial artery terminates in the plantar arteries. The pero-

# RIGHT SIDE

# LEFT SIDE

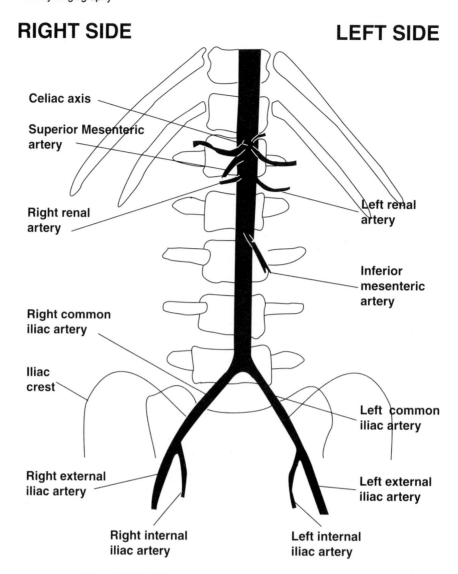

**Figure 26 – 1.** Major arterial branches of the abdominal aorta.

neal artery is an extension of the popliteal and feeds the tarsal vessels.

## INDICATIONS

Angiography of the abdominal or the pelvic arteries is indicated when there is a need to assess the nature, number, and course of the great vessels extending from the aorta. The procedure is employed to rule out the presence of aneurysms, congenital anomalies, stenosis, or occlusions. Abdominal angiography is also used for vascular interventional therapy.

Angiography of the lower extremities is indicated in cases of tumors or arteriosclerosis obliterans, nonhealing ulcers, rest pain, and poor circulation. Vascular pathologic conditions caused by arteriosclerosis obliterans may be demonstrated as emboli, arteriovenous malformations, or occlusions.

## EQUIPMENT

For abdominal angiography, the equipment is similar to that for any standard angiography procedure and includes a rapid film changer, an automatic injector, and the normal accessory equipment required for a femoral puncture. Angiography of the lower extremities requires similar basic routine angiographic equipment. For digital subtraction angiography (DSA), a DSA unit is required.

There are two basic types of tables employed for lower extremity angiography. The original type is a special femoral table that uses a long (72″) source-image distance and four to six cassettes of the 36″ × 14″ size. The cassettes are unique in that the screen speed varies. The different screen speeds help compensate for the different thicknesses of the extremity, producing a more uniform radiographic density on the radiograph. The fast portion of the screen (speed) is

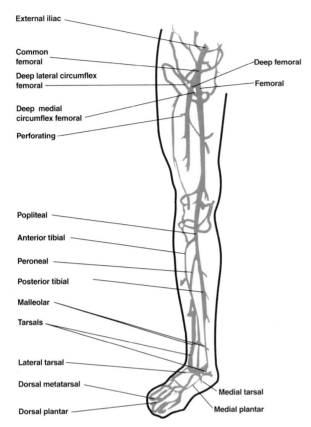

**Figure 26 – 2.** Major arterial branches of the lower extremity (From Johnsrude et al.: A Practical Approach to Angiography, ed. 2. Little, Brown, & Co., Boston, 1987, with permission).

Labels (top to bottom, left): External iliac, Common femoral, Deep lateral circumflex femoral, Deep medial circumflex femoral, Perforating, Popliteal, Anterior tibial, Peroneal, Posterior tibial, Malleolar, Tarsals, Lateral tarsal, Dorsal metatarsal, Dorsal plantar. (right): Deep femoral, Femoral, Medial tarsal, Medial plantar.

placed under the thickest part of the lower extremity (thigh), and the slow portion of the screen is located under the ankle area. Another method employed to compensate for the various thicknesses of the extremity is the use of a wedge filter (Fig. 26 – 3). The thickest part of the filter is placed over the thinnest part of the leg. Although this type of table is the original method used to perform lower extremity angiography, it is no longer in use. It is mentioned here as historic information.

The second and most common table is the movable tabletop or "stepping" table (see Fig. 12 – 13). Filming is accomplished with a rapid film changer positioned under the tabletop. Most stepping tables are designed with a minimum of four stopping positions. The distance the table moves between each step (exposure) can be programmed by the technologist. Usually the tabletop moves four or five times in increments of 10″. The operator selects the technical factors, for example, kVp, mA, and time and sets the appropriate film programming sequence.

## PREPROCEDURAL CARE AND CAUTIONS

In addition to the normal angiographic preparation, angiography of the lower extremities requires assessment of the iliac, femoral, and pedal pulses. If the femoral or iliac pulse on the catheterization side is absent, the contralateral side should be punctured. If bruits and scar tissue are present at the catheterization site, puncturing that area is contraindicated. It is also recommended that the contralateral side be employed if the affected leg is ischemic.

The angiographer should be aware that the injection of contrast medium in the lower extremities is painful. Using nonionic, low osmolarity contrast agents has been helpful in reducing pain. Also, an injection of 2 percent lidocaine prior to contrast medium injection has been somewhat successful in alleviating pain, but there seems to be some controversy regarding the effectiveness of lidocaine. Some authors suggest that it is counterproductive. The effectiveness of employing lidocaine should be evaluated by each angiographer.

## APPROACHES

Three approaches for abdominal angiography include the percutaneous femoral, translumbar, and axillary. Of these, the percutaneous femoral approach is the most common. However, sometimes the femoral approach cannot be used for the lower leg because of the tortuosity of the vessels. In this case, the angiographer must decide on either the less common translumbar or axillary approach.

## CATHETERS

When the abdominal aorta is the area of interest, an end-hole, multiple-side-hole catheter is used. The catheter is positioned at the level of T-12. Other abdominal

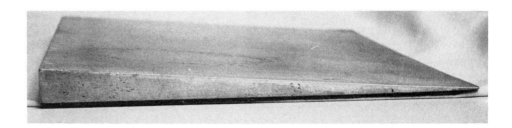

**Figure 26 – 3.** Wedge filter.

catheters include a pigtail catheter and a ring catheter with multiple side holes.

If the lower extremities are to be studied, an end-hole, multiple-side-hole catheter is employed at the level of L-4. In selective extremity angiography, a sharp, curved catheter is introduced into the common iliac artery from the contralateral femoral artery. An alternate technique for selective extremity catheterization is through the use of a bilateral femoral injection. In this method, catheters with only one end hole are placed in each femoral artery. The catheters are connected by a Y Luer-Lok to fill both catheters simultaneously with one injection.

## CONTRAST MEDIA

Demonstration of the abdominal aorta requires an injection of 40 to 50 ml of 50 to 60 percent concentration of either ionic or nonionic contrast media. The rate of injection is 20 to 25 ml/sec with a total injection time of 1.5 to 2 seconds. Angiography of the lower extremities requires a lesser amount of contrast medium. The recommended dosage for examination of the lower extremity is 20 to 30 ml of contrast medium for unilateral extremity angiography and 50 to 70 ml of contrast medium for bilateral angiography at a rate of 8 to 10 ml/sec.

Since patients having angiography of the extremities often have poor circulation, it may be difficult to visualize vessels distal to the popliteal artery. Therefore, it may be necessary to find a means of improving the flow of contrast medium to the distal end of the extremity. Several methods have been developed to increase the distal blood flow, including the use of drugs (tolazoline or bradykinin), work hyperemia (exercise), the Valsalva maneuver, and blood pressure cuffs.

Drugs dilate the vessels, increasing blood flow to the feet. The Valsalva maneuver and work hyperemia increase aortic pressure, facilitating the blood flow to the distal aspect of the extremity. A blood pressure cuff can also be used to increase the blood flow. Positioning the pressure cuff above the knee level and inflating it 50 mg above the systolic pressure for 3 minutes decreases blood flow. Upon cuff deflation, there is an increased flow of blood to the feet. It is difficult to assess the effectiveness of these methods to increase distal blood flow. A review of the literature indicates that these methods may have some success, but it is evident that a safe, reliable, and effective method needs to be developed.

## POSITIONING AND FILMING

Imaging may be performed using a routine angiography or DSA technique. Research indicates that the quality of both methods is equal for upper arterial filming. However, intra-arterial DSA is more effective in demonstrating the distal (pedal) arteries. Although DSA is the modality of choice for distal imaging, it does have disadvantages, including a small field size, the inability to perform biplane filming, and the presence of motion artifacts. DSA is advantageous because it reduces patient pain and less contrast medium is needed for injection. However, some angiographers argue that although less medium is necessary for imaging, DSA often requires multiple injections because of the limited field size; thus, the total amount of contrast medium is the same.

Rapid serial filming of the abdominal aorta is performed with the patient in the supine position at the recommended rate of 2 frames/sec for 3 seconds, followed by 1 frame/sec for 3 seconds, and then 1 frame every other second for 6 seconds. Care should be taken to demonstrate both the proximal and distal ends of obstructed vessels. If there is a need to improve the visualization of the bifurcation or common iliac vessels, oblique views may be taken. A right posterior oblique position demonstrates the right iliac artery, and a left posterior oblique view demonstrates the left iliac artery.

Filming of the lower extremity is performed with the patient in the supine position with the feet internally rotated 30 degrees. Because of the varying thickness of the lower extremities, the x-ray tube heel effect should be employed to its advantage by placing the cathode end of the x-ray tube toward the thickest part of the extremity (thigh).

Other methods for producing radiographs of uniform density include the use of a wedge filter, special cones, special cassettes, or a stepping tabletop. The film rate depends on the patient's circulation and the speed of tabletop shifting. The majority of patients undergoing examinations of the lower extremity have reduced blood circulation rates. A suggested filming rate is 2 frames/sec for 4 seconds, followed by 1 frame/sec for 8 seconds. If work hyperemia or the Valsalva technique is employed, the circulation rate should increase, reducing the filming time.

## COMPLICATIONS

The complications in abdominal and lower extremity angiography are limited to those normally associated with percutaneous or translumbar punctures. However, there have been some research studies that indicate there may be an increased rate of femoral thrombosis in patients with atherosclerotic obstructive disease.

## SOME ANGIOGRAPHIC FINDINGS

The major angiographic findings include aneurysms (Fig. 26–4), arteriovenous malformations, tumors, and atherosclerosis. The patterns of atherosclerosis vary according to the stage of the disease. Atherosclerosis is most commonly found in vessels that have sharp bends or at bifurcations. The most common areas of vascular involvement are the femoral artery (58 percent) and the iliac arteries (34 percent). The deep femoral artery is the chief collateral artery when the femoral is occluded.

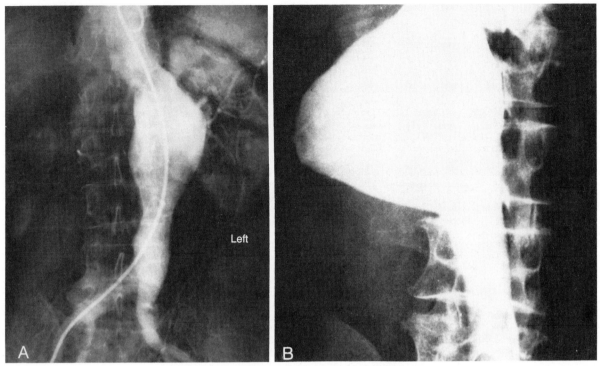

**Figure 26–4.** (*A*) Abdominal aneurysm; (*B*) ruptured aneurysm.

## REVIEW QUESTIONS

1. The abdominal aorta bifurcates at about the level of the _____ lumbar.
   A. second
   B. third
   C. fourth
   D. fifth

2. The _____ artery feeds blood to the pelvis and pelvic organs.
   A. internal iliac
   B. external iliac
   C. common femoral
   D. deep femoral

3. For rapid serial angiographic filming of the lower extremity, a _____ is required.
   A. stepping table
   B. pigtail catheter
   C. cineradiograph
   D. millimeter camera

4. Select the answer below that is *not* a reason to catheterize the contralateral side for abdominal and lower extremity angiography.
   A. affected leg is ischemic
   B. scar tissue is present on involved side
   C. iliac pulse is absent on affected side
   D. artery on involved side is movable

5. To help alleviate the pain of a lower extremity contrast medium injection, _____ may be administered prior to contrast medium.

   A. atropine
   B. Valium
   C. 2 percent lidocaine
   D. dextrose

6. For abdominal aortography, the tip of the catheter is placed at the level of _____.
   A. T-10
   B. T-12
   C. L-2
   D. L-4

7. To visualize the abdominal aorta, an injection volume of about _____ ml is suggested.
   A. 40 to 50
   B. 60 to 80
   C. 90 to 110
   D. greater than 110

8. _____ may be used to increase the blood flow to the lower extremities.
   A. Two percent lidocaine
   B. Dextrose
   C. Tolazoline
   D. A diuretic

9. When performing a lower extremity angiogram, the _____ method of filming is most effective in demonstrating the distal arteries.
   A. DSA
   B. rapid film changer
   C. cineradiography
   D. millimeter

10. List at least three indications for performing abdominal angiography.

## BIBLIOGRAPHY

Abrams, H: Angiography, Vol 2, ed 3. Little, Brown & Co, Boston, 1983.

Almén, T: Peripheral angiography with metrizamide. Diagn Imaging 48(4):206, 1979.

Blakeman, BM, Littooy, FN, and Baker, WH: Intra-arterial digital subtraction angiography as a method to study peripheral vascular disease. J Vasc Surg 4(2):168, August 1986.

Dardik, H, et al: Primary and adjunctive intra-arterial digital subtraction arteriography of the lower extremities. J Vasc Surg 3(4):599, April 1986.

Eisenberg, R, Mani, R, and Hedgcock, M: Pain associated with peripheral angiography: Is lidocaine effective? Radiology 127(1):109, April 1978.

Gordon, I and Westcott, J: Intraarterial lidocaine: An effective analgesia for peripheral angiography. Radiology 124(1):43, July 1977.

Holder, J and Dalrymple, G: Choosing a contrast material for aortofemoral runoff angiography. Radiology 128(3):787, September 1978.

Huff, JA, Kasemeyer, B, and Lutjen, G: Bilateral femoral angiography: A step by step approach. Radiol Technol 6(1):35, October 1989.

Johnsrude, I, Jackson, D, and Dunnick, NR: A Practical Approach to Angiography, ed 2. Little, Brown & Co, Boston, 1987.

Kandarpa, K: Handbook of Cardiovascular and Interventional Radiologic Procedures. Little, Brown & Co, Boston, 1989.

Kauffmann, G, et al: Indications and use of abdominal angiography in trauma. Cardiovasc Radiol 2(1):35, 1979.

Kogutt, M and Jander, H: Use of a curved multi-hole catheter for abdominal and femoral arteriography. Radiology 128(3):817, September 1978.

Luzsa, G: X-ray Anatomy of the Vascular System. JB Lippincott Co, Philadelphia, 1974.

Maeda, M, et al: Evaluation of peripheral vascular disease by intravenous digital subtraction angiography with the Fuji computed radiography (FCR) system. Digit Bilddiagn 7(1):15, March 1987.

Meschan, I: An Atlas of Anatomy Basic to Radiology. WB Saunders, Philadelphia, 1975.

Novelline, R, et al: Recent advances in abdominal angiography. Adv Intern Med 21:417, 1976.

Nunn, D: Complications of peripheral arteriography. Am Surg 44(10):664, October 1978.

Rees, R, et al: Angiography in extremity trauma: A prospective study. Am Surg 44(10):661, October 1978.

Snopek, A: Fundamentals of Special Radiographic Procedures. WB Saunders, Philadelphia, 1992.

White, R: Fundamentals of Vascular Radiology. Lea & Febiger, Philadelphia, 1976.

Widrich, W, Singer, R, and Robbins, A: The use of intraarterial lidocaine to control pain due to aortofemoral arteriography. Radiology 124(1):37, July 1977.

Wojtowycz, M: Handbook in Radiology, Interventional Radiology, and Angiography. Year Book Medical Publishers, Chicago, 1990.

# CHAPTER 27

# Upper Extremity Angiography

*Marianne R. Tortorici, EdD, ARRT(R)*

Angiography of the upper extremity is very similar in technique to angiography of the lower extremity, although it is performed less frequently. It is an important procedure for the diagnosis and therapy (interventional) of vascular pathologies of the upper extremities. This chapter concentrates on the diagnostic aspect of the procedure. The reader is referred to Chapter 29, Vascular Interventional Angiography, for a discussion of the therapeutic aspects of the procedure.

## ANATOMY

The anatomy of the vascular system of the upper extremity begins with the subclavian arteries. The left subclavian artery arises directly from the aortic arch, and the right subclavian originates at the brachiocephalic, or innominate, artery. The superior branches of the subclavian arteries are the vertebral, the thyrocervical, and the costocervical. The thyrocervical gives rise to the inferior thyroid, superficial cervical, and suprascapular arteries. The only inferior branch of the subclavian artery is the internal mammary artery. At the border of the first rib, the subclavian continues to become the axillary artery.

The axillary artery has several branches, which include the thoracoacromial, lateral thoracic, subcapsular, and anterior and posterior humeral circumflex. At the lateral border of the teres major muscle, the axillary artery becomes the brachial artery.

The profunda brachialis, ulnar collateral, and supratrochlear arteries are the main branches of the brachial artery. The brachial artery ends at the cubital fossa, where it bifurcates into the ulnar and radial arteries.

The radial artery originates lateral to the neck of the radius and terminates in the palm of the hand. It anastomoses with the ulnar artery to form the deep palmar arch. The radial artery gives rise to the radial recurrent, muscular, and several other branches. The ulnar artery gives rise to the ulnar recurrent, common interosseous, anterior interosseous, and muscular branches. The deep palmar arteries, branches of the radial and ulnar arteries, give rise to the metacarpal arteries, which join the palmar and digital arteries. Figure 27–1

**255**

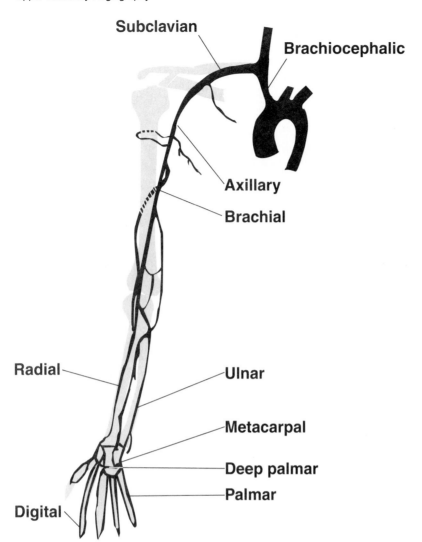

**Figure 27–1.** Major arterial branches of right upper extremity (From Abrams, H: A Practical Approach to Angiography, ed 3. Little, Brown, & Co., Boston, 1983, with permission).

represents a diagram of the major arteries of the upper extremity.

## INDICATIONS

Angiography of the upper extremities is indicated in cases of occlusive diseases, arteriovenous malformations, tumors, thoracic outlet syndrome, and trauma. Common occlusive diseases include atherosclerosis, aneurysms, embolus, Raynaud's disease, and Raynaud's phenomenon.

Atherosclerosis is usually found in the proximal portion of the upper extremity. Digital subtraction angiography (DSA) is very useful in visualizing distal atherosclerosis.

There are many causes of aneurysms. The most common cause of aneurysms is trauma. Some types of aneurysms include mycotic, congenital, and poststenotic. Aneurysms located in the subclavian arteries are often a result of thoracic outlet syndrome.

Most emboli in the upper extremity originate from the heart and are seen in patients with atrial fibrillation or myocardial infarction. Mitral stenosis is usually a predisposing cause of emboli. Small emboli usually affect the digits, causing gangrene. Larger emboli may become trapped at the bifurcation of the brachial artery.

Raynaud's disease has no known etiology. Symptoms include cold, numb digits. In the later stages, the patient may experience cyanotic digits with throbbing pain. Raynaud's disease usually is bilateral and occurs primarily in women. It rarely results in tissue loss.

Unlike Raynaud's disease, Raynaud's phenomenon has an underlying systemic or local disease present. There are numerous diseases that may demonstrate Raynaud's phenomenon. Among these are lead or arsenic poisoning, trauma, drug intoxication, carpal tunnel syndrome, arteriosclerosis, primary pulmonary hypertension, thoracic outlet syndrome and thermal injury.

Arteriovenous malformations may be congenital or in the form of a fistula. Most fistulas are a result of trauma.

The most common tumor is the hemangioma, which is usually located in the hand. These tumors are caused by the abnormal vascular development of the capillaries.

Thoracic outlet syndrome occurs when the blood supply is obstructed. There are numerous causes of thoracic outlet syndrome, most of which result in compression of the vessels by muscles, ribs, or ligaments. These are often seen at the brachial plexus.

Trauma to the upper extremity is often seen in the form of fractures, dislocations, penetrating wounds (gunshot or stab wounds), and temperature effects (frostbite). Most trauma occurs at the brachial artery site.

## EQUIPMENT

The equipment employed for angiography of the upper extremity includes a rapid film changer and the routine accessory equipment associated with a percutaneous catheterization (see Chapter 16, Guide Wires and Catheters, and Chapter 17, Supplementary Catheterization Equipment). Since some upper extremity angiography is best performed using digital subtraction, a DSA unit should be available. Catheter placement requires the use of an image intensifier.

## PREPROCEDURAL CARE AND CAUTIONS

Preprocedural care for upper extremity angiography employs the normal angiographic preparation. It is extremely important to assess the strength of the axillary, brachial, and radial pulses. Weak pulses may indicate some form of pathology or vascular injury. Checks should also be made to detect the presence of bruits.

Sometimes vessel vasospasm exists in the upper extremity. This may be caused by the catheter, pathology, or external room temperature. If vasospasm is present, it can inhibit the ability to visualize the vessels, especially the distal arteries. To improve the flow of blood and contrast medium, the arteries may be dilated by warming the extremity or by using vasodilators. The extremity may be warmed by using a heating pad, an infrared light, or warm compresses. Common vasodilators employed are tolazoline, phentolamine, and reserpine. Tolazoline is injected intra-arterially over 10 to 15 seconds immediately before filming. The recommended dosage is 25 mg diluted in 10 to 15 ml of normal saline or 5 percent dextrose. With phentolamine, 2 to 4 mg is injected intra-arterially 30 seconds before filming. Reserpine's effect maximizes within 40 minutes after injection. It is injected slowly intra-arterially using 0.5 to 1.0 mg diluted in 10 to 15 ml of normal saline or 5 percent dextrose.

Injection of contrast medium into the extremities is painful. Using nonionic, low osmolar contrast medium is preferred over ionic agents, since the nonionics reduce the amount of pain the patient experiences. In the lower extremity, lidocaine may be injected prior to the contrast medium injection to reduce the pain. However, this practice is not recommended for the upper extremity because lidocaine may enter the brain, causing complications.

## APPROACHES

Approaches to the upper extremity include percutaneous puncture of the femoral, brachial, or axillary arteries. The femoral approach is the most popular approach. In this approach, the catheter is manipulated through the abdominal aorta to the thoracic aorta for selective catheterization of the subclavian artery. On the right side, this requires the catheter to pass through the brachiocephalic, or innominate, artery. On the left side, the catheter is passed directly into the left subclavian and advanced to the axillary and brachial arteries. In this selective catheterization, care needs to be taken to avoid catheterizing the common carotid artery. The catheter may be advanced to the axillary or brachial artery for better visualization of the distal arteries.

The brachial or axillary catheterization method (brachial preferred) is useful if the femoral approach is not feasible. A drawback to the brachial method of catheterization is that the ulnar or radial artery may have a high origin above the puncture site, preventing visualization of these vessels during contrast medium injection.

## CATHETERS

A brachiocephalic catheter with only an end hole is most commonly employed for the femoral approach. In this approach, a Judkins Headhunter I or soft wall Mani-type catheter is used for the average adult. Elderly patients may require the use of a Sidewinder II catheter. Straight end-hole catheters are employed for punctures of the axillary or brachial arteries. Regardless of the type of catheterization method, a small thin-wall catheter should be employed to decrease the possibility of obstructing the vessel.

## CONTRAST MEDIA

A 45 to 60 percent concentration contrast medium is employed for injection. The concentration depends on the method of filming; a lower concentration is needed for DSA filming. The amount of contrast medium employed for visualization of the distal arm and the forearm is 15 to 24 ml. The medium is hand injected over a period of 2 to 4 seconds. A higher dosage and longer injection time are needed to visualize the distal arteries. To alleviate the pain associated with the injection of the contrast medium, nonionic medium may be employed.

## POSITIONING AND FILMING

A rapid serial film changer or DSA may be employed for upper extremity filming. It is important to visualize the upper extremity vessels from the subclavian to the

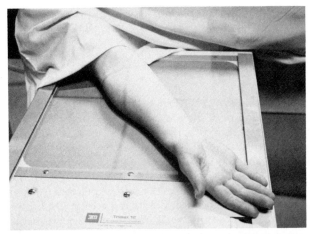

**Figure 27 – 2.** Anterior-posterior projection of upper extremity demonstrating diagonal placement of the arm on the film changer.

digital arteries. This requires multiple injections and overlapping filming. For example, the first set of films may be performed to visualize the subclavian to brachial vessels. A second injection may be used to demonstrate the brachial to digital vessels.

For upper extremity filming using a rapid serial film changer, the arm is abducted about 45 degrees and the central ray is directed toward the midpoint of the part of interest, e.g., center approximately 2″ distal to the elbow joint to visualize the brachial to digital vessels. The patient's arm is placed in anatomic position (palm of hand supinated) diagonally over the film changer (Fig. 27 – 2). The distal vessels of the extremity are often difficult to visualize unless magnification angiography is employed.

The filming sequence depends on the catheter location and area of interest. For subclavian or axillary catheter placement proximal to the first rib, the recommended rate is 2 frames/sec for 4 to 6 frames and 1 frame/sec for 6 frames. This programming results in 10 to 12 total frames. If the hand is the area of interest, there is a 2-second delay and filming is at a rate of 1 frame/sec.

When the catheter is placed in the midbrachial artery proximal to the bifurcation, the filming rate is 1 per second for 6 frames and 1 every other second for 4 seconds.

## COMPLICATIONS

Some of the more common complications most often encountered in upper extremity angiography are arterial spasm, arterial thrombosis, injection of contrast medium into the wrong vessel, local hematoma, and nerve root damage. Arterial spasm is usually caused by catheter manipulation. This may be alleviated by injecting a vasodilator. Arterial thrombosis is most commonly seen with the brachial catheterization method. This is often related to multiple catheter changes and the use of a large French size catheter. Catheter recoil may inadvertently cause the injection of contrast medium into the thyrocervical or costocervical vessels. These arteries feed the vessels of the spinal cord. If contrast medium enters the spinal cord, it may cause complications. Local hematoma and nerve root damage are the most common complications of axillary catheterization. The incidence of hematoma may be decreased by using small catheters and firm pressure over the puncture site until the bleeding has stopped. Injury caused to the nerve roots is usually the result of needle or hematoma pressure on the nerve.

## SOME ANGIOGRAPHIC FINDINGS

The major angiographic findings of upper extremity angiography include arteriovenous malformations, tumors, and atherosclerosis. The patterns of atherosclerosis vary with the stage of the disease. Atherosclerosis of the upper extremity usually involves the subclavian artery. If the proximal end of the subclavian artery is occluded or narrowed, the subclavian artery will "steal" blood from the vertebral arteries or other branches of the subclavian. This occurs because the narrowing of the subclavian artery results in a decrease of pressure at its distal end. This in turn results in a backflow of blood from the vessel of higher pressure, the vertebral vessel, to the vessel of lower pressure, the subclavian vessel. Figure 27 – 3 illustrates some angiographic findings.

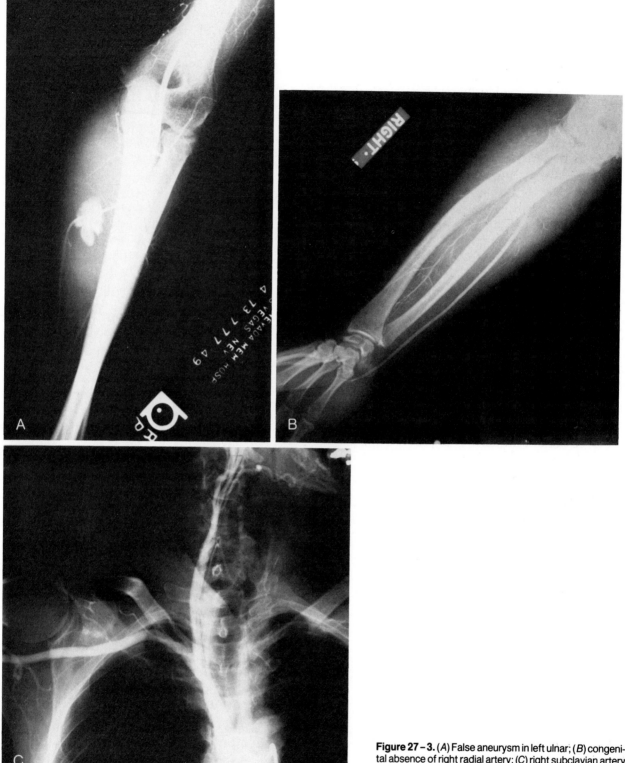

**Figure 27 – 3.** (*A*) False aneurysm in left ulnar; (*B*) congenital absence of right radial artery; (*C*) right subclavian artery ''stealing'' blood.

# REVIEW QUESTIONS

1. The left subclavian artery rises _____.
   A. directly from the aortic arch
   B. from the innominate artery
   C. from the carotid artery
   D. inferior to the brachiocephalic artery

2. The _____ artery is an inferior branch of the sub-clavian artery.
   A. vertebral
   B. thyrocervical
   C. mammary
   D. costocervical

3. The lateral border of the teres major muscle marks the beginning of the _____ artery.
   A. subclavian
   B. axillary
   C. brachial
   D. ulnar

4. The brachial artery terminates at the _____.
   A. teres major muscle
   B. cubital fossa
   C. palmar arch
   D. first rib

5. Aneurysms of the subclavian artery most often occur as a result of _____.
   A. atherosclerosis
   B. congenital disorders
   C. Raynaud's disease
   D. thoracic outlet syndrome

6. Most emboli of the upper extremities originate from the _____.
   A. lung
   B. brain
   C. heart
   D. aorta

7. _____ have (has) no known etiology.
   A. Emboli
   B. Raynaud's disease
   C. Arteriovenous malformations
   D. Fistulas

8. Hemangioma is often located in the _____.
   A. bifurcation of the brachial artery
   B. hand
   C. brachial plexus
   D. wrist

9. The angiographic catheter, pathology, and exter-nal room temperature may cause _____.
   A. emboli
   B. occlusion
   C. aneurysm
   D. vasospasm

10. _____ is a useful technique in dilating the blood vessels.
    A. Lidocaine
    B. Warm compresses
    C. Saline
    D. Use of large catheters

11. Tolazoline, phentolamine, and reserpine are _____.
    A. vasodilators
    B. anesthetics
    C. vasoconstrictors
    D. interventional drugs

12. The _____ approach is the most common upper ex-tremity catheterization method.
    A. axillary
    B. brachial
    C. femoral
    D. subclavian

13. Distal upper extremity arteries are better visual-ized if the catheter is placed in the _____ artery.
    A. subclavian
    B. innominate
    C. radial
    D. brachial

14. If the ulnar and radial arteries have a high point of origin, the _____ catheterization method should be avoided.
    A. subclavian
    B. axillary
    C. brachial
    D. femoral

15. Elderly patients undergoing upper extremity angi-ography may require use of a _____ catheter.
    A. Sidewinder II
    B. Judkins Headhunter 1
    C. Mani-type
    D. cobra

16. Distal artery visualization of the upper extremity require a _____ dose and _____ injection time than the proximal arteries.
    A. higher, shorter
    B. higher, longer
    C. lower, longer
    D. lower, shorter

17. To visualize the upper extremity from the subcla-vian to digital arteries often requires _____.
    A. a large film
    B. long exposure time
    C. multiple injections
    D. few frames per second

18. Filming of the distal upper extremity arteries of the hand requires _____.
    A. a 2-second film exposure delay
    B. a decrease in contrast medium volume
    C. a high concentration of contrast medium
    D. high rate of film exposures

19. Multiple catheter changes and use of a large French catheter in the brachial approach of upper extremity angiography may cause _____.
    A. hematoma

B. arterial thrombosis
C. vasodilation
D. infection

20. _____ are (is) a common complication of axillary catheterization.
   A. Emboli
   B. Arterial spasm
   C. Arthritis
   D. Nerve root damage

## BIBLIOGRAPHY

Abrams, H: A Practical Approach to Angiography, Vol 3, ed 3. Little, Brown & Co, Boston, 1983.

Johnsrude, I, Jackson, D, and Dunnick, NR: A Practical Approach to Angiography, ed. 2. Little, Brown & Co, Boston, 1987.

Kadir, S: Diagnostic Angiography. WB Saunders, Philadelphia, 1986.

Luzsa, G: X-ray Anatomy of the Vascular System. JB Lippincott, Philadelphia, 1974.

Meschan, I: An Atlas of Anatomy Basic to Radiology. WB Saunders, Philadelphia, 1975.

Wojtowycz, M: Handbook in Radiology, Interventional Radiology, and Angiography. Year Book Medical Publishers, Chicago, 1990.

# PART FOUR

# INTERVENTIONAL PROCEDURES

# CHAPTER 28

# Cardiac Interventional Angiography

*Dennis A. Bair ARRT(R)(CV)*
*Carol A. Mascioli ARRT(R)(CV)*

Cardiac intervention is the field of radiology representing various therapeutic procedures dedicated to the treatment of numerous heart diseases and abnormalities. At the printing of this text, cardiac intervention is still relatively new and is expanding dramatically. Percutaneous transluminal coronary angioplasty (PTCA) is the oldest cardiac interventional procedure and has provided the foundation for the development of additional therapeutic methods. Common cardiac interventional procedures discussed in this text include directional coronary atherectomy (DCA), introduction of intravascular stents and various thrombolytic agents, and numerous pediatric cardiac interventions. Prior to the development of these interventional techniques, surgery was the only alternative to medical therapy for coronary artery disease and other cardiac abnormalities. While many of these technologies are still under investigation for their long-term results, initial data appear promising. Cardiac intervention is so extensive that numerous textbooks and journal articles have been written on this subject. The purpose of this chapter is to provide an overview of cardiac interventional radiology.

## PERCUTANEOUS TRANSLUMINAL CORONARY ANGIOPLASTY

Percutaneous transluminal coronary angioplasty was developed by Andreas Gruntzig and is a modification of the technique he used for peripheral artery angioplasty. PTCA employs a balloon catheter to increase the blood flow in a vessel. The method requires that a deflated balloon catheter be positioned at the area of vessel narrowing and inflated to expand that area. Advances in the design of coronary angioplasty balloons and guide wires have decreased the difficulty of this procedure and increased the technical success, while the overall technique described by Gruntzig remains relatively unchanged.

It is believed that the success of PTCA can be attributed to the pressure of the balloon on the vessel wall,

**265**

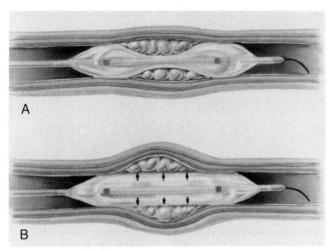

**Figure 28–1.** Mechanism of coronary angioplasty: (*A*) A balloon is inflated, showing indentation of the balloon by the plaque; (*B*) total inflation of balloon resulting in widening of the arterial lumen. (Courtesy of Medi-tech, a division of Boston Scientific Corporation, Watertown, MA.)

which causes a controlled injury, or dissection, of the artery with subsequent overstretching of the arterial wall. The tunica intima and media are torn, the atherosclerotic plaque is fractured, and the adventitia is stretched beyond its elastic recoil point. This causes a widening of the arterial lumen and subsequent increase in blood flow (Fig. 28–1).

## Indications

Indications for PTCA include stable or unstable angina pectoris, acute myocardial infarction, and previous coronary artery bypass surgery. These conditions, in conjunction with documented coronary artery stenosis, provide the basis for deciding to use angioplasty as a therapeutic tool.

## Contraindications

Contraindications to PTCA include left main coronary artery disease, an excessive amount of myocardium dependent on the artery to undergo angioplasty, poor contractile function of the myocardium supplied by other vessels, multivessel disease, and location or etiology of lesion to undergo angioplasty.

## Risks and Complications

Complications during PTCA occur at an overall rate of about 4 to 5 percent. These complications can be broken down into major and minor categories. The major complications include:
1. coronary artery occlusion
2. myocardial infarction
3. neurologic deficit

4. renal failure
5. death

The minor complications include:
1. side branch occlusion
2. ventricular arrhythmias
3. heart blocks
4. hematoma at the puncture site
5. pericardial tamponade

These complications can also occur during other interventional cardiac procedures, such as directional coronary atherectomy and intravascular stents.

## Approaches

The approaches used for therapeutic catheterization are the same as those used for any angiographic procedure. However, unlike routine vessel catheterization, which employs a catheter and guide wire, angioplasty uses a guiding catheter, a balloon catheter, and a steerable guide wire (Fig. 28–2). The guiding catheter is positioned at the ostium (opening) of the coronary artery. After the guiding catheter is positioned, the steerable guide wire is manipulated past the area of stenosis, and the balloon catheter is advanced to the location of the vessel narrowing (Fig. 28–3). The vessel is dilated or opened by inflating the balloon at the narrowing. Initial success of PTCA is quite high, while the long-term (2- to 5-year follow-up) success results in approximately 70 to 75 percent patency. Although angioplasty is very successful, several problems may occur. These include elastic recoil, re-stenosis caused by intimal proliferation, and abrupt closure of the artery. Attempts to solve these problems have led to the innovation of several new technologies. Common new technologies currently being used are evaluated in the following sections of this chapter.

## DIRECTIONAL CORONARY ATHERECTOMY

Directional coronary atherectomy (DCA) has emerged as a possible improvement to PTCA. The overall concept of atherectomy involves the removal or

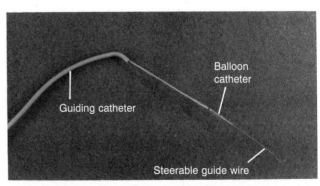

**Figure 28–2.** Coronary angioplasty equipment.

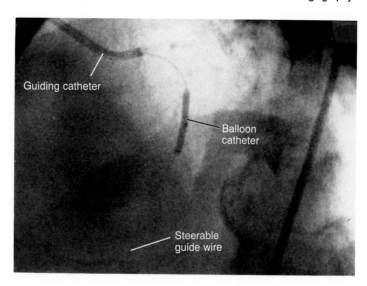

**Figure 28–3.** Radiograph of coronary angioplasty, demonstrating the equipment inside the coronary vessel.

extraction of the atheromatous material from the vessel (Fig. 28–4). This method differs significantly from angioplasty, which opens vessels by injuring the arterial layers, fracturing the plaque, and stretching the artery beyond its elastic recoil point. Advocates of DCA believe that it causes less injury to the artery and has a longer period of success than angioplasty.

Indications for DCA include proximal and middle segmental lesions in the coronary arteries, primary lesions without previous PTCA, and lesions with a high risk morphology for PTCA. DCA has also been used on areas of restenosis after PTCA. The limiting factor of DCA is the stiffness of the equipment, which prohibits the use of DCA in distal lesions, diffusely diseased ar-

teries, total occlusions, and arteries with severe angulation. Figures 28–5 through 28–7 demonstrate three of the systems currently being used and under evaluation. These are the Simpson Atherocath (Devices for Vascular Intervention, Inc., Redwood City, CA), the Transluminal Extraction Catheter (Interventional Vascular Technologies, Inc., San Diego, CA), and the Rotablator (Heart Technology, Bellevue, WA).

## INTRAVASCULAR STENTS

The use of intravascular stents in coronary arteries is an experimental method of intervention that shows

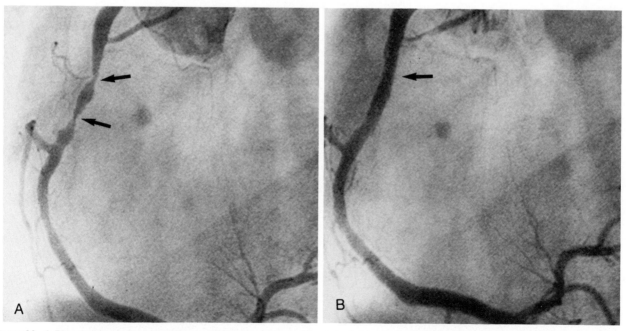

**Figure 28–4.** Directional coronary atherectomy: (*A*) Preatherectomy, demonstrating constricted vessel (*arrows*); (*B*) postatherectomy with Simpson Atherocath, demonstrating vessel dilatation (*arrow*).

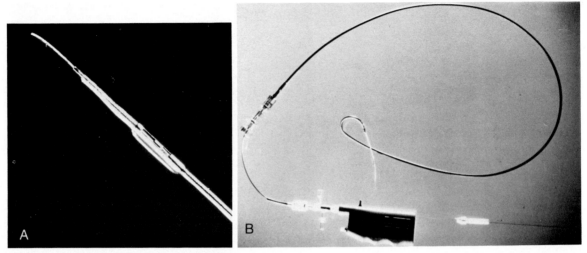

**Figure 28-5.** (*A*) Directional coronary atherectomy Simpson Atherocath tip; (*B*) directional coronary atherectomy, entire Simpson Atherocath system.

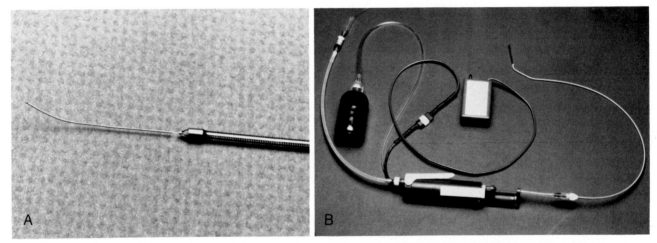

**Figure 28-6.** (*A*) Directional coronary atherectomy transluminal extraction catheter tip; (*B*) entire transluminal extraction catheter system.

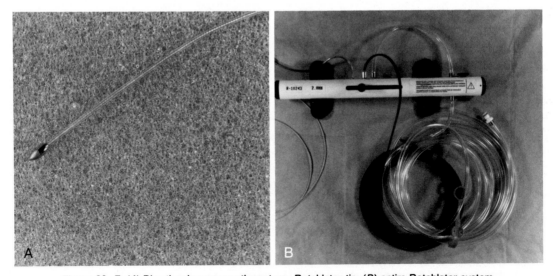

**Figure 28-7.** (*A*) Directional coronary atherectomy Rotablator tip; (*B*) entire Rotablator system.

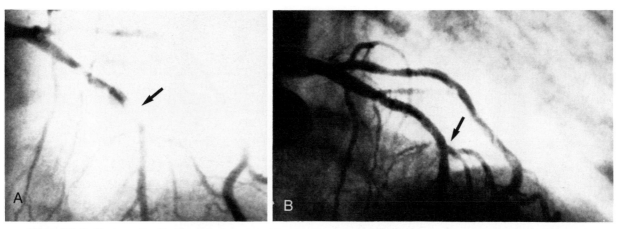

**Figure 28–8.** Gianturco-Roubin Flex Stent placement in coronary artery: (A) Prestent placement; (B) Poststent placement.

promising results. Intravascular stents provide a scaffolding or bridging to physically hold the arterial lumen open. One use of this procedure is to repair elastic recoil resulting from angioplasty. Other indications for intravascular stents include abrupt closure of an artery after angioplasty, uncontrolled dissection, unsatisfactory angioplasty results, and prevention of restenosis (Fig. 28–8). Three major designs for intravascular stents in current evaluation and use are the balloon expandable, self-expandable, and thermal memory stents. Figure 28–9 shows examples of different types of stents. Intravascular stents for coronary artery use are not Food and Drug Administration (FDA)–approved and, therefore, not commercially available. Investigation of these devices continues, and long-term results are not yet available in the United States.

## THROMBOLYTIC AGENTS AND RISKS

Formation of thrombus within a coronary artery can cause an acute myocardial infarction, or heart attack. The use of thrombolytic agents such as streptokinase, urokinase, and tissue plasminogen activator during acute myocardial infarction appears to improve survival when administered early in the course of the infarction. The mechanism of action is different for each of these agents, but all activate the body's own clot-dissolving system to break down the blockage (Fig. 28–10) that is causing the acute myocardial infarction episode. The exact mechanism of each agent is beyond the scope of this text. These agents can be administered directly into the affected artery or administered intravenously. Intravenous administration can be accom-

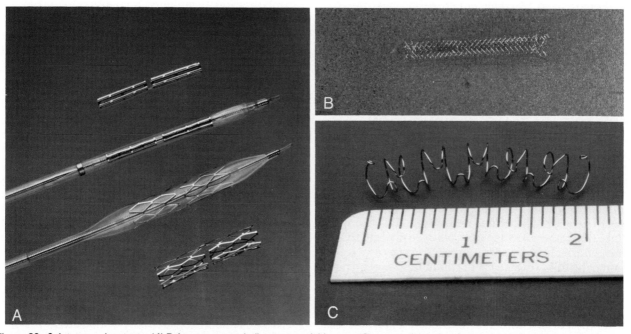

**Figure 28–9.** Intravascular stents: (A) Palmaz coronary balloon-expandable stent (Courtesy of Johnson & Johnson Interventional Systems, Warren, NJ); (B) Wallstent, a self-expandable stent (Courtesy of Schneider (USA) Inc., Minneapolis, MN); and (C) Gianturco-Roubin Flex Stent, a metallic balloon expandable stent (Courtesy of Cook Incorporated, Bloomington, IN).

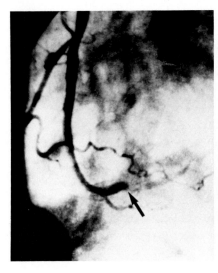 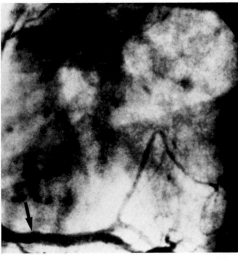

**Figure 28–10.** Thrombolysis in coronary arteries: (*A*) Prethrombolysis; (*B*) postthrombolysis.

plished while the patient is in the ambulance en route to the hospital or in the emergency department. Intra-arterial administration through a catheter into the affected coronary artery must be performed in the cardiac catheterization facility to determine the exact location of blockage. Both techniques have similar efficacy, but the use of intravenous thrombolytic therapy allows for more rapid administration and decreases the need for a dedicated cardiac catheterization facility.

Directional coronary atherectomy, intravascular stents, and thrombolytic therapy all carry risks associated with their uses. Many of these risks and complications are similar to PTCA, but there are some differences with the use of thrombolytic therapy. The following represents a list of complications associated with thrombolytic agents used for acute myocardial infarction:

1. hemorrhage, bleeding (puncture site, gastrointestinal, intracranial, and hemopericardium)
2. distal embolization
3. new thrombus formation on the infusion catheter
4. recurrent ischemia or myocardial infarction
5. in rare instances, death

## PEDIATRIC CARDIAC INTERVENTION

Prior to the development of cardiac interventional angiography, congenital and pediatric abnormalities were correctable only by surgery. Open heart surgery in infants and young children carries a risk of death, and many of these congenital abnormalities require a series of surgeries that extend well into adolescence. To reduce this risk, many attempts have been made to treat these abnormalities by percutaneous cardiac catheterization. The following is a list of common successful pediatric cardiac interventional procedures:

1. atrial balloon or blade septostomy
2. dilatation of aortic coarctations
3. embolization of atrial or ventricular septal defects
4. embolization of patent ductus arteriosus
5. embolization of pulmonary arteriovenous fistulae
6. valvuloplasty of all cardiac valves

Atrial septostomy is performed when there is a need for an atrial septal defect to allow for mixing of arterial and venous blood supplies. One example of this need is in the case of transposition of the great vessels where the infant is born highly cyanotic. A catheter is placed across the foramen ovale in the intra-atrial septum, and a larger opening is produced by cutting the septum or pulling an inflated balloon across the septum, causing a tear.

Coarctation of the aorta involves a narrowing of the descending aorta, causing upper extremity hypertension and left ventricular hypertrophy. Balloon dilatation of the narrowed segment results in a resolution of these symptoms. Surgical management is the initial treatment of choice for coarctation, while balloon dilatation of postoperative, recurrent coarctation has proved very successful.

Embolization techniques for closure of atrial and ventricular septal defects is experimental, and surgery remains the treatment of choice for these defects. The technique involves the use of umbrella closure devices. Clinical application of these interventional techniques continues, and many angiographers are optimistic about their impact in the future.

Embolization of a patent ductus arteriosus involves the closure of a communication between the aorta and the pulmonary artery that has failed to close after birth. Although polyvinyl plugs, coils, and umbrella closure devices have been used successfully, surgical ligation is the treatment of choice because of its low mortality and morbidity rates.

In congenital heart disease, pulmonary arteriovenous fistulae and abnormalities often appear to help compensate for the changes in cardiac circulation. After successful corrective surgery of the primary condition, these abnormalities can hinder the patient's return to health. Using standard embolization techniques, embolization of these vessels has proved quite successful.

Cardiac balloon valvuloplasty is indicated for symptomatic patients who decline surgical valvular replacement or who are not surgical candidates because of pre-existing medical conditions that may increase the risk of mortality. Aortic, mitral, and pulmonary valvuloplasty are the most common of these procedures. Valvuloplasty is considered successful when hemodynamic pressure measurements show improvement after balloon inflation.

Contraindications to valvuloplasty include moderate to severe insufficiency of the stenotic valve, unstable angina, and left atrial thrombus when the transseptal approach is used.

Complications of balloon valvuloplasty include increased valvular insufficiency, cardiac tamponade, myocardial infarction, cerebral vascular accident (CVA), arrhythmias, hypotension, and, in rare instances, death.

## FUTURE CONSIDERATIONS

The key to determining the number and variety of cardiac interventional procedures that will be available in the future may in the long term be results of the current technologies under evaluation. Correlating these technologies with the results will determine which of these technologies is effective and where the next improvements and innovations might occur.

## REVIEW QUESTIONS

1. Cardiac intervention is a relatively ____ field.
   A. new
   B. old
   C. stagnant
   D. unchanging

2. PTCA is the abbreviation for ____.
   A. percutaneous therapeutic cardiac atherectomy
   B. permanent transient cardiac arrhythmia
   C. percutaneous transluminal coronary angioplasty
   D. post-traumatic cardiac aneurysm

3. The mechanism of balloon angioplasty involves ____.
   A. extraction of the plaque
   B. squeezing the fluid from the plaque
   C. stretching the artery
   D. rupturing the artery

4. The coronary artery angioplasty system consists of a ____.
   A. guiding catheter
   B. balloon catheter
   C. guide wire
   D. all of the above

5. Coronary angioplasty has a 2- to 5-year success rate of approximately ____ percent patency.
   A. 30 to 40
   B. 50 to 60
   C. 70 to 75
   D. 85 to 90

6. Directional coronary atherectomy differs from coronary angioplasty by ____ the atheromatous material.

   A. vaporizing
   B. dissolving
   C. compressing
   D. removing

7. One indication for the use of an intravascular stent might be ____.
   A. good angioplasty result
   B. good flow distal to angioplasty area
   C. uncontrolled dissection
   D. dilated vessel

8. Which of the following is not a thrombolytic agent?
   A. heparin
   B. urokinase
   C. streptokinase
   D. tissue plasminogen activator

9. Acute blockage of a coronary artery causes a(n) ____.
   A. arrhythmia
   B. myocardial infarction
   C. bradycardia
   D. tachycardia

10. Congenital and pediatric cardiac abnormalities can be treated with the use of ____.
    A. medications
    B. surgery
    C. interventional cardiac catheterization
    D. all of the above

## BIBLIOGRAPHY

Abrams, HL: Angiography, Vol 3, ed 3. Little, Brown & Co, Boston, 1983.

Cope, C, Burke, DR, and Meranze, S: Atlas of Interventional Radiology. JB Lippincott, Philadelphia, 1989.

Becker, GL, et al: Angioplasty induced dissections in human iliac arteries: Management with Palmaz balloon-expandable stents. Radiology 176:31–38, July 1990.

Grossman, W and Baim, DS: Cardiac Catheterization, Angiography, and Intervention, ed 4. Lea & Febiger, Philadelphia, 1991.

Hinohara, T, et al: Directional atherectomy: New approaches for treatment of obstructive coronary and peripheral vascular disease. Circulation 81(3):(IV)79–90, March 1990.

Kandarpa, K: Handbook of Cardiovascular and Interventional Radiologic Procedures. Little, Brown & Co, Boston, 1989.

Kerns, MJ: The Cardiac Catheterization Handbook. Mosby-Year Book, St Louis, 1991.

The TIMI Study Group: The thrombolysis in myocardial infarction (TIMI) trial. N Engl J Med 312:932–936, April 1985.

Muller, DW, et al: Quantitative angiographic comparison of the immediate success of coronary angioplasty, coronary atherectomy, and endoluminal stents. Am J Cardiol 66:938–942, October 1990.

Palmaz, JC, et al: Intraluminal stents in atherosclerotic iliac artery stenosis: Preliminary report of a multicenter study. Radiology 168:727–731, July 1988.

Soto, B, Kassner, EG, and Baxley, WA: Imaging of Cardiac Disorders: Vol 2, Acquired Disorders. JB Lippincott, Philadelphia, 1992.

Umans, VA, et al: Comparative quantitative angiographic analysis of directional coronary atherectomy and balloon angioplasty. Am J Cardiol 68:1556–1562, December 1991.

Umans, VA, et al: Comparative angiographic quantitative analysis of the immediate efficacy of coronary atherectomy with balloon angioplasty, stenting, and rotational ablation. Am Heart J 122:836–843, September 1991.

# CHAPTER 29

# Vascular Interventional Angiography

*William F. O'Donnell Jr., AS, ARRT(R)*
*Marianne R. Tortorici, EdD, ARRT(R)*

For 80 years, radiology served primarily as a diagnostic discipline. However, in the 1960s the development of cardiovascular interventional angiography expanded radiology to include therapy. This new branch of radiology uses specialized catheters to perform various therapeutic procedures that formerly required surgical intervention. Thus, cardiovascular interventional angiography is appealing, because it reduces the trauma to the patient and lessens the length of hospitalization, reducing cost. Interventional procedures range from such simplistic procedures as nephrotomy tube placement, used to drain obstructed kidneys, to the rarer and more complex approaches, such as the placement of an occlusion balloon in an aneurysm of a vessel in the brain.

Interventional radiology is divided into two areas, vascular and nonvascular. Although the equipment and methods for these procedures are similar, there are differences. Thus, this text addresses each area in its own chapter.

This chapter is dedicated to vascular interventional angiography and summarizes eight common vascular interventional procedures: balloon angioplasty, vascular stents, thrombolysis, embolization, retrieval, transjugular interhepatic portosystemic shunt (TIPS), atherectomy, and inferior vena cava (IVC) filter. For vascular interventional procedures of the heart, refer to Chapter 28, Cardiac Interventional Angiography. Balloon angioplasty, atherectomy, vascular stent placements, and thrombolysis are procedures used to increase blood flow, while embolization decreases blood flow. TIPS is useful in decreasing portal hypertension. Retrieval is a method of foreign body removal from a blood vessel. IVC filters help prevent pulmonary emboli. Since in-depth discussion of the procedures addressed in this chapter is beyond the scope of this text, each procedure is presented in a short, concise format.

## BALLOON ANGIOPLASTY

The most common interventional procedure is balloon angioplasty, which employs a balloon catheter to

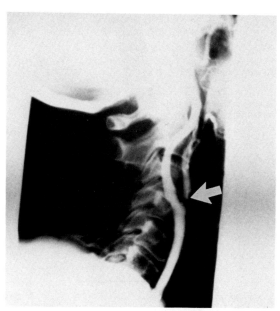

**Figure 29-1.** Angiogram showing a stenotic vessel.

## Technique

Angioplasty is performed using a modified Seldinger technique (see Chapter 19, Catheterization Methods and Patient Management). In this approach, an introducer sheath is placed into the vessel over the wire (Fig. 29–2) to provide a means for catheter exchange. The introducer enables the angiographer to exchange several catheters with minimum trauma to the entry site. A dilator is used to enlarge the vessel so that the sheath can be positioned over the guide wire.

An introducer sheath consists of a long, thin-walled tube that is open at one end and has a diaphragm at the opposite end. The size of the introducer sheath is determined by the length and inside diameter of the thin-walled tube. As with catheters, the length of the introducer is measured in centimeters, and the inside diameter is determined using the French scale. The diaphragm prevents bleeding by providing a seal around the catheter and covering the opening of the introducer when the catheter is removed. An arm is also attached to one side of the diaphragm end, which provides a means to flush the system, thus preventing blood clot formation. In balloon angioplasty, the introducer sheath is used to exchange the angiographic catheter used for the angiogram with a balloon catheter. The balloon catheter has two lumina, one for the guide wire and the other for balloon inflation and deflation. Balloon diameters range from 2 mm (for coronary vessels) to 20 mm (for large vessels). Their length varies from 1 to 10 cm. A balloon that is 1 mm larger in diameter than the proximal end of the stenotic vessel and slightly longer than the narrowing should be employed. Balloons may have radiopaque markers at each end or at the most distal end of the balloon. Balloons with radiopaque markers at each end are used to assess the balloon's location in the vessel. The balloon portion of the catheter is advanced over the guide wire into the narrow area of the vessel so that the radiopaque markers are at either end of the stenosis. Figures 29–3 through 29–5 represent a summary of balloon angioplasty technique. Figure 29–3 is a diagram of an oc-

enlarge a narrowed vessel lumen (stenosis). The stenosis may be a result of a variety of disease processes. To assess the need for a balloon angioplasty, an angiogram (Fig. 29–1) is performed to determine the extent, location, and number of stenotic areas.

## Indications

Balloon angioplasty is indicated for patients with relatively few stenotic areas that are easily accessed and are surrounded by a relatively normal outer vessel wall. If possible, 1 to 2 days prior to the examination, the patient should be placed on some form of antiplatelet therapy to reduce possible blood clotting. A common therapy is 300 mg of aspirin four times/day.

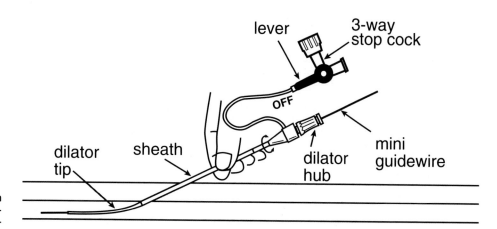

**Figure 29-2.** Introducer sheath in vessel (Courtesy of Medi-tech, a division of Boston Scientific Corporation, Watertown, MA).

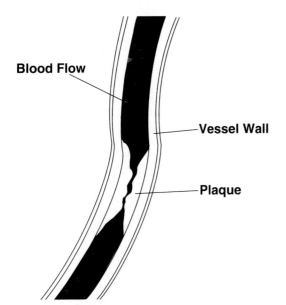

**Figure 29 – 3.** Occluded artery (Courtesy of Abbott Laboratories, North Chicago, IL).

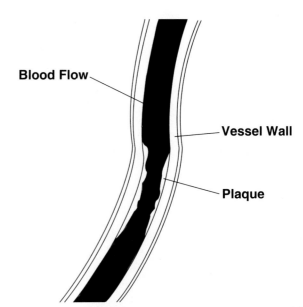

**Figure 29 – 5.** Post – balloon angioplasty of a vessel (Courtesy of Abbott Laboratories, North Chicago, IL).

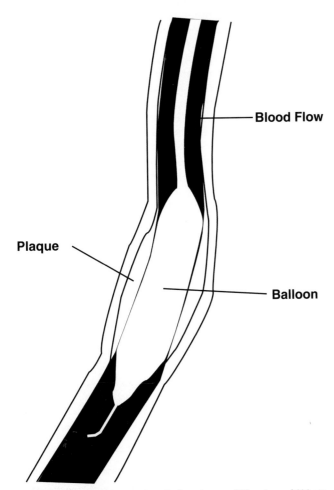

**Figure 29 – 4.** Inflated angioplasty balloon in vessel (Courtesy of Abbott Laboratories, North Chicago, IL).

cluded vessel. When the balloon is in the correct position (within the occlusion), it is inflated (Fig. 29 – 4) under fluoroscopic observation to the manufacturer's recommended maximum pressure using a mixture of equal portions of sterile water and contrast medium. Employing high concentration contrast medium is discouraged, because it may crystallize, causing problems in balloon deflation. During balloon inflation, it is possible to visualize a "waist" (hour-glass shape) in the narrow area. It is not unusual to have to perform several inflations before the vessel is adequately dilated (Fig. 29 – 5). The length of time the balloon is inflated varies relative to vessel location and may be as long as 1 minute with an average of 20 to 40 seconds. Some physicians prefer to use a high pressure inflation for a short time, while others use lower pressure for a longer time.

Regardless of the method, it is generally agreed that once the stenosis "gives," there is no advantage in increasing pressure. As the pressure in the balloon is increased, the material that has caused the narrowing responds according to its composition. If the material is soft plaque, the material is "spread thinly" over the wall of the vessel during balloon inflation. During balloon inflation of hard plaque, both the plaque material and the vessel wall tend to crack during the vessel lumen widening. As a result of this trauma, thrombosis may occur when platelets are released and form a clot. To prevent this, 3000 to 5000 units of heparin may be injected at the site of dilatation and the patient started on anticoagulants. This practice may vary from one angiographer to another. When the vessel appears dilated to the appropriate size, another angiogram is performed at that time to document and verify the results.

Because the wall of the vessel may be damaged when

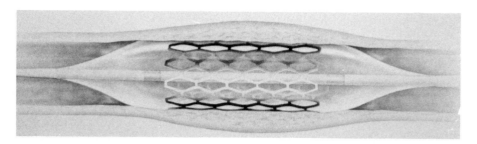

**Figure 29-6.** Angioplasty Palmaz balloon-expandable stent (Courtesy of Johnson & Johnson, Warren, NJ).

the atheromatous plaque is crushed by the balloon, the guide wire may dig into the vessel wall, raising a flap across the lumen and blocking the blood flow. To prevent this, the guide wire should remain across the lesion when exchanging the balloon catheter with the postdilation angiographic catheter.

It is also a common practice to compare the preprocedural arterial pressure above and below the dilation site with postprocedural pressures. Preprocedural pressure readings greater than 10 mm Hg peak systolic are an indication for angioplasty. It is not unusual for the postdilation angiogram to demonstrate improvement while a significant pressure gradient still persists.

## Complications

Complications of balloon angioplasty are rather uncommon. Complications that may occur at the angioplasty site include a tear in the artery wall, which can lead to extravasation; a tear in the artery, resulting in a dissection; a clot formation blocking the vessel; perforation; false aneurysm; arteriovenous fistula; embolic showering (when plaque is broken away, it flows to smaller vessels, occluding them); and lifting a flap, blocking vessel blood flow. Complications at the puncture site include hematoma and bleeding.

## VASCULAR STENTS

A stent is a device placed in a vessel to enlarge the lumen and provide a "scaffolding" to hold the vessel

open. The stent remains in the vessel and acts as a support for the vessel wall. Several types of vascular stents are commercially available. Some are implanted in the vessel using an angioplasty balloon (Fig. 29-6), while others are self expanding (Fig. 29-7). The self-expanding stents are most often installed after the narrowing has been opened with a balloon angioplasty. Stents are most often limited to the torso, because they may become crimped if they are placed in the extremities, causing a vascular blockage. At present, research is attempting to determine whether stents can be safely used in smaller vascular areas.

## Indications

Since approximately 25 to 30 percent of balloon angioplasties are unsuccessful or do not have optimal results, another method of dilation may be needed. There are also occasions when a flap on the inside of a vessel may partly block the flow of blood. In these instances a stent may be indicated.

## Technique

The technique for placement of a stent varies relative to the stent's design. One design uses a cover. In this system, a covered stent is placed over a guide wire and positioned to the area of interest. Once positioned, the cover is retracted from the stent, allowing the stent to self-expand. When the stent delivery system is removed, a balloon catheter is positioned inside the stent

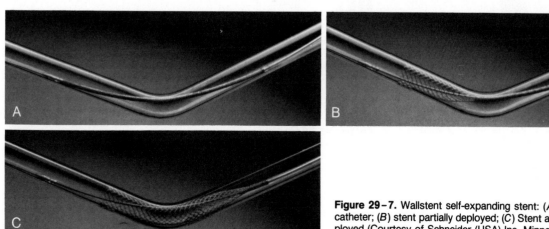

**Figure 29-7.** Wallstent self-expanding stent: (*A*) Stent mounted on catheter; (*B*) stent partially deployed; (*C*) Stent almost completely deployed (Courtesy of Schneider (USA) Inc, Minneapolis, MN).

and inflated to ensure that the ends of the stent are fully expanded.

Another common type of stent is mounted over a balloon catheter and then advanced over a guide wire to the involved area. Once in place, the balloon is inflated to expand the stent.

## Complications

Bleeding, infection, clot formation, premature placement or misplacement of stent, vessel dissection, and deployment problems are possible complications of stent placement. Another complication is crimping of the stent, which would result in occlusion of the vessel. Therefore, stents are limited to large vessels, for example, vessels of the torso.

## THROMBOLYSIS

Thrombolysis is a procedure in which the clot, or thrombus, is destroyed, or lysed. This is accomplished by injecting a clot-dissolving agent through a specially designed catheter (Fig. 29-8). Urokinase, a natural enzyme having few reactions, is the most common agent used. Heparin is often used in conjunction with urokinase to prevent immediate clot formation. A disadvantage of urokinase is that it is very expensive and difficult to extract.

## Indications

Angiographic findings may reveal a vessel blocked by a clot. If the clot is acute, a thrombolysis procedure is indicated.

## Technique

The technique varies with the patient's condition and the angiographic findings. For example, if a long segment of the vessel is blocked, the treatment differs from that used for a more focal occlusion. Consequently, manufacturers offer an array of catheters and guide wires to accommodate various pathology needs. Two common methods using specialized catheters are the pulse spray and infusion techniques.

Before performing thrombolysis, blood-clotting studies are completed by the laboratory to determine a baseline coagulation profile. During the procedure, a guide wire is positioned through the soft clot. In the pulse spray method, a catheter with side holes is advanced over the wire as far into the clot as possible. The side holes of the catheter are used to deliver small boluses of the dissolving agent (Fig. 29-9) directly into the clot using a 1-ml syringe and at a rate of 0.2 ml every 20 seconds. The catheter is advanced approximately 2 cm, and the bolus injection is repeated. This process continues until the catheter is at the tip of the clot.

The infusion method uses a catheter placed in the artery and connected to a pump to administer a slow infusion of the dissolving agent (Fig. 29-10) over a period of hours. Frequently, the dissolving agent is infused overnight, and occasionally for several days. As the dissolving agent lyses the clot, the catheter is advanced in the vessel so that the enzyme concentration is greatest at the clot. It is possible that as a result of catheter manipulation, the clot may flow to a distal vessel, causing a blockage, so care must be used. During this injection period, the patient is kept in a nursing unit for observation and monitoring. When the injection is completed, a follow-up angiogram is performed to evaluate vessel patency.

As the clot dissolves, the initial cause of clot forma-

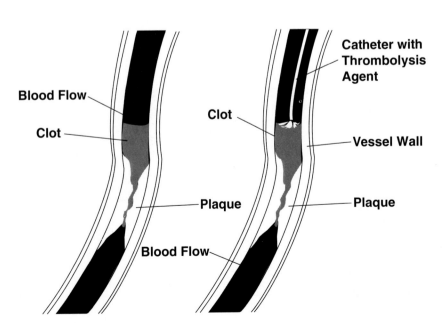

**Figure 29-8.** Occluded vessel being lysed (Courtesy of Abbott Laboratories, North Chicago, IL).

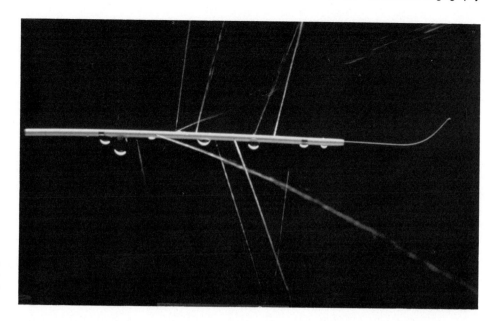

**Figure 29-9.** Thrombolysis pulse spray catheter (Courtesy of Meditech, a division of Boston Scientific Corporation, Watertown, MA).

tion may become evident and should be treated by the most appropriate method, for example, balloon angioplasty. Another example is a clot that may have formed because of small vessel disease. In this case, small vessels become blocked, and since the flow in the major vessels has nowhere to go, they too become blocked.

## Complications

Infection and bleeding are possible complications of thrombolysis. A major concern is bleeding, because urokinase and heparin contribute to this condition. Thus, patients with brain tumors or stomach ulcers, or those who have had recent surgery, should not be considered for thrombolysis.

Another complication occurs when clot particles from a partially dissolved clot break off the vessel wall and block the distal vessels. Although this is very painful for the patient, the condition is usually transient. However, there are recorded instances of losing a limb as a result of this complication.

## EMBOLIZATION

Embolization is a procedure that is used to form a thrombus or block the flow of blood in a vessel. Emboli-

zation uses the human body's natural ability to form an embolus over a foreign body (e.g., fibered coils) placed in a vessel. Also, small particles can be injected into the small vessels to mechanically obstruct them.

## Indications

Arteriovenous malformations (AVM), hemorrhage, and extravasation from damaged vessels are indications for embolization. Before removing an organ or tumor, embolization should be considered to decrease the loss of blood during surgery. Also, embolization is indicated for some aneurysms (Fig. 29-11).

## Technique

There are numerous embolic materials or agents available (Fig. 29-12). Those most commonly used include, but are not limited to, spheres of varying sizes, dehydrated alcohol, fibered coils, boiling contrast medium, glue, Gelfoam, and occlusion balloons. Substances such as Gelfoam, collagen fibers, and balloon catheters are temporary, since they are either removed from, or absorbed by, the body. Other agents, such as coils, spheres, occlusion balloons, dehydrated alcohol, and boiling contrast medium, are considered long

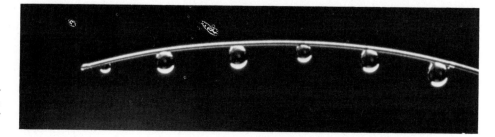

**Figure 29-10.** Thrombolysis infusion catheter (Courtesy of Medi-tech, a division of Boston Scientific Corporation, Watertown, MA).

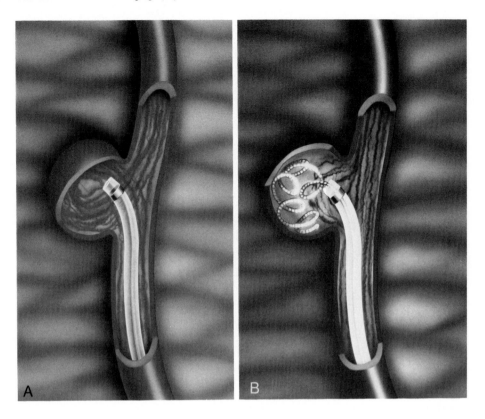

**Figure 29–11.** (*A*) Catheter positioned in aneurysm; (*B*) coils used to embolize the aneurysm (Courtesy of Target Therapeutics, Fremont, CA).

term, since they remain in the body or their effects are permanent. The physician determines the most appropriate material based upon the individual case.

When a catheter is placed in the vessel to be embolized, the embolic material is injected or advanced into the vessel through the catheter. Care must be taken to ensure that the flow of blood does not carry the embolic material into a nontarget vessel. When the embolic agent is in place, contrast medium injections are used to ensure that the blood flow is completely blocked.

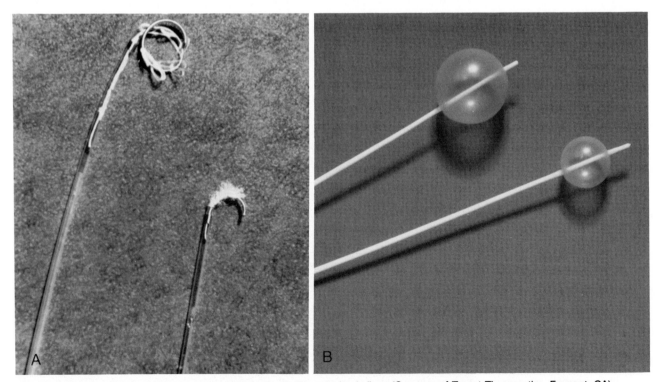

**Figure 29–12.** Two embolic agents: (*A*) Fibered coil; (*B*) occlusion balloon (Courtesy of Target Therapeutics, Fremont, CA).

When occluding an AVM or a vessel that has been bleeding, the patient rarely feels any discomfort. However, pain medication should be considered in cases in which an organ or tumor vessel is to be embolized, since the resulting ischemia is often painful. Use of boiling contrast medium or alcohol is also painful.

## Complications

As always, infection, bleeding, and ischemia are potential problems. When performing embolization procedures, the greatest concern is to ensure that the embolic agent is introduced at the intended site only. If a balloon is used and overinflated, it may rupture the vessel. Performing embolization of the head and neck area may cause a clot to flow to the head, resulting in an infarction or hemiplegia.

## RETRIEVAL

As the name implies, retrieval is a procedure used to recover foreign object(s) from blood vessels.

## Indications

Retrieval is indicated when a broken catheter, guide wire, or other foreign body is free or lodged within the vascular system. If the object is located on the venous side, it can flow to the heart or lungs. Foreign bodies on the arterial side can flow into a distal vessel, causing an obstruction.

## Technique

Retrieval of foreign objects from the vascular system is limited by the design of the retrieval mechanism employed. Fortunately, there are many designs offered by commercial companies, which include, but are not limited to, grasping forceps (Fig. 29–13A), retrieval baskets (Fig. 29–13B, balloon-tip retrieval catheters, goose-neck snares (Fib. 29–13C), and hook-shaped catheters. One of the more common and simplest devices is the loop snare. This device is a catheter with a long wire made into a loop that extends through the distal end of the catheter lumen. The ends of the wire pass through the catheter so that a snare is formed by pulling on the ends of the wire. To use a snare, it is manipulated so that the foreign object is secured in the wire loop, the snare is withdrawn into the catheter, and the entire system is pulled from the vessel with the foreign object entrapped in the snare. This system has some limitations, since the wire loop manipulations are limited to advancement and retraction.

Another common device, which offers more maneuverability than the loop snare, is the goose-neck snare. This snare includes a spring wire, which, when advanced and retracted, returns to its original shape. Another advantage is that the loop can form a 90-degree angle with the catheter providing a secure "hold" on the foreign body. Once the foreign object is in the snare, the entire device is removed from the blood vessel.

Also available are basket loops, which are employed in a similar fashion as the other loops, though they are most often used in nonvascular retrieval procedures.

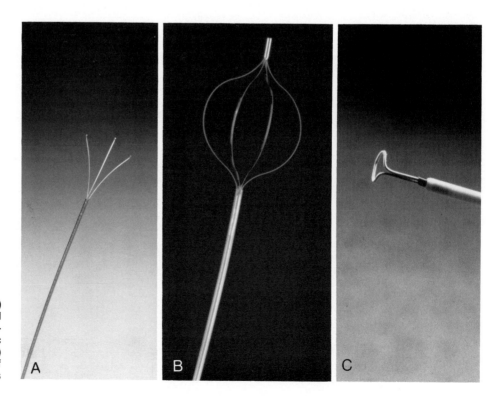

**Figure 29–13.** Retrieval tools: (A) Grasping forceps and (B) retrieval baskets; (A and B Courtesy of Meditech, a division of Boston Scientific Corporation, Watertown, MA); (C) goose-neck snare (Courtesy of Microvena Corporation, Vadnais Heights, MN).

## Complications

Complications of retrieval include bleeding, vessel perforation, and thrombosis. Another complication may result when a foreign body dislodges and flows to a more detrimental location while attempting to remove it.

If the retrieval device must pass through the heart, care must be taken to avoid causing arrhythmia. This disruption in the normal heart rhythm may result in death.

## TRANSJUGULAR INTERHEPATIC PORTOSYSTEMIC SHUNT

A therapy for managing variceal hemorrhage in the liver is a transjugular interhepatic portosystemic shunt (TIPS) procedure. In this procedure, the portal system is decompressed by shunting blood flow from the portal vein to the hepatic vein. In the early years of this procedure, long-term success was not achieved because the shunt would gradually close. However, the introduction of the expandable metal stent has created more favorable results.

### Indications

The primary indication for TIPS use is variceal bleeding caused by portal hypertension, ascites, and primary cirrhosis. This condition is marked by an increase in portal pressure.

## Technique

To perform a TIPS, the right jugular vein is cannulated, and a guide wire and catheter are manipulated into the hepatic vein. A transjugular needle is passed through the catheter into the hepatic vein. The needle is advanced beyond the end of the protective catheter, through the hepatic vein and liver parenchyma into the portal vein (Fig. 29–14). This process is observed under fluoroscopy using contrast medium injections.

When the needle is in place, a guide wire is advanced through the needle into the portal vein and the needle is withdrawn. Balloon catheters are advanced over the guide wire, creating a dilated tract through the liver tissue forming a shunt from the portal vein to the hepatic vein. At this point, a metallic stent is placed in the newly formed tract and expanded.

The metallic stent has been the key to success since historically the shunt would gradually close. Even with the stent in place, the shunt may close off because of neointimal hyperplasia within the stent. This complication is rare and can be reversed percutaneously. Pressure readings can be taken before and after the stenting to document the reduction in pressure.

## Complications

Intraperitoneal hemorrhage is of great concern with this procedure. This complication can be decreased by avoiding transhepatic cannulations before the TIPS procedure and by limiting the intrahepatic excursions of the transjugular needle for each needle pass. Each

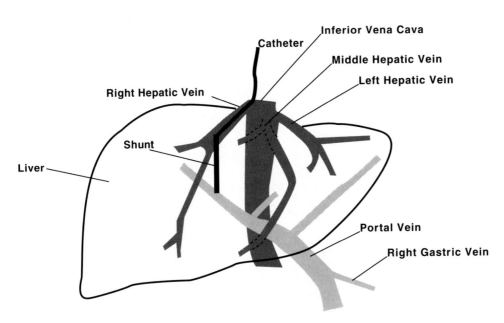

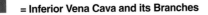 = Inferior Vena Cava and its Branches

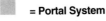 = Portal System

**Figure 29–14.** Location of transjugular interhepatic portosystemic shunt (TIPS).

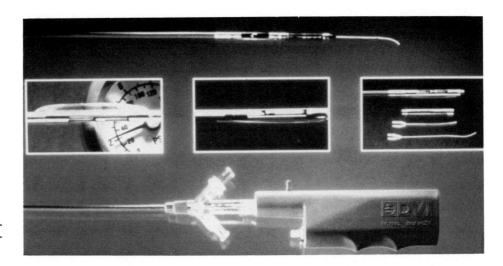

**Figure 29–15.** Simpson atherectomy system (Courtesy of Mallinckrodt Medical, St. Louis, MO).

needle pass should be within the liver tissue, since it is this surrounding tissue that tamponades the bleeding. The main hepatic vein lacks surrounding tissue to aid in the arrest of bleeding; thus, only intrahepatic veins are cannulated.

Thrombosis is also a potential complication. An ultrasound examination on the day following the procedure is advised to assess possible thrombus formation.

Hepatic encephalopathy is a treatable side effect of TIPS. This side effect appears to increase as the amount of shunted blood increases. As less blood passes through the liver, ammonia levels can increase in the blood, ultimately affecting the brain. Disorientation, confusion, tremors, and death may result.

## ATHERECTOMY

Atherectomy is an uncommon procedure during which plaque is cut away from the vessel wall by means of a specially designed catheter (Fig. 29–15). Although atherectomy is uncommon, it is most often performed in the extremities. This procedure is rarely used in the trunk since stents can be used to keep vessels open. The restenosis rate seems to be higher with atherectomy than with angioplasty or stents.

## Indications

In noncoronary vessels, the most common indication for atherectomy is where the narrowed area expands and contracts with an angioplasty balloon (is unable to remain open). Other indications include an eccentric plaque and a narrowing at an anastomosis.

## Technique

Several kinds of atherectomy devices are commercially available. Some use a guide wire, while others are passed through a guiding catheter. Since design and operation vary from one manufacturer to another, only procedural steps common to all types of devices are discussed here.

The procedure involves placing the cutting device next to the involved plaque (Fig. 29–16). When the device is properly positioned, it is activated. If the device uses a wire, the plaque may be removed as the

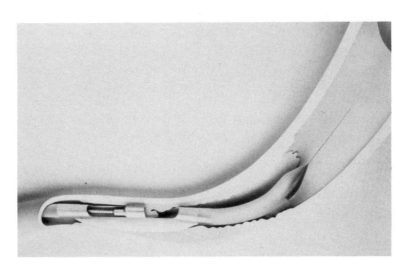

**Figure 29–16.** Atherectomy catheter in vessel (Courtesy of Peripheral Systems Group, Mt. View, CA).

**282** Vascular Interventional Angiography

catheter rotates and is advanced along the wire. The removed plaque is evacuated, along with blood, during this process. If a guiding catheter is used, a balloon may be inflated to push the cutter toward the plaque to stabilize it while the cutter is advanced to remove the plaque. The entire device must be withdrawn from the patient to remove the plaque that was cut away.

## Complications

Complications associated with atherectomy are the same as those seen with angioplasty. Additionally, cutting through the wall of the vessel and clot formation on the wall of a vessel immediately following atherectomy procedure are potential complications. Large

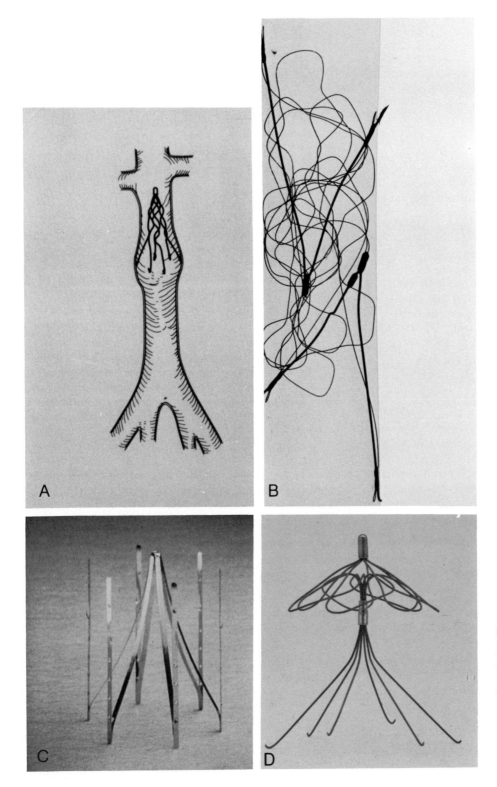

**Figure 29–17.** IVC filters; (A) Greenfield filter (Courtesy of Medi-tech, a division of Boston Scientific Corporation, Watertown, MA); (B) Bird's Nest vena cava filter (Courtesy of Cook Incorporated, Bloomington, IN); (C) LGM vena cava filter (Courtesy of B. Braun Vena Tech, Evanston, IL, distributor, and B. Braun Celsa, Chasseneuil, France, device manufacturer); (D) Simon Nitinol filter (Courtesy of Nitinol Medical Technologies, Boston, MA).

atherectomy devices may increase the number of hematomas at the puncture site.

## INFERIOR VENA CAVA FILTER PLACEMENT

Inferior vena cava (IVC) filters, either wire frame or metal mesh (Fig. 29–17), are placed in the IVC to prevent clots that may be formed in the lower extremity from flowing to the lungs and causing pulmonary emboli. The filter traps the clots, and the intrinsic lytic system dissolves them. The IVC filter is permanent and removable only by surgery; thus, careful consideration and patient assessment should occur to determine the viability of the IVC filter over other procedures.

### Indications

Placement of an IVC filter is indicated when the patient cannot be placed on anticoagulants to treat pulmonary emboli and when pulmonary emboli are not relieved by anticoagulants.

### Technique

There are two percutaneous approaches that can be used to place an IVC filter: a right jugular vein or femoral vein puncture. The approach selected depends on the patient's condition, filter design, and physician's preference.

The femoral approach is more common, since there is no need to manipulate a catheter through the heart. If this approach is used, an ultrasound examination should be performed prior to catheterization to rule out the presence of a clot, which could dislodge and flow toward the lungs during the installation of the filter. If a clot is seen on the ultrasound scan or the angiogram, the jugular approach should be used to place the filter.

The Seldinger technique is used to gain access to the femoral vein and perform an IVC angiogram. The angiogram is used to ensure that the placement of the filter is inferior to the renal veins. The size of the IVC can also be approximated from this angiogram, which is important since filter installation is limited by vessel size. Sizes usually range from 28 to 40 mm. The specific technique used to implant the filter is in accordance with the manufacturer's instructions. However, a general technique used to install the filter is to introduce a guide wire via the Seldinger technique and position it in the IVC. Loaded in its catheter, the filter is passed over the guide wire and positioned in the IVC. Once positioned, the filter is released, and the catheter and guide wire are removed. The filter is equipped with hooks that anchor it to the vessel wall.

In the jugular approach, the Seldinger technique is used on the right jugular vein, and the filter is positioned through the heart and into the IVC. Care must be taken when passing the filter through the heart. Regardless of the approach, once a filter has been placed, a radiograph should be taken to document its position.

### Complications

Even though filters have hooks that dig into the vessel wall, filters have been known to migrate into the heart and lungs. The patient should be observed for the first 2 to 3 days to assess possible postinsertion thrombosis. Infection is also a potential complication. A long-term complication of concern is occlusion of the IVC.

## REVIEW QUESTIONS

1. The most common interventional procedure is _____.
   A. balloon angioplasty
   B. IVC
   C. embolization
   D. thrombolysis

2. Balloon angioplasty employs a balloon catheter to _____ a vessel.
   A. filter
   B. restrict
   C. enlarge
   D. occlude

3. A common antiplatelet therapy for balloon angioplasty is _____ four times a day.
   A. 300 mg aspirin
   B. 150 mg urokinase
   C. 200 mg streptokinase
   D. 50 mg Vistaril

4. Balloon angioplasty uses an introducer sheath to _____.
   A. introduce the guide wire
   B. exchange catheters
   C. expand the balloon
   D. deflate the balloon

5. A common diameter size for a balloon catheter used for coronary vessels is _____.
   A. 5 mm
   B. 5 cm
   C. 2 cm
   D. 2 mm

6. When selecting a balloon for balloon angioplasty, it is best to use one with a diameter that is _____ than the proximal end of the stenotic vessel.
   A. 1 mm larger
   B. 1 mm smaller
   C. 1 cm longer
   D. 1 cm smaller

7. An average balloon inflation time is _____ seconds.
   A. 1 to 10
   B. 11 to 20
   C. 20 to 40
   D. 41 to 60

8. _____ is a complication associated with stents.
   A. Vessel dilation
   B. Stenosis
   C. Increased blood flow
   D. Crimping

9. _____ is a procedure in which the clot is decomposed or lysed.
   A. Stent
   B. Embolization
   C. Thrombolysis
   D. TIPS

10. Urokinase is used during _____.
   A. balloon angioplasty
   B. thrombolysis
   C. retrieval
   D. embolization

11. A(n) _____ is useful to perform before thrombolysis.
   A. angioplasty
   B. anticoagulation therapy
   C. chest x ray
   D. coagulation profile

12. _____ is useful in decreasing or stopping blood flow in a vessel.
   A. Embolization
   B. Balloon angioplasty
   C. Thrombolysis
   D. Stent

13. _____ is (are) a temporary embolization material.
   A. Spheres
   B. Gelfoam
   C. Coils
   D. Alcohol

14. List three types of retrieval devices.

15. _____ is indicated for variceal bleeding caused by portal hypertension.
   A. Stent
   B. Balloon angioplasty
   C. Embolization
   D. TIPS

16. A(n) _____ is used to prevent clots from flowing to the lungs.
   A. loop basket
   B. TIPS
   C. IVC filter
   D. snare

17. _____ is a procedure by which plaque is cut away from the vessel wall.
   A. TIPS
   B. Atherectomy
   C. Angioplasty
   D. Retrieval

18. Atherectomy devices may use a guide wire or a _____.
   A. transducer
   B. torque device
   C. guiding catheter
   D. metal vessel tubing

19. Care needs to be taken not to _____ when performing an atherectomy.
   A. rotate the catheter
   B. cut through the vessel
   C. underinflate the balloon
   D. constrict the vessel too much

## BIBLIOGRAPHY

Abrams, H: Angiography, Vol 3, ed 3. Little, Brown & Co. Boston, 1983.

Johnsrude, I, Jackson, D, and Dunnick, NR: A Practical Approach to Angiography, ed 2. Little, Brown & Co, Boston, 1987.

Kandarpa, K: Handbook of Cardiovascular and Interventional Radiologic Procedures. Little, Brown & Co, Boston, 1989.

Snopek, A: Fundamentals of Special Radiographic Procedures. WB Saunders, Philadelphia, 1992.

Wojtowycz, M: Handbook in Radiology, Interventional Radiology, and Angiography. Year Book Medical Publishers, Chicago, 1990.

# CHAPTER 30

# Nonvascular Interventional Radiology

*William F. O'Donnell Jr., AS, ARRT(R)*
*Marianne R. Tortorici, EdD, ARRT(R)*

Nonvascular interventional radiology is a therapeutic branch of radiology that replaces some procedures previously performed in surgery. These interventional procedures use a percutaneous approach to drain body fluids, inject medications, perform biopsies, or place tubes in organs and cavities of the body. Equipment to perform percutaneous access is commercially available from various manufacturers and varies slightly in design. Figure 30–1 is an example of one type of system.

Although most nonvascular interventional procedures are performed in an angiographic room, they may also be monitored with an ultrasound, computed tomographic, or fluoroscopic unit. This chapter concentrates on the routine angiographic methods and does not address the techniques used by other imaging modalities. Thus, discussion is limited to nephrostomy, percutaneous biliary drainage (PBD), percutaneous abscess drainage, percutaneous needle biopsy, and gastrostomy tube placement.

## PERCUTANEOUS ACCESS METHODS

### Modified Seldinger

A modified Seldinger technique is used for several nonvascular interventional procedures. In this technique, following local anesthesia, the skin is nicked to accommodate the size of the interventional device. A 21 gauge needle with stylet is advanced through underlying tissue to the area of interest (e.g., kidney). The stylet is removed, and a reflux of fluid (urine if kidney, bile if liver, and so on) from the needle indicates that it is in the proper location. If there is no backflow of fluid, a tube can be attached to the needle and gentle aspiration applied, via syringe, as the needle is slowly withdrawn. After the fluid is aspirated, a contrast medium is injected to visualize the area of interest under fluoroscopy to assure proper needle placement.

When the 21 gauge needle is in the desired area, a guide wire (usually 0.018) is advanced through the needle into the selected area and the needle is removed over the guide wire. A lock sheath and dilator-cannula

**285**

**The .018" guidewire is advanced fully through the needle.**

21 ga. Diagnostic Needle                                          .018" Wire

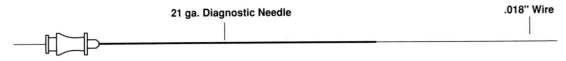

**After removing the needle, the locked sheath and dilator/cannula assembly is advanced over the .018" guidewire.**

6Fr Sheath                                  4Fr Dilator        .018" Wire

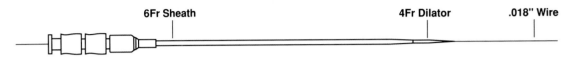

**The dilator/cannula assembly is removed and the .038" guidewire is advanced through the 6Fr sheath.**
**The .018" guidewire acts as a "safety" wire.**

6Fr Sheath                                              .018" Wire

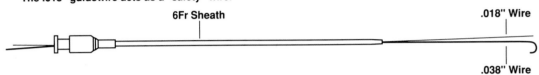

.038" Wire

**Figure 30–1.** AccuStick System used in percutaneous puncture for interventional procedures (Courtesy of Medi-tech, a division of Boston Scientific Corporation, Watertown, MA).

assembly is then placed over the top of an 0.018 guide wire, which enlarges the vessel. When the dilator is removed, a larger guide wire, such as a 0.038, is threaded through the sheath. It is over this larger guide wire that dilators of increasing size are used to enlarge the opening to the desired diameter. Once enlarged, the appropriate drainage catheter, stent, and so on, are introduced over the guide wire.

## Trocar Technique

The trocar method is usually employed in drainage procedures for large pathologies that are not located in a critical structure. The trocar, which consists of a cutting stylet, is inside a cannula which is inserted in a catheter (Fig. 30–2). It is introduced percutaneously into the area of interest, such as an abscess. Once in the area of interest, the stylet is removed. The cannula is held in place while the catheter is positioned in the desired area (a guide wire may be introduced through the cannula to guide the catheter). Contrast medium may be injected to confirm the position. After the position of the catheter is verified, a syringe is attached to the cannula to aspirate the abscess. After aspiration, the cannula is removed, and the catheter is sutured in place to allow the abscess to drain.

## NEPHROSTOMY

### Indications

A percutaneous nephrostomy is a procedure used to drain an obstructed kidney or ureter, remove a stone, or infuse drugs for therapeutic reasons. In this proce-

dure, a catheter is introduced through the skin and kidney parenchyma to the renal pelvis or other target area. After proper placement of the catheter, the specific intervention proceeds, for example, drainage or stone removal.

### Contraindication

Nephrostomy is a relatively safe procedure. However, it is contraindicated where a patient has a clotting deficiency.

### Technique

For a posterior approach, the patient is placed prone on the x-ray table with the side of interest slightly elevated. If the patient has a transplanted kidney, the supine position is used for an anterior approach because most transplanted kidneys are placed in the lower quadrant of the abdomen. The posterior approach allows for puncture through the greater curvature of the kidney and into the renal pelvis. Needle entry is usually 2 to 3 cm below the 12th rib. To facilitate catheter placement into the calyx, it is best to enter a middle or lower posterior calyx from a posterolateral angle. Puncture of a superior calyx is preferred for stone removal. Ultrasound guidance may be used to indicate the appropriate depth of the needle and angle of the needle. Occasionally, contrast medium is administered intravenously to visualize the kidney under fluoroscopy. However, if the kidney is obstructed, the contrast medium may not be visualized. Contrast medium is useful in identifying the anatomy and distending the calyx.

When percutaneous access to the kidney pelvis has

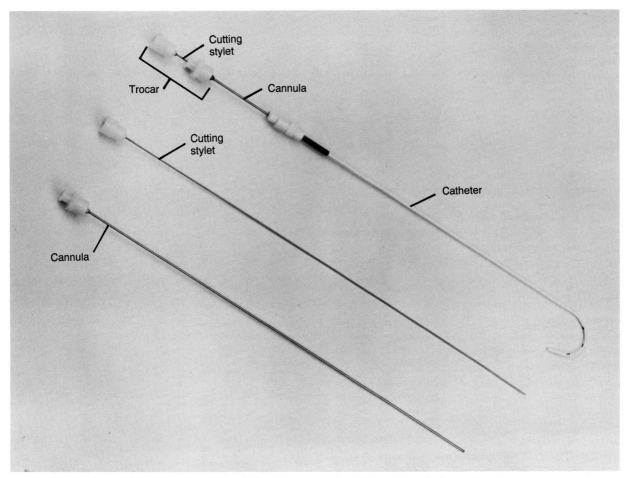

**Figure 30–2.** Trocar setup (Courtesy of Medi-tech, a division of Boston Scientific Corporation, Watertown, MA).

been accomplished, the pathology present determines the specific techniques that follow. For example, if there is a stricture of the ureter, a stent (Fig. 30–3) may be introduced into the ureter to restore the flow of urine from the kidney to the bladder. If the stricture does not permit access to the bladder, a nephrostomy drain tube (Fig. 30–4) may be inserted and left in place. Other common interventions include the use of a bal-loon catheter to treat ureteral strictures and a basket catheter, or other appropriate device, to remove stones.

## Complications

The most common and transient complication of nephrostomy is microscopic hematuria. Other less

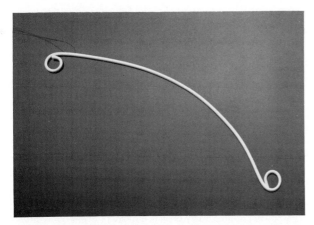

**Figure 30–3.** Percuflex double J stent used for nephrostomy (Courtesy of Medi-tech, a division of Boston Scientific Corporation, Watertown, MA).

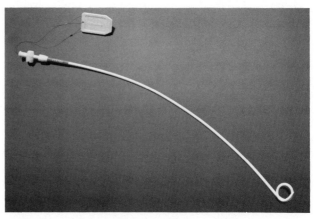

**Figure 30–4.** VTC nephrostomy drainage catheter (Courtesy of Medi-tech, a division of Boston Scientific Corporation, Watertown, MA).

common complications include hemorrhage, pneumothorax, infection, peritonitis, urine extravasation, catheter dislodgment, catheter obstruction, and perirenal bleeding.

## PERCUTANEOUS BILIARY DRAINAGE

### Indications

Percutaneous biliary drainage (PBD) is indicated in patients with unresectable malignant disease. The procedure is palliative. Other, less popular, uses of PBD are for the treatment of biliary obstruction, suppurative cholangitis, postoperative or post-traumatic biliary leakage, and stone removal.

### Contraindications

PBD is contraindicated in patients with asymptomatic jaundice, ascites, advanced cirrhosis, and impaired coagulation. It is also contraindicated in patients with diffuse hepatic metastases or liver failure, or in those who have a life expectancy of less than 1 month.

### Technique

It is common for patients undergoing PBD to have infected bile. Therefore, antibiotics should be administered at least 1 hour before the procedure. For the procedure, the patient is placed supine on the x-ray table with the right arm positioned over the head. Needle puncture may be made from the right, the left, or both sides of the liver, depending on the location of the obstruction. Left-sided puncture is useful when separate ductal obstructions or hilar obstructions are present. For the right-sided puncture, a fine needle (22 gauge) is used with entry on the right lateral upper portion of the abdomen and below the 10th rib to avoid puncturing the lung or pleura. After needle placement, contrast medium may be injected under fluoroscopic observation to ensure that the needle is in the biliary duct. Upon successful cannulation of the duct, the appropriate treatment is administered.

A common PBD technique is to secure internal or external drainage. Internal drainage (Fig. 30–5) requires that a catheter or stent be positioned through the common bile duct into the duodenum. External drainage (Fig. 30–6) is achieved by securing a catheter located through the common bile duct into the duodenum and to the external surface of the patient. Since catheter displacements have resulted in death, it is critical that the catheter be appropriately secured for external drainage. Other treatment methods include endoprostheses (in which a stent or catheter is used for biliary strictures) and direct irradiation of neoplasms with an injection of an appropriate radioisotope.

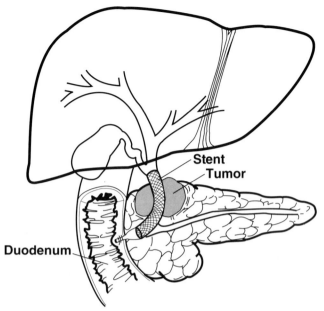

**Figure 30–5.** Wallstent for internal biliary drainage (Courtesy of Schneider (USA) Inc, Minneapolis, MN).

### Complications

Since many patients already have bile infection, sepsis is the most common complication associated with PBD. Hemobilia is another common complication. Other complications include catheter obstruction, catheter displacement, cholangitis, and bile peritonitis. If a lung or the pleural lining is punctured, a pneumothorax or hemothorax may occur.

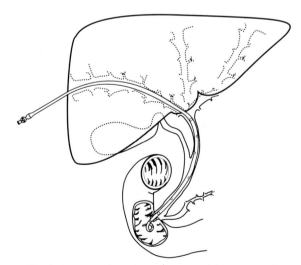

**Figure 30–6.** External biliary drain (Courtesy of Schneider (USA) Inc, Minneapolis, MN).

## PERCUTANEOUS ABSCESS DRAINAGE

### Indications

An abscess is a localized collection of pus, which may occur internally or externally in any area of the body. There are many causes of an abscess, for example, a breach of sterility during surgery. As part of the body's defense, the breached area is "walled off" and resolved. Most internal abscesses are life threatening and infectious. An abscess is best identified by means of computed tomography (CT), ultrasound, or radionuclide scan. Depending on the size and location of the abscess as well as the patient's condition, abscesses may be percutaneously drained or surgically treated. Since surgical treatment is more invasive than the percutaneous method, the chance of spreading the purulent material increases substantially with the surgical method. Therefore percutaneous drainage is the method of choice. However, patients with large and extensive abscesses that may involve organs are more appropriately treated by surgical means.

### Contraindications

The primary contraindication for percutaneous drainage of an abscess is when a major organ, blood vessel, or the pleural space must be transgressed. Other contraindications include coagulation deficiency and an intrahepatic echinococcal cyst, which may be fatal if leakage occurs.

### Technique

Percutaneous drainage of an abscess may be performed by means of needle aspiration or by catheter drain placement. The physician assesses the patient's physical condition to determine the best approach. In general, needle aspirations are performed on small abscesses (less than 5 cm).

#### NEEDLE ASPIRATION

In needle aspiration, a 22 gauge needle is most often sufficient; however, if the material to be aspirated is too viscous, an 18 gauge needle may be used. After the needle is positioned, a small amount of fluid is aspirated for a Gram's stain and culture tests. If the results of the tests indicate an infection, antibiotics may be injected. If the tests indicate that the material is purulent, the abscess is drained and the needle removed.

#### CATHETER DRAINAGE

Catheter drainage may be performed using the Seldinger or the trocar technique (see "Percutaneous Access Methods" section of this chapter). There are different types and sizes of catheters available for drainage. The single-lumen style is the most common. A large-size catheter is often preferred since it provides better drainage for viscous material. Suction may be needed depending on the location of the abscess, the viscosity of the fluid, and the type of catheter employed. Suction may cause the wall of the abscess to adhere to a catheter with side holes (side walling). To prevent side walling, a double-lumen sump drain (Fig. 30–7) catheter (which allows room air to flow into the abscess while suction is applied) is used.

Once the catheter is in place, the purulent material is aspirated and a contrast medium injection is performed. The resulting sinogram serves as a baseline and is useful in demonstrating fistulae. The catheter is left in place for several days with output monitored daily. A drainage output greater than 50 ml after 4 days indicates a possible fistula or other problem requiring investigation. When the output approaches zero, this indicates that the abscess is drained and the catheter may be removed.

### Complications

Complications of percutaneous abscess drainage include septic shock, fistula formation, and bleeding.

## PERCUTANEOUS NEEDLE BIOPSY

### Indications

A biopsy is performed to determine whether a mass is benign or malignant. Biopsies may be performed in a variety of areas, with the lungs, kidneys, pancreas, and liver the most common organs biopsied.

### Contraindications

In general, a biopsy is contraindicated in patients exhibiting coagulation deficiency. Lung biopsy is contraindicated in patients with suspected vascular lesions or pulmonary hypertension. Renal biopsies should not be performed in patients with severe hypertension or atrophic kidneys or in those with a cyst, tumor, or vascular malformation of the kidney.

### Technique

A biopsy is a technique used to obtain a sample tissue for analysis. A needle is required to remove the sample from the area of interest. There are a variety of needles that may be employed to obtain a tissue sample.

Correct positioning of the needle may be achieved by monitoring with CT, ultrasound, or fluoroscopy. Most biopsies of pulmonary masses or large mediastinal lesions are monitored with fluoroscopy or CT scan.

Although the specific technical methods vary

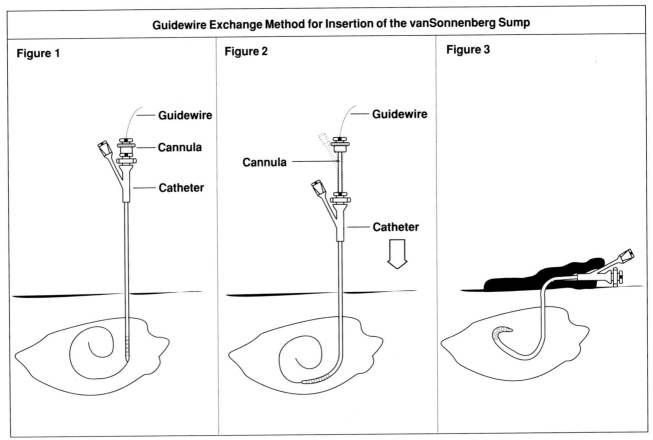

**Guidewire Exchange Method for Insertion of the vanSonnenberg Sump**

| Figure 1 | Figure 2 | Figure 3 |

**Figure 30–7.** VanSonnenberg sump drain (Courtesy of Medi-tech, a division of Boston Scientific Corporation, Watertown, MA).

slightly, after needle placement, the needle is rotated to cut the tissue sample and then is withdrawn from the patient. It is important to handle the sample using sterile technique procedures. Samples may be placed on a glass slide or in formalin for Gram's stains or culture assessment as indicated.

## Complications

Complications vary with the area biopsied. Pulmonary biopsy complications include pneumothorax, hemothorax, air embolization, and hemoptysis. Kidney biopsy complications include hematuria, perinephric hematoma (usually transient), and ureter obstruction.

## GASTROSTOMY TUBE PLACEMENT

### Indications

Gastrostomy tube placement is a procedure in which a tube is placed, percutaneously, through the stomach into the duodenum (Fig. 30–8). The most common reason for gastric tube placement is for long-term feeding, necessitated by neurologic disorders, usually caused by a stroke. Patients who have a gastrostomy tube in place are unable to eat on their own; otherwise

they have normal gastrointestinal function. Other indications for gastrostomy include a pharyngeal or esophageal fistula, oropharyngeal-esophageal neoplasm, aspiration, and mechanical blockage. Gastrostomy may also be performed for short-term decompression therapy.

## Contraindications

As a long-term treatment, gastrostomy is contraindicated in the presence of gastric outlet, or intestinal, obstruction. Patients with ascites, severe neurologic impairment, gastroesophageal reflux, or poor gastric emptying should have the tube placed in the jejunum to decrease the possibility of reflux or aspiration. Gastrostomy should not be performed as a means of "quick cure" for gastrointestinal problems. If percutaneous access to the stomach is unlikely, for example, if the patient has an enlarged liver, then gastrostomy is contraindicated.

## Technique

Patients having gastrostomy should fast for at least 8 hours before the procedure. It is important to identify the location of the liver and colon to avoid accidentally

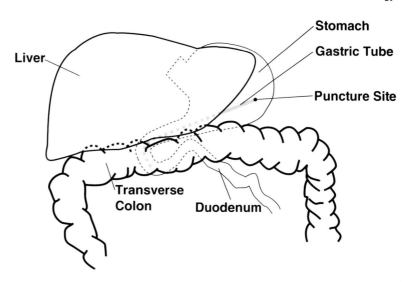

**Figure 30–8.** Position of gastrostomy tube.

puncturing them. The liver border can be located by ultrasound or CT. Because the bowel tends to have gas in it, fluoroscopy is useful in pinpointing the colon. Also, administering dilute barium the day previous to the examination sometimes proves useful in identifying the colon.

Prior to percutaneous puncture, a nasogastric tube is placed in the stomach to aspirate gastric fluids and inflate the stomach. Stomach insufflation is useful in locating the colon because the air is easily visualized under fluoroscopy.

An area in the epigastric region below the costal margin and left of the midline is chosen for the percutaneous puncture. The puncture site varies depending on the type of tube employed and the patient's size and age. When the puncture site is prepared, a local anesthetic is administered. The skin is nicked to accommodate the needle and tube. The Teflon sheath needle is rapidly advanced about 2″ so that it rests inside the stomach. The needle is removed, and an injection of contrast medium confirms that the sheath is placed correctly. Also, at this time, any gastric fluid may be aspirated through the sheath. A guide wire is advanced through the sheath. Dilators are used to enlarge the puncture site. After dilation, the gastronomy tube is threaded over the guide wire and may be advanced to various levels of the upper gastrointestinal tract, including the stomach, duodenum, and jejunum. The tube should be anchored internally (either by a locking or a balloon catheter) and externally.

After the gastronomy tube placement, the patient is monitored closely to ensure that there are no complications, such as peritonitis.

## Complications

Great care must be taken during needle placement to avoid puncture of the liver, colon, posterior wall of the stomach, or other vital structures. Also, since the stom-

ach is not a well-anchored organ, care must be taken to avoid placing the tube or dilators into the abdominal wall. This may result if the stomach is not well anchored or if it is insufficiently distended with air.

## REVIEW QUESTIONS

1. A(n) _____ percutaneous access for nonvascular interventions is usually employed for large pathologies that are not located in a critical structure.
   A. trocar
   B. 22-gauge needle
   C. Seldinger
   D. aspiration

2. Needle entry for nephrostomy is usually 2 to 3 cm below the _____ rib.
   A. 6th
   B. 8th
   C. 10th
   D. 12th

3. During nephrostomy, puncturing a superior calyx is preferred for _____.
   A. drainage
   B. drug infusion
   C. stone removal
   D. dilation of a ureter

4. List two reasons why the use of contrast medium during a nephrostomy procedure is advantageous.

5. List four complications that may occur with nephrostomy.

6. PBD is usually a _____ procedure.
   A. diagnostic
   B. palliative
   C. curative
   D. screening

7. _____ should be given 1 hour before a PBD.
   A. Sedatives
   B. Plenty of fluids

C. A fatty meal
D. Antibiotics

8. Left-sided liver puncture for a PBD is useful when _____ is (are) present.
   A. a dilated gallbladder
   B. benign tumors
   C. a hilar obstruction
   D. stones

9. During PBD, the distal end of the catheter for internal drainage is located in the _____.
   A. pancreas
   B. duodenum
   C. common duct
   D. gallbladder

10. _____ is the most common complication of PBD.
    A. Sepsis
    B. Pneumothorax
    C. Hemothorax
    D. Tube displacement

11. Surgical treatment and drainage of an abscess is indicated when _____.
    A. the abscess is small
    B. the percutaneous attempt fails
    C. an organ is involved
    D. the pus leaks into the body cavity

12. List two situations in which a percutaneous drainage procedure is contraindicated.

13. When performing a percutaneous abscess drainage via needle aspiration, a _____ is used to determine the need to administer antibiotics.
    A. Seldinger technique
    B. Gram's stain
    C. trocar test
    D. sump drain

14. _____ may occur when suction is used for percutaneous abscess drainage.
    A. A fistula
    B. Hemorrhage
    C. Distention
    D. Side walling

15. A _____ is useful in demonstrating a fistula of an abscess when performing a percutaneous drainage.

A. sinogram
B. sump pump
C. trocar test
D. double-lumen catheter

16. State the primary reason for performing a biopsy.

17. _____ is a complication associated with kidney biopsy.
    A. Hematuria
    B. Hemothorax
    C. Air embolization
    D. Hemoptysis

18. The most common reason for gastric tube placement is for long-term feeding, necessitated by _____.
    A. fistulae
    B. neoplasms
    C. poor diet
    D. neurologic disorders

19. _____ is a contraindication of gastrostomy.
    A. Esophageal fistula
    B. Oropharyngeal neoplasm
    C. Ascites
    D. Difficulty ingesting food

20. _____ is a method used to identify the colon for gastrostomy.
    A. Insufflation of air in the stomach
    B. Aspiration of fluid in the stomach
    C. Decompressing the stomach
    D. Palpating the rectus abdominis muscle

## BIBLIOGRAPHY

Abrams, H: Angiography, Vol 3, ed 3. Little, Brown & Co, Boston, 1983.

Kandarpa, K: Handbook of Cardiovascular and Interventional Radiologic Procedures. Little, Brown & Co, Boston, 1989.

Snopek, A: Fundamentals of Special Radiographic Procedures. WB Saunders, Philadelphia, 1992.

Wojtowycz, M: Handbook in Radiology Interventional Radiology and Angiography. Year Book Medical Publishers, Chicago, 1990.

# PART FIVE

# SPECIALIZED IMAGING

# CHAPTER 31

# Fundamentals of Mammography

*Janice C. De'Ath, ARRT(R)(M)*
*Patrick J. Apfel, MEd, ARRT(R)*

Mammography is a radiographic study of the human breast. Although it is most commonly performed on women, the male breast is also examined, but on a much less frequent basis. Equipment for this procedure has developed over the years from conventional radiographic rooms to dedicated mammography units designed to produce high quality images with low radiation dosages. The medium for recording mammographic images has progressed from nonscreen film, to xeroradiographic paper (and image processing), and currently to single-emulsion film combined with one intensifying screen. The objective of using a dedicated mammography x-ray unit and single-screen imaging is to optimize quality and reduce radiation exposure to the patient.

Mammography is currently the best diagnostic tool to detect cancers of the breast. It is capable of revealing growths as early as 2 years before they are large enough to be palpated during physical examination. Since early detection is essential to the successful treatment of the disease, the American Cancer Society (ACS) along with the American College of Radiology (ACR) have developed specific recommendations and guidelines for mammography departments.

In 1992, the Mammography Quality Standards Act (MQSA) was enacted. This act became effective on October 1, 1994, and requires that all facilities conducting mammography (except agencies of the Department of Veterans Affairs) become certified by the Food and Drug Administration (FDA). Following initial certification, a yearly site inspection is required to meet MQSA guidelines for continuing certification. The major accrediting agency approved and used by the FDA is the ACR. However, Arkansas, California, and Iowa have their own accrediting agencies approved by the FDA.

Mammographers are an essential and integral part of the mammography diagnostic imaging and patient care team. Among the skills the mammographer must possess are patient care and rapport, knowledge of breast anatomy, equipment usage, and quality control. The mammographer is the individual most closely associated with both the patient and the equipment. Thus, the mammographer plays an important role in making contributions to imaging and the proper diagnosis of each patient. Although the radiologist is responsible for the radiologic image quality as well as interpretation of the films, the mammographer must take some responsibility for undetected breast cancers because of suboptimal film quality. The latitude in the various parameters in mammography, including positioning, technique, compression, and processing, is much narrower than in conventional radiographic procedures.

Mammography is one of the few areas in radiology in which film quality is the primary factor affecting proper patient diagnosis. In 1991, the American Registry of Radiologic Technologists offered the first national mammography certification examination. At the printing of this text, many states have passed legislation requiring mammographers to hold a current license in the discipline. The intent of licensure is to ensure that mammographers have adequate knowledge to perform a diagnostic mammogram. Many licensures require mammographers to participate in continuing education. This trend toward licensure, equipment regulations, and continuing education is designed to ensure that a patient will benefit from the latest mammographic technology and a quality examination conducted by a qualified mammographer.

Since most mammography is performed on women, this chapter deals with mammography of the adult female breast. It should be noted that examination of the male breast is similar to the female imaging procedure. Also discussed in this chapter are regulations that were in effect at the time of the printing of this text and the criteria a mammographer should follow to ensure that every patient receives an optimum mammogram. It should be noted that providing all the essential information needed to pass state and national certification examinations is beyond the scope of this chapter.

### INDICATIONS

Statistically, breast cancer is the leading cancer in women. There is disagreement among professionals regarding the age and frequency at which mammography should be performed on women. Since one third of breast cancers are found in women between the ages of 35 to 49 years, the American Cancer Society recommends that asymptomatic women undergo a baseline mammogram between the ages of 35 and 40 years. The baseline examination, which is the initial set of routine mammography films, is compared to subsequent studies, which the society recommends be performed on a 1- to 2-year basis for women 40 to 49 years old (women with high risk factors may require annual examinations) and on an annual basis for women aged 50 and above. These guidelines are continually reviewed and changes may occur after the publication of this text. Although the risks and benefits from screening mammography are not precisely known, the radiation risk is negligible when compared with the proven benefits from early detection. Mammography cannot prevent breast cancer, but early detection of the disease increases the survival rate and decreases the death rate. Though only

an interim measure, mammography screening does represent a major step in the control of breast cancer. Certain studies have shown that patients participating in yearly mammography screening programs have a 25% lower death rate from breast cancer than those who do not participate in a screening program.

### BASIC ANATOMY

In the adult female, breast size can vary from individual to individual. The average breast extends approximately from the level of the second or third rib to the level of the sixth or seventh rib. The breasts lie external to the pectoralis muscles and are attached to them by a fascia (fibrous tissue). Ligaments of Cooper (a collection of fibrous bands of tissue) attach the breast to the skin. External structures of the breast include the areola, which is the rounded area at the tip of the breast and is usually red to brown in color; the nipple, which protrudes from the center of the areola; and the inframammary crease, formed by the junction of the inferior breast with the chest wall. Although, externally, the breast appears to cover the anterior and lateral aspects of the chest wall, breast tissue further extends toward the sternum and into the axillary area. That portion extending into the axillary area is commonly called the tail of the breast and is important radiographically since that is where a large number of breast cancers are located.

Internally, the breast consists of glandular (mammary), connective (fibrous), and adipose (fat) tissues. Figure 31 – 1 illustrates the anatomy of the breast. The

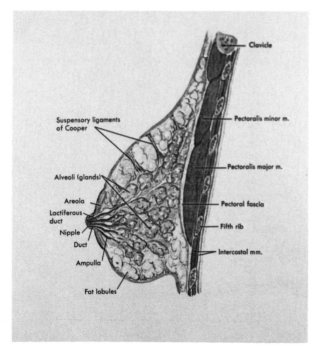

**Figure 31–1.** Basic female breast anatomy. (From Anthony, CP and Thibodeau, GA: Textbook of Anatomy and Physiology, ed 10. Mosby, Philadelphia, p 629, with permission.)

glandular tissues of the breast occupy a central location and are composed of 15 to 20 lobes of tissue extending toward the areola. The tissue lobes are divided into lobules of connective tissue with small clusters of glandular tissue (alveoli) embedded in them. During pregnancy, cells within the alveoli multiply (causing breast enlargement) in preparation for milk production. Lactation (milk production) occurs in the alveoli following delivery. The milk produced during lactation flows from the alveoli through multiple ducts, which empty into a single duct for each lobe. The ducts continue on to the nipple of the breast, where they open to the external surface (15 to 20 openings are present in the nipple). Just before opening onto the surface of the nipple, each duct forms an ampulla or expanded area to temporarily store milk. The ducts and lobules are the sites for the two major types of breast cancers: ductal carcinoma or adenocarcinoma, and lobular carcinoma (which is less common than ductal carcinoma).

Fibrous tissue surrounds the breast below the skin and infiltrates the breast between the glandular tissue lobes, thus connecting them together. Posteriorly, the fibrous tissue of the breast and the fibrous tissue overlying the anterior surface of the pectoralis muscle form a space between them known as the retromammary space. Intervening fibrous tissue loosely connects the breast to the anterior chest wall.

Adipose tissue surrounds the breast and is present in the spaces between the lobes of glandular tissue. The amount of adipose tissue present accounts for the differences in breast size, since it represents the greatest amount of tissue within the breast. It is evident, then, that breast size does not affect the amount of milk production.

Blood vessels, lymphatic vessels, and nerves supply each breast. Veins in this area are typically larger than arteries, and some can be visualized on a finished radiograph of the breast. Since the breast is composed of soft tissues, it is often difficult to delineate the various tissues of the breast on a film. The many markings, including vessels, ducts, and tissues seen on a radiograph of the breast, that cannot be distinctly identified, are referred to as trabeculae.

As a woman ages, her breast undergoes involution with a significant reduction in the number of breast lobules and a relative increase in the fatty tissue of the breast. The age at which and the extent to which this involution occurs will vary among patients.

## EQUIPMENT

During the past 20 years, there have been many significant technologic improvements in mammographic x-ray equipment and in screen film recording systems. Currently, mammography is performed using dedicated mammographic x-ray equipment. Among other features, these units have specially designed tube targets, smaller focal spots, and significantly improved breast compression devices. Other dedicated accessory equipment includes cassettes and screen film combinations. Film processing has also improved tremendously

over the years. These equipment, screen film, and processing improvements now make it possible to obtain mammograms of higher quality at a significantly lower radiation dose to the patient compared with that required for mammography 20 years ago.

## Dedicated X-ray Equipment

Although mammography can be performed using conventional x-ray equipment, dedicated units specifically designed for the examination are currently employed (Fig. 31–2). Since the area of interest is composed of soft tissue structures and the pathologies involved are basically soft tissue, the radiographic equipment must be capable of producing high quality (detailed) films. The kilovolt (peak) range of a dedicated mammography unit is usually between 25 and 40 kVp. Since the tissues comprising the breast have similar densities, lower kilovoltage is necessary to optimize radiographic contrast. There are over 30 commercial companies that provide dedicated mammographic x-ray units. Inherent in the design of all of these units are appropriate beam quality, grid capability, breast compression devices, and automatic exposure control.

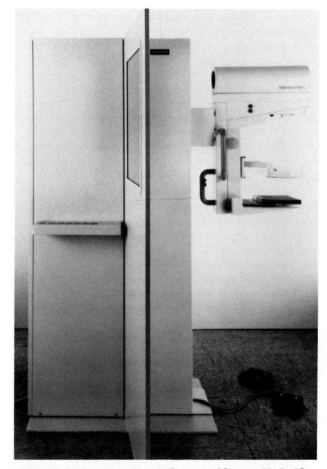

**Figure 31–2.** Mammographic unit (Courtesy of Siemens Medical Systems, Inc., Iselin, NJ).

The mammographic tube contains a rotating target made of molybdenum. This material produces lower energy photons necessary to increase radiographic contrast. Some of the differences that distinguish these units from each other are focal spot size, geometry (focal spot to object and object to receptor distances), magnification capability, x-ray beam quality, design of the compression device, and price of the unit.

## Dedicated Processing

Since the rate of cure for breast cancer increases with the ability to see small pathologies on the radiograph, the quality of the image is vital for proper diagnosis. Consequently, processing conditions must be closely controlled and monitored. As with the mammographic units, there are many processors commercially available. It is recommended that imaging departments purchase processors from a company having a good, long-standing reputation in the processing of the mammographic image.

To assure the highest quality, processing must be optimized in conjunction with a proper film screen combination. There are two methods of processing mammography film. The first, and preferred, method is to use a processor specifically designed to run mammogram films. The second, and less desirable, method is to attach an extended cycle switch on a processor used for conventional radiographic processing. In both methods the film manufacturer's rigid standards must be followed as to immersion time, replenisher rates, temperature, and types of processor chemicals.

Single-emulsion mammography film requires a longer development time. Developer immersion of 42 to 47 seconds is recommended by several film companies. The recommended ideal developer temperature for single-emulsion film is 95°F. Some major film company suppliers are promoting a single-emulsion film for use in a standard 90-second processor without sacrificing image quality.

Processor quality control must be performed daily. Every mammography department should follow the guidelines set up by the ACR. The most effective method of processor monitoring is sensitometry, which assesses image density, contrast, and fog. This method employs a sensitometer to produce a series of penetrometer steps at different levels of gray through black. A densitometer is used to record the densities of the penetrometer steps. These data provide a means of inferring the response of the film and processing to radiographic exposures. On a daily basis, the processor should be monitored and data recorded in order to detect any changes.

## Phantom Images and Quality Control

A mammographic phantom is used to assure that radiographic density, contrast (density difference), uniformity, and image quality produced by the x-ray imaging system and film processor are maintained at optimum levels. The phantom is equivalent to a 4- to 5-cm breast. It contains appropriate breast-simulated details ranging from visible to invisible fibers, spots, and specks on the mammographic image. The ACR Accreditation Program does specify which type of phantom is acceptable for testing purposes. Additional guidelines by the ACR include exposing and interpreting the phantom, which, as with the sensitometry strip, should be explicitly followed and data accurately recorded.

## PREPROCEDURAL CARE

The only pre-examination care for mammography is that the patient's skin area be clean and free of any powders or deodorants in the axilla and breast areas. Some deodorants and powders leave a residue on the skin that mimics microcalcifications on the film.

When working in a facility where patients are referred and taken by appointment, the patient must be asked if, and where, she had a previous mammogram. It is recommended that patients with previous mammograms at another facility be advised to bring the previous study to the mammography appointment. The importance of the previous study cannot be overstressed. Since breast tissue varies immensely from patient to patient, the radiologist can make a much more accurate diagnosis of a current study if the previous films are readily available.

Once the patient has arrived, she is asked to complete a history form (Fig. 31–3). This information is useful in alerting the mammographer and radiologist to any area of concern, past surgeries, and family history. Of particular importance is whether or not the patient is in a high risk category. Some factors in the high risk category include (from highest to lowest risk factor) individuals who have a history of breast cancer in the family (particularly of the mother or a sister); those who have borne children late in life; and those who are obese. The form should also include diagrams of both breasts since both breasts are routinely radiographed. The mammographer should indicate on these drawings the specific area of complaint and also identify any scars or moles. This is useful in providing the radiologist with information as to the area the patient and her referring physician have concerns about, thus enabling the radiologist to address that area in the report. If the patient has a palpable lump, the mammographer should inform the radiologist, who often elects to perform a physical examination on the patient.

## POSITIONING AND FILMING

Prior to positioning a patient, the mammographer should evaluate the patient's body build and individual anatomy. Every mammogram must be tailored to the physical characteristics of the patient. Another important process prior to positioning the patient is for the mammographer to explain the procedure and the value of breast compression. Compression is used to

# MAMMOGRAPHY QUESTIONNAIRE

NAME_____ DATE OF BIRTH _____ PHONE # _____

DOCTOR_____ DATE _____

### Are you currently experiencing any of the following?

| | | | | |
|---|---|---|---|---|
| Breast Tenderness | No _____ | Yes _____ | Right_____ | Left _____ |
| Lumps | No _____ | Yes _____ | Right_____ | Left _____ |
| Nipple Discharge | No _____ | Yes _____ | Right_____ | Left _____ |
| Nipple Retraction | No _____ | Yes _____ | Right_____ | Left _____ |
| Surgery on Breasts | No _____ | Yes _____ | Right_____ | Left _____ |
| Implants in Breasts | No _____ | Yes _____ | When _____ | |
| Previous Mammogram | No _____ | Yes _____ | When _____ | |
| | Where _____ | | | |

Number of Pregnancies?_____  Age at first Pregnancy? _____

Did you Breast-Feed your child/children?   Yes _____ No _____

Age when you had your first Period?   _____

Have you gone through Menopause or had an hysterectomy?   Yes _____ No _____ When _____

Are you presently taking any hormones or birth control pills?   Yes _____ No _____

Type _____

Have you or any member of your family had Breast Cancer?   Yes _____ No _____

Relation_____

Other complaints or explanation of any problems with your breasts _____

RIGHT                    LEFT

**Figure 31–3.** Example of mammography questionnaire (history form).

even out the thickness of the breast tissue. To achieve adequate compression of the breast, the compression force should range between 25 and 40 pounds. Proper compression achieves the following: improved radiographic contrast; diminished motion unsharpness; uniform radiographic density; reduction of radiation exposure; and separation of superimposed breast tissue. This allows for accurate assessment of the density of any mass that may be present. A relaxed patient results in much easier and accurate positioning. If a patient is extremely fearful of the compression either from a bad experience or from inaccurate hearsay, it is wise to manually compress rather than use the automatic compression control.

The two most common routine projections are the craniocaudad and mediolateral oblique of each breast. It is important to remember that the chest wall is curved and that the Bucky and cassette are flat. Consequently, it is important to position the patient so that the maximum amount of posterior breast tissue is visualized.

The mediolateral oblique and craniocaudad projections are essential and are usually the only projections used for screenings. These standard projections may be supplemented with localizing, 90-degree, true lateral, mediolateral, or lateromedial projections. The appropriate lateral projection should be chosen to assure the shortest object to image receptor distance, to limit the amount of geometric unsharpness, which improves image quality. Other angled, rotated, coned, and magnified views also are helpful in mammography when additional information is required about a specific area in the breast.

## Craniocaudad Projection

The craniocaudad projection (Fig. 31–4) is important for examining the subareolar, central, and medial portions of the breast. The following are steps for craniocaudad positioning:
1. The patient must be erect and facing the image receptor (grid or cassette).
2. Adjust the height of the image receptor so that the breast lies comfortably upon it. The edge of the cassette should rest in the patient's inframammary crease.

3. Check the height from both the medial side and the lateral side to ensure that both sides of the breast are in contact with, and are included on, the image receptor.
4. Place the breast on the film so that it is centered with the nipple in profile. Positioning from the medial side helps to ensure that the breast is perpendicular to the chest wall. This step is of the utmost importance to guarantee complete compression with the minimum amount of discomfort to the patient.
5. Have the patient turn the head away from the side being examined and lean forward. Placing your hand on the patient's back throughout the procedure keeps the patient from backing away from the receptor, especially as soon as the compression device begins to lower, and is reassuring and comforting to most patients.
6. Unless the patient is tense, use the automatic compression control to compress the breast. For tense patients, it is best to compress manually. As compression is applied, the arm of the affected side should be extended downward along the patient's side. It may be advantageous to have the patient turn the palm of the hand forward while making sure to keep the shoulder relaxed.
7. Palpate the lateral and medial borders simultaneously and test the tautness of the tissue. The skin should be firm.
8. Position the central ray so that it is at the base of the breast.
9. After the patient is positioned and compression is accomplished, ask the patient to hold her breath. Make the exposure, then release the compression device as quickly as possible. To expedite a quick compression release, most modern units have a release near the control panel.

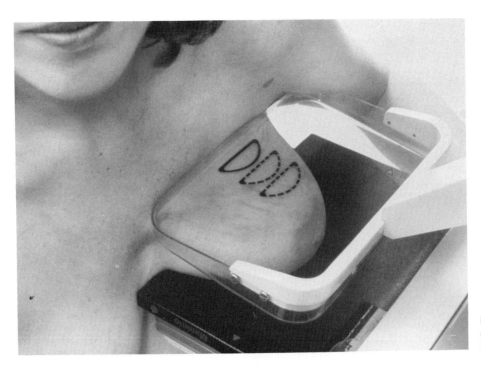

**Figure 31–4.** Positioning for craniocaudad projection (Courtesy of AGFA Corporation, Ridgefield Park, New Jersey).

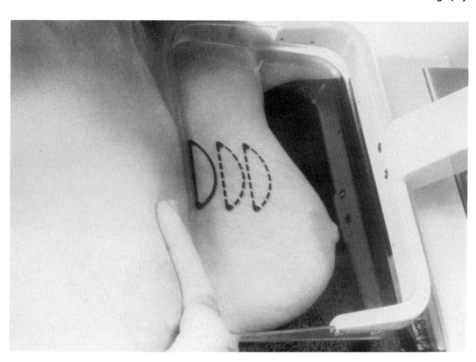

**Figure 31–5.** Positioning for mediolateral oblique projection (Courtesy of AGFA Corporation, Ridgefield Park, New Jersey).

## Mediolateral Oblique Projection

A mediolateral oblique projection best demonstrates the lateral juxtathoracic portion of the breast, especially the axillary tail. The following are steps used to position the breast for the mediolateral projection (Fig. 31–5):

1. Rotate the x-ray assembly so that the image receptor is perpendicular to the patient's pectoral muscle.
2. Direct the central ray to the inferolateral position with the angle varying relative to the patient's build. For tall, thin women, 60 degrees is recommended; an average woman would require approximately 45 degrees; and a pendulous-breasted woman would need about 40 degrees.
3. Position the patient so that the hip on the side of the breast being radiographed is aligned with the bottom of the image receptor.
4. Using the hand on the side of the breast being imaged, have the patient grasp the handlebar on the side of the tube assembly.
5. Raise the height of the image receptor until as much of the axillary area as possible will be included on the finished radiograph.
6. Have the patient bend slightly at the waist and relax against the image receptor.
7. The patient's breast is positioned in a lateral position with the nipple in profile.
8. Prior to compression, it is important to pull the posterior portion of the breast forward onto the image receptor.
9. Compress the breast until it is taut. The upper, outer edge of the compression device should be just inferior to the clavicle.
10. After the patient is positioned and compression is accomplished, ask the patient to hold her breath. Make the exposure, then release the compression device as quickly as possible.

## RADIOGRAPHIC FINDINGS

Mammography can demonstrate a variety of cancerous and noncancerous abnormalities or changes in breast tissue. However, the most important purpose of mammography is to locate breast cancer. There are numerous types and varying degrees of breast cancers. Mammographic demonstration of these cancers will vary from tiny groups of microcalcifications to large, invasive tumors. Some of the most obvious cancers seen on a mammogram are termed stellate lesions. Radiographically, these are presented as a radiating structure with ill-defined borders (Fig. 31–6). Less obvious cancers may be demonstrated as tiny groups of microcalcifications. These microcalcifications are usually numerous and grouped as seen in the biopsy specimen in Figure 31–7. It is noteworthy to mention that this particular malignancy would probably not have been detected for about 2 years, or more, without mammography. Classic malignant masses have spiculated borders, are reproducible on two views, and are usually denser than the surrounding breast tissue. The radiologist is responsible for deciding which lesions should be followed up with additional views or biopsy. Secondary findings in the breast, such as skin dimpling or thickening, nipple retraction, asymmetry, or a newly developed tissue density, will often provide supplemental support for the suspicion of breast cancer. Other types of malignancies include inflammatory breast cancer,

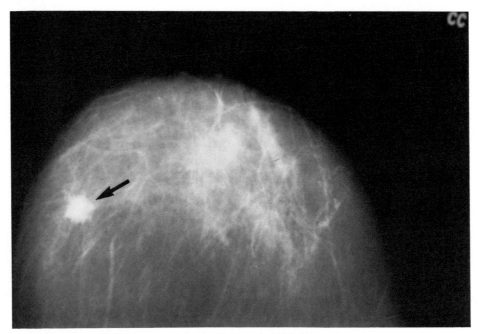

**Figure 31–6.** Stellate lesion.

Paget's disease, intraceptic carcinoma, ductal carcinoma, medullary carcinoma, colloid carcinoma, and invasive lobular carcinoma.

Noncancerous findings are also identifiable on the images. These findings may include fibrocystic changes (Fig. 31–8), cysts, adenosis, papillomatosis, fibroadenoma, lipoma, mastitis, benign calcification, and fatty breasts (Fig. 31–9).

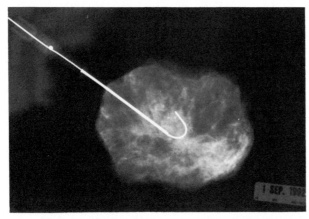

**Figure 31–7.** Microcalcifications (biopsy specimen).

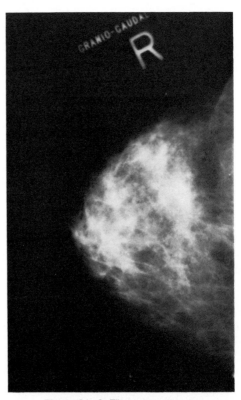

**Figure 31–8.** Fibrocystic changes.

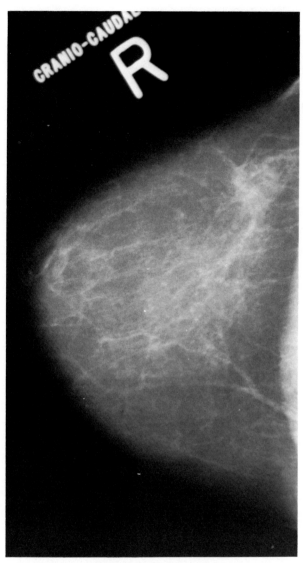

**Figure 31–9.** Fatty breast.

## REVIEW QUESTIONS

A. 20
B. 30 to 35
C. 35 to 40
D. 45

1. Mammography can detect growths as early as ＿＿ years before they are large enough to be palpated.
   A. 1
   B. 2
   C. 3
   D. 4

4. Some studies reveal that women who have a yearly mammogram have a death rate ＿＿ percent lower than those who have not been examined.
   A. 10
   B. 15
   C. 25
   D. 50

2. In mammography, the ＿＿ is the primary factor affecting proper diagnosis.
   A. breast density
   B. mammographer
   C. radiologist
   D. film quality

5. The highest risk factor for cancer of the breast is ＿＿.
   A. obesity
   B. a history of maternal breast cancer
   C. bearing children late in life
   D. difficult pregnancies

3. The American Cancer Society recommends that women have a baseline mammogram done at age ＿＿ (in years).

6. The ＿＿ portion of the breast extends into the axillary area.
   A. main
   B. medial
   C. inferior
   D. tail

7. Lactation occurs in the ＿＿ tissue of the breast.
   A. alveolar
   B. areolar
   C. adipose
   D. fibrous

8. The retromammary space lies between ＿＿ and ＿＿.
   A. Cooper's ligaments, the breast
   B. the pectoralis major muscle, the breast
   C. alveolar, connective tissue
   D. glandular tissues, adipose tissue

9. In the breast, arteries are larger than veins and sometimes visualize on a finished radiograph.
   A. true
   B. false

10. The many indistinct markings, including vessels, ducts, and tissues, visualized on breast radiographs are termed ＿＿.
    A. ampullae
    B. trabeculae
    C. lobes
    D. alveoli

11. The American College of Radiology recommends that processor quality assurance for mammography be performed ＿＿.
    A. before each examination
    B. daily
    C. every two days
    D. once a week

12. State the preprocedural care for mammography.

13. Breast compression primarily helps to produce a mammogram _____.
    A. with high radiographic contrast
    B. with even radiographic density
    C. with high radiographic density
    D. without artifacts

14. The common routine series for mammography includes _____.
    A. AP and lateral
    B. craniocaudad and mediolateral
    C. craniocaudad and mediolateral oblique
    D. craniocaudad and lateromedial

15. The mediolateral oblique projection of the breast demonstrates the _____.
    A. anterior portion of the breast
    B. anterior chest wall
    C. tail of the breast
    D. medial aspect of the breast

16. The craniocaudad projection of the breast demonstrates the _____.
    A. subareolar area
    B. central area
    C. medial portion
    D. all answers are correct

17. For the craniocaudad projection of the breast, the central ray should be directed to the _____.
    A. nipple
    B. midportion of the breast
    C. tail of the breast
    D. base of the breast

18. During mammography, the patient may continue breathing normally since respiration has no effect on the study.
    A. true
    B. false

## BIBLIOGRAPHY

ACR Mammography Accreditation Program. ACR, 1991.

Bontrager, KL: Textbook of Radiographic Positioning and Related Anatomy, ed 3. Mosby Yearbook, St. Louis, 1993.

Guyton, AC: Anatomy and Physiology. Saunders College Publishing, Philadelphia, 1985.

Johnson, E, et al: Human Anatomy. Saunders College Publishing, Philadelphia, 1985.

Quality Assurance in Mammography (a training guide). AGFA Corporation, Ridgefield Park, New Jersey, 1990.

Reitherman, RW: Film-Screen Mammography Interpretation Workshop (a seminar), Phoenix, Arizona, 1991.

Special Touch (pamphlet). American Cancer Society, Inc., 1987

# CHAPTER 32

# Fundamentals of Computed Tomography

*Angie Alford, AS, ARRT(R)(M)*
*Patrick J. Apfel, MEd, ARRT(R)*

In the years since the discovery of the x ray, its use in medicine has led to developments of more sophisticated x-ray technologies, including the field of computed tomography (CT). CT is the process of creating a cross-sectional tomographic plane or "slice" of any body part. In lay terms, the process can be compared to taking an uncut loaf of bread, slicing it up in various thicknesses, and observing each slice separately.

The first successful clinical demonstration of CT was conducted by Godfrey Hounsfield, an English physicist, in 1967 at the Central Research Laboratory of EMI, Ltd., in England. He combined computer technology with conventional radiography to develop the first CT system. In 1973, the first CT units were installed in the United States at the Mayo Clinic and Massachusetts General Hospital. The original scanner had many disadvantages and was used only for neurologic work. The types of x-ray tubes and detectors used to acquire the complex series of motions and to collect the absorption data resulted in very long scan times. Dr. Robert Ledley developed the first scanner capable of visualizing any section of the body in 1974, at Georgetown University Medical Center. Original scans took as long as 5 minutes, or more, per image. Since its development in the early 1970s, CT technology has progressed and improved in the areas of data gathering techniques and image reconstruction. Today's generation of scanners can scan the entire anatomic area of interest in much less than 5 minutes.

Computed tomography combines x-radiation and radiation detectors coupled with a computer to create a multidimensional image of any part of the body. The image is reconstructed by the computer using x-ray measurements collected by the detectors at multiple points around the periphery of the part being scanned. This image is then viewed on a display monitor. It is composed of thousands of picture elements, or pixels, each having its own characteristic x-ray absorption value in direct relationship to the actual tissue density. The resulting image depends upon several factors including the nature of the x-ray source, the number and array of detectors, the quantity and speed of the measurements, and the reconstruction technique. This chapter presents discussions of the principles, data gathering techniques (generations), system components, image reconstruction, and contrast agents used in CT. Procedures, anatomic areas, and disease conditions demonstrated by CT are also presented.

It should be noted that CT technology is constantly improving, so that by the publication date of this text, new advancements may have occurred. This chapter is designed to present the basic concepts of CT technology. For more details on CT technology, the reader is referred to texts listed in the bibliography of this chapter.

## PHYSICAL PRINCIPLES

In CT the patient is irradiated with a closely collimated x-ray beam, and the resulting remnant radiation is measured by a detector that transmits the data to a computer. The signal from the detector is processed by the computer, and through manipulation of the data, the image is reconstructed and visualized on the display monitor. Mathematical equations, or algorithms, are used to reconstruct the image. The image can then be photographed as a hard copy and/or archived for later use. Algorithms are partially responsible for image quality. Selection of an inappropriate reconstruction algorithm by the operator can result in image graininess and loss of detail.

An x-ray image can demonstrate anatomy and convey diagnostic information because of the variation in tissue densities, which results in different linear attenuation coefficients. These, in turn, give rise to differences in transmitted x-ray intensities, resulting in subsequent variations in film densities.

Computed tomography demonstrates a transaxial tomogram of the body; thus, the body is always referred to in the X and Y axis. Coronal, sagittal, oblique, diagonal, and three-dimensional images can be produced through computer reformatting of the information obtained from the original transaxial scans. Producing optimal images requires the CT technologist to have a significant knowledge of physics, equipment, and science coupled with cross-sectional anatomy.

## GENERATIONS

Data gathering techniques have developed in stages termed generations. Simply put, this defines the age of a particular unit with the generation number referring to the fundamental tube-detector structure. Some newer scanners use existing generation designs (e.g., third-generation configuration), but because of advanced engineering, the technology has improved. As a result, some manufacturers have ceased using the term "generation" when describing these newer scanners. The authors of this text have chosen to use a generation number for the first four types of tube-detector configurations discussed in this section. Those CT scanners beyond the fourth generation are described by their technological improvements. The first-generation scanner was designed specifically to look at the brain. The first system, by EMI, scanned in a "translate-rotate" technique (Fig. 32–1) in which the x-ray tube and two detectors were paired parallel to each other and passed across the patient during the exposure (translation). The tube produced a thin beam of radiation, and the data resulting from the measurement of the remnant radiation by the detectors, at the initial angle, were transmitted to the computer to be processed. Then the tube and detector would move as little as 1 degree to another angle (rotate), and the pro-

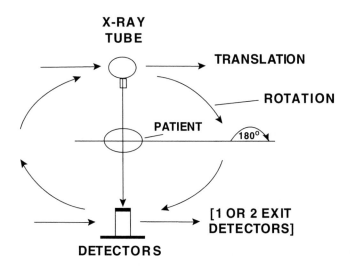

**1° ROTATIONAL INCREMENTS**

**Figure 32–1.** First-generation scanner: translate-rotate configuration. The x-ray tube and detectors move across the patient during the exposure (translation). The tube produces a thin beam of radiation. When the exposure is complete, the tube and detectors return to the first position, rotate 1 degree, and a second exposure is made. The sequence is continued through 180 degrees. (Courtesy of GE Medical Systems, Milwaukee, WI.)

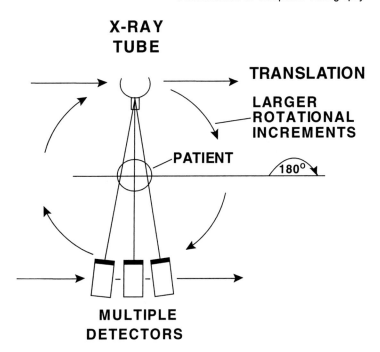

**Figure 32-2.** Second-generation scanner: translate-rotate multiple detector configuration. The tube and detector movements are the same as for the first-generation scanner (see Fig. 32-1). However, the tube produces a fan-shaped beam, there are multiple detectors (up to 30), and rotation angles are increased to 5 to 10 degrees. (Courtesy of GE Medical Systems, Milwaukee, WI.)

cess would be repeated until 180 degrees were scanned and enough information was gathered. With two detectors, two images were produced at a scan time of about 5 minutes. A third detector was used to sample the unattenuated beam for a reference.

It soon became evident that if more detectors were used, the scan time could be greatly reduced. This gave rise to the second-generation scanners. They were still considered a "translate-rotate" system (Fig. 32-2), but incorporated up to 30 detectors separated by absorbent materials designed to reduce scatter radiation and improve the image. This generation of scanners implemented a pie-shaped, or fan, beam of radiation passing linearly across the patient and then rotating with repeat exposure and rotation cycles. Because there were multiple detectors, translation increased to 5 degrees or more. Therefore scanning times per slice were reduced to 20 seconds, allowing for full-body scans.

Both the first- and second-generation scanners have become obsolete and are no longer in use.

Third-generation systems soon followed with the development of the "rotate-rotate" system (Fig. 32-3). In this system, the x-ray tube emits a fan beam of radiation that is in direct alignment with a series of up to 850 detectors. The tube and detectors rotate simultaneously a full 360 degrees around the patient. Scan times were reduced to 1 to 8 seconds per slice or image. Many systems used today are of this configuration. An advantage of this system is the closeness of the detectors to the patient, which reduces magnification. A disadvantage of this design is that if a detector malfunctions, it becomes evident on the visual image as a distinct line, representing a deficiency of information on the image.

The 1980s saw the birth of the "rotate-fixed" (Fig. 32-4), or fourth-generation, scanner. It featured a ring of detectors fixed in a full 360-degree array with the x-ray tube rotating within the ring. Originally equipped with 600 detectors, the new fourth-genera-

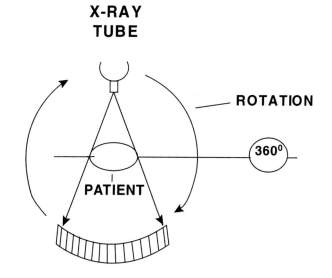

**MULTIPLE DETECTOR ARRAY**

**Figure 32-3.** Third-generation scanner: rotate-rotate configuration. The x-ray tube and multiple detectors (up to 850) rotate around the patient a full 360 degrees for each slice of tissue. The x-ray beam is fan-shaped. (Courtesy of GE Medical Systems, Milwaukee, WI.)

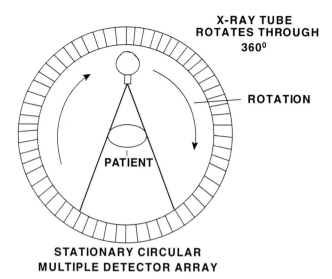

X-RAY TUBE
ROTATES THROUGH
360°

ROTATION

PATIENT

STATIONARY CIRCULAR
MULTIPLE DETECTOR ARRAY

**Figure 32–4.** Fourth-generation scanner: detector ring configuration. The x-ray tube rotates through 360 degrees, per tissue slice, within a ring of up to 4800 stationary detectors. (Courtesy of GE Medical Systems, Milwaukee, WI.)

tion scanners have as many as 4800 detectors, each separated by a radiation absorption material to reduce scatter. An advantage of this type of configuration is that several detectors can become dysfunctional without this being evident on the image. Disadvantages are magnification (due to the increased ratio of the source object distance to the object receptor distance) and the higher cost incurred because of the number of detectors.

In the 1990s one of the more recent developments is the helical, or spiral, scanner. This scanner differs from older generations in that it uses a constantly revolving x-ray source while the patient is moved in a continual motion through the x-ray beam. Data acquisition in this type of scanner is termed spiral, or helical (i.e., like a coiled spring) because of the movement of the patient through the beam as it rotates around the patient. These motions allow data acquisition from a volume of tissue rather than the slice-by-slice technique of older scanners. Advantages of this system include speed and three-dimensional reconstruction. In the older generation scanners, the tube and table (patient) motions were synchronized, but not continuous, and data were collected from individual slices of tissue. Configurations for the helical scanner can vary. One example, featuring helical data acquisition, is similar to the third-generation scanner with the tube and detectors aligned and moving in a rotate-rotate system. Continual tube motion is possible because of an improvement in engineering and design termed "slip-ring" technology, which does away with the high tension cables to the x-ray tube. Helical data acquisition allows for faster scanning time and a reduction in the amount of contrast medium (when used). Further, image reconstruction can be achieved at any thickness, and surgical and radiation

therapy planning are possible because of improved image quality.

Another system is the cardiovascular computed tomography (CVCT) scanner, which as the name implies, can be used to scan the heart. The CVCT scanner does not use a conventional x-ray tube but encircles the patient with detector (crystal photodiodes) and tungsten (target) rings (Fig. 32–5). An electron beam is produced and directed over the length of the tungsten rings. The beam is then deflected by electromagnetic coils to strike these rings and produce an x-ray beam, which penetrates the patient to reach the detector rings. With a scan time as short as one tenth of helical scanners, this scanner is very fast, making examination of the heart possible. Additionally, because of the multiple tungsten target rings and detector rings, several image slices can be produced simultaneously. Because of the speed of the CVCT, it is also known as an Ultrafast scanner. Other applications include the head, thorax, and abdomen.

## SYSTEM COMPONENTS AND FUNCTIONS

The three main components in a CT system are the gantry, the couch, and the operator's console (Fig. 32–6). While the gantry and couch are positioned in the scanning room, the console is located in a separate control room. Discussion of the basic system components is limited to those used in conventional scanners (up to fourth generation) and does not include CVCT type systems.

### Gantry

During a CT scan the patient is recumbent on the couch, which is suspended within the opening of the gantry. The gantry contains the major hardware needed to produce the image: the x-ray tube, collimators, and detectors.

#### THE X-RAY TUBE

In structure, the x-ray tube is very similar to the conventional x-ray tube; however, it is designed for high output and heat capacity. Heat is dissipated through the use of high speed, rotating anodes. A small focal spot size (less than 1 mm) can be employed to improve spatial resolution.

#### COLLIMATORS

Collimation is required during scanning to decrease scatter radiation, reduce patient exposure, and improve image quality. Unlike conventional radiography, CT uses two collimators. One, the fine beam collimator, is the prepatient collimator. Located in the tube housing, it limits the area of the patient that intercepts the useful beam and thereby determines the slice thickness and patient dose. In reducing scatter, it improves

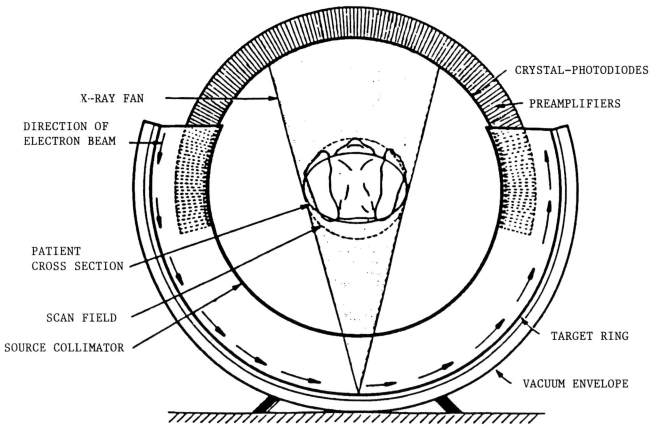

X-RAY FAN

DIRECTION OF
ELECTRON BEAM

PATIENT
CROSS SECTION

SCAN FIELD

SOURCE COLLIMATOR

CRYSTAL-PHOTODIODES

PREAMPLIFIERS

TARGET RING

VACUUM ENVELOPE

**Figure 32-5.** CVCT type (Ultrafast) scanner configuration. The patient is suspended within stationary multiple target rings and detector array (crystal-photodiode) rings. An electron gun produces an electron beam that is directed within the target rings. The electron beam is deflected by electromagnetic coils to the target rings. The resulting x-ray beam is collimated into a fan shape. (Courtesy of Imatron Inc., San Francisco, CA.)

contrast resolution. Improper adjustment of the prepatient collimator may result in an unnecessary radiation to the patient if the field is too large. The postpatient collimator, or predetector collimator, restricts scatter radiation reaching the detectors. As the name indicates, the postpatient, or predetector, collimator is positioned between the patient and the detector array.

This collimator, along with the prepatient collimator, aids in determining slice thickness.

## DETECTORS

During an exposure, photons passing through the patient as remnant radiation are received by the detec-

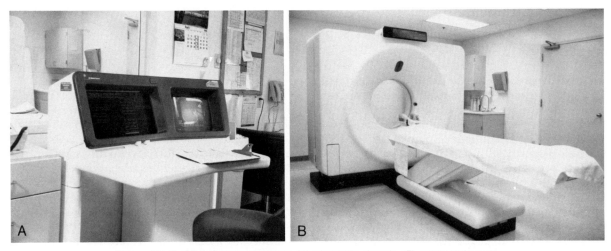

**Figure 32-6.** CT system components: (A) operator's console; (B) gantry and couch.

tors. When a detector receives radiation, the photons interact with the detector and produce a small current as an output analog signal. This signal is proportional to the radiation intensity. The analog signal is changed to digital during the image reconstruction process. The greater the absorption capabilities of the detector, the better the quality of the image.

There are two basic types of detectors, the solid-state and the gas (ionization chamber) detector. The solid-state detector contains a crystal scintillation material, which when stimulated by x-ray photons, produces light photons. These detectors have an absorption capability of 90 to 100 percent. A disadvantage of the solid-state detector is that the operator must compensate for light afterglow during image reconstruction. The ionization chamber (gas) detector is filled with xenon, a heavy, odorless, and colorless gas, and is limited in use to the rotate-rotate scanner. This detector exhibits no afterglow, characteristic of the solid-state detector, but absorbs only 50 to 60 percent of the x-ray photons. While xenon detectors are not as sensitive as solid-state detectors, they are still in use because they are cost efficient and easy to calibrate. Most newer scanners are equipped with solid-state detectors.

## Couch

The patient positioning and support couch is one of the most important components of the scanner. It must be constructed of a material (usually a carbon fiber) that does not interfere with the x-ray beam transmission and patient imaging. It must be strong enough to handle the force imposed on it, because of leverage, when it is suspended within the gantry during a patient scan. The couch should be motor driven to move smoothly and accurately within the gantry. It should be capable of automatic indexing (usually in millimeters) so that the operator does not have to enter the room during the entire scan, except for patient care purposes. Located on the front of the gantry are digitized couch-positioning controls including horizontal, vertical, in, out, and tilt table movements and a laser positioning light. These are used to aid the operator in producing the most accurate scan possible.

## Console

The control console is available in a variety of styles. Older models required two consoles: one dedicated to operating the scanner, and the other to printing and archiving. These units required a separate room just for the computer. Current models require a single console, which performs all functions and has the computer built into the base of the unit. The decrease in size makes it possible to place the equipment in smaller rooms. Separate remote consoles can be added to allow two technologists to work simultaneously or to allow the radiologist to view the scanned images in the reading room. If image manipulation is required on remote consoles, a separate computer is advantageous to re-

duce interference or to slow the operation of the main computer. Using fiber optics, modern scanners can be connected to any location (e.g., a radiologist's home).

## CONTROLS

The operator's console is the control system for running the CT unit. Controls for kV, mA, scan time, slice thickness, algorithms, and many other variables (e.g., image size) may be selected. Couch indexing is also controlled by the console. These can all be preprogrammed and initialized by calling up certain "protocols" for a given procedure. All of these factors influence the quality of the image, but a discussion of the proper technique settings for the various areas of the body is beyond the scope of this text. The console is also equipped with a regular keyboard to log in patient information and control the various functions of the computer.

## IMAGE PRINTING

Once the CT images are acquired, the images are printed onto x-ray film for a hard copy. The original camera used for printing was the matrix, or multiformat, camera. This camera photographed the monitor image and transposed it onto film via an enlarger. Images can be displayed from groups of 2 to 24 images per film. Image size and the number of images per film depend on the size of the film used (i.e., 8″ × 10″ or 14″ × 17″). The drawbacks of this equipment are that only one copy can be made at a time and that film jams are common since there is a series of rollers between the sending and receiving magazines. Also, density settings tend to "drift," often making it impossible to get the image on the film to look exactly like the image on the monitor. Currently, the multiformat camera is being replaced by the laser camera. With the laser camera, images are stored in the computer memory bank (buffer) and, upon command, printed by means of laser photography. Any number of images can be displayed on a single 14″ × 17″ film, and any number of copies can be produced at one time. Each copy is an original. Processors can be docked (attached) to both the multiformat and the laser camera, making the finished product available without leaving the control room.

## ARCHIVING

Archiving is another important feature of all CT units. Patient files can be retrieved from whatever archiving system is in use. Several systems are available. Currently, the most efficient archiving device is the optical disk, which can store several thousand images on a single disk. Many patient examinations can be stored in a relatively small amount of space, and retrieval is immediate. Most older systems use magnetic tape, which can store approximately 200 images per tape. Retrieval is slower since files are sequential and the tape must be searched to locate an individual patient file. A great deal of space is required to store the tapes. Magnetic tapes can be written over, and after several months, the tapes can be reused, thereby cutting the cost factor of buying and storing new tapes. However, care must be taken to avoid erasing examinations that may need to be stored (e.g., for legal reasons).

## IMAGE QUALITY

During both the scanning and the reconstruction process, the CT operator can make adjustments to affect the quality of the image, including the contrast, detail, and amount of image noise.

## Contrast

Although the image one sees displayed on the CT monitor appears solid, it is actually a matrix made up of a series of small squares, or picture elements, known as pixels, that are arranged in rows and columns. The pixels are two-dimensional representations of voxels (small volumes) of the slice of the tissue scanned (see Chapter 14, Digital Imaging Techniques, for detailed information). In this type of image, each pixel has uniform brightness.

Each pixel within an image matrix has a numeric value, or CT number, related to the density of the voxel it represents. Water is used as a reference with a CT number of 0. Tissues with a greater density than water are assigned a positive CT number, and those with densities less than water are given a negative CT number. The numbers are in Hounsfield units (linear attenuation coefficients) ranging from +1000 to −1000, but these must be adjusted by the operator to be displayed on the CT monitor as a maximum of 256 shades of gray (the maximum possible for the number of shades available on current monitors). Dense tissues would have a positive CT number and appear light on an image, while less dense tissues would have a negative CT number and appear darker on an image. The relationship between the CT number and the gray scale is adjustable; therefore, during reconstruction of the image, the operator can regulate contrast through a process termed windowing. A window is a range of CT numbers producing the full gray scale range (i.e., from black to white). The central number is the window level, and the numbers above and below it are the window width. By narrowing the window width, a high contrast image can be obtained. This is especially helpful when imaging soft tissues of similar densities. A wide width produces a low contrast image. The window level and width are generally chosen relative to the anatomy or pathology being imaged. In practice, in an effort to extract the maximum diagnostic information, multiple window levels and widths may be used when producing anatomic images. For example, head images for trauma are often filmed at three separate settings: one to demonstrate bony detail, a second to accent a possible subdural hematoma, and a third to demonstrate soft tissue differences between white and gray brain matter.

Compared to routine radiography, CT provides superior imaging of soft tissue structures with similar densities. Several factors make this possible, including the ability to adjust window level and width, the direct viewing of anatomy (i.e., without overlying tissues), and a greater reduction of scatter radiation as compared to routine radiography.

## Detail

Image detail can be controlled during scanning by using a small focal spot, reducing the detector aperture (in units where this is possible), and reducing the slice thickness. Before reconstruction, choosing an appropriate filter algorithm and matrix size will improve detail. The operator must choose an appropriate reconstruction filter algorithm. This algorithm is a mathematical filter that is used to remove abnormal deviations produced during the scanning process and affecting image quality. A reduction in the voxel size results in greater detail. This can be accomplished by increasing the matrix size. Typical matrix sizes are 64, 128, 256, and 512. A 512 matrix has 512 pixels in each row and column. The more pixels per matrix, the smaller the pixels in the field or view.

## Noise

Image noise or mottling results in decreased visibility in low contrast areas. This can be controlled by increasing the amount of radiation to the patient or by increasing the slice thickness (voxel size) during the scan. It must be realized, however, that increasing radiation increases patient dose and increasing the voxel size decreases image detail.

## Artifacts

Artifacts in the form of streaks or other configurations are possible on a CT image. These may be caused by patient movement, faulty detectors, or the presence of metal within the area scanned. Although filter algorithms may reduce artifacts, they cannot be totally subtracted from the image.

## CONTRAST MEDIA

Originally, with CT, most physicians believed there would no longer be a need to enhance different internal organs with contrast media. However, it was soon realized that by using contrast agents, it was easier to delineate organs that had similar densities. Dilute barium sulfate is a common oral contrast medium used to enhance visualization of the stomach, small intestine, and large intestine. It is given from 24 hours to 30 minutes before the scan, depending on the facility protocol and the organ(s) to be opacified. Routine abdominal scanning requires approximately 16 ounces of the barium suspension. The time the barium is administered prior to the scan varies with the level of the GI tract to be examined. For example, if the stomach is of interest, barium is administered immediately before the procedure. If the lower bowel or colon is of interest, barium may be given any time from the evening before the examination or up to 4 to 6 hours before the examination. Fasting for at least 3 hours prior to the scan is also recommended.

Other contrast agents used are the intravenous (IV), water-soluble contrast media. These media may be ionic or nonionic. These contrast media highlight vascular organs such as the liver, spleen, kidneys, and heart including the aorta. Generally speaking, ionic contrast media must be given carefully, and patients must be screened for possible reaction to iodine before administration. Nonionic contrast media are generally reserved for high risk patients and for patients who have experienced reactions to the ionic contrast media (but only after suitable premedications). High risk patients include: children; the elderly; patients with allergies, asthma, chronic pulmonary or heart disease; patients with a high BUN-creatinine ratio (indicating some form of renal failure); those with only one kidney; and diabetics. Intravenous contrast media injections may be administered in one of two ways, by manual injection or by mechanical power injection. Coupled with the newer scanners, the power injector optimizes IV contrast enhancement because of the constant flow rate achieved.

## DIAGNOSES AND OTHER APPLICATIONS

Computed tomography provides for the diagnosis of a multitude of patient conditions including cancer and metastases (Fig. 32–7). Ultrasound and CT scans are the methods of choice for detecting abdominal aneurysms. Computed tomography can locate the exact level, diameter, and extent of an aneurysm (Fig. 32–8). Kidney hydronephrosis and cystic lesions are also easily diagnosed by CT. Masses are easily biopsied, and cysts (Fig. 32–9) can be drained under the guidance of CT. Computed tomography of the brain is used for a wide variety of pathologies, including trauma such as skull fractures (Fig. 32–10), subdural hematoma (Fig. 32–11), cerebral bleeds and CVA, or stroke.

Another use of CT is in screening for osteoporosis in women and in staging the disease. Computed tomography is making strides in the area of three-dimensional imaging. Surgeons are able to use CT reconstruction for surgical planning before walking into the operating room. This has been especially helpful in facial reconstruction as well as in the lumbar and knee areas.

In some cases CT may be preferred over magnetic resonance (MR) scanning. For example, claustrophobic patients are better suited to CT because the greater diameter of the gantry opening presents a less confined feeling. While an MR scan has become the study of choice in some instances, CT is preferred for studies of the chest and abdomen (because these areas can be scanned while the patient momentarily holds his or her

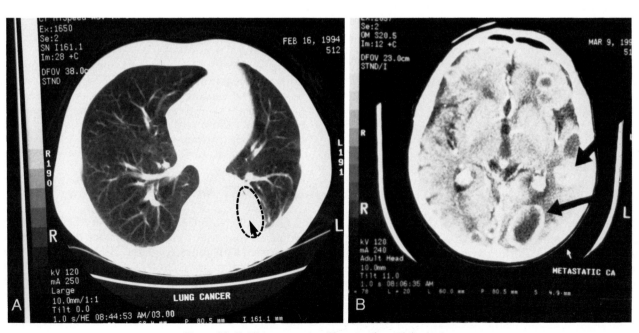

**Figure 32–7.** (*A*) Lung cancer; (*B*) metastases to the brain.

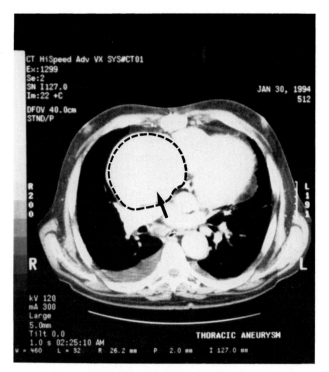

**Figure 32-8.** Thoracic aneurysm.

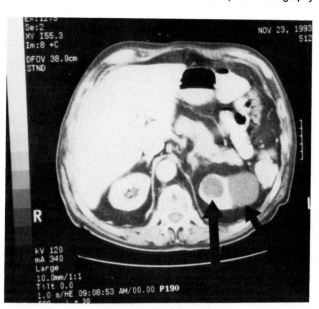

**Figure 32-9.** Renal cysts.

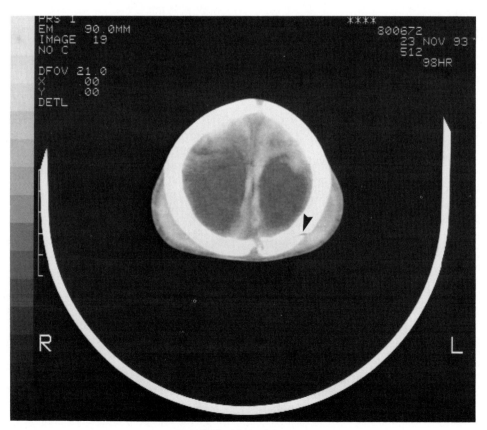

**Figure 32-10.** Skull fracture.

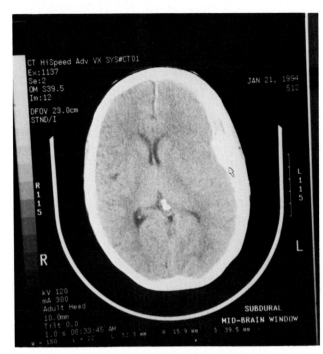

**Figure 32–11.** Subdural hematoma.

breath) and for patients who have had trauma to the head. Patients with pacemakers or metal implants cannot have an MR scan and need to be evaluated by means of CT.

## REVIEW QUESTIONS

1. The rotate-rotate CT system was used by the _____-generation scanner.
   A. first
   B. third
   C. fourth
   D. fifth

2. A tungsten ring is used in the _____, rather than an x-ray tube.
   A. first generation
   B. third generation
   C. fourth generation
   D. CVCT

3. A detector ring with a 360-degree detector array and tube rotating within the ring describes a _____-generation CT scanner.
   A. second
   B. third
   C. fourth
   D. fifth

4. The translate-rotate CT system was used by the _____-generation scanner(s).
   A. first
   B. second
   C. third
   D. A and B

5. Scanning time for a single slice in the first-generation scanner was approximately _____.
   A. 60 seconds
   B. 90 seconds
   C. 3 minutes
   D. 5 minutes

6. Scanning time for a single slice in the third-generation scanner is approximately _____ seconds.
   A. 60
   B. 30
   C. 1–8
   D. less than 1

7. The component of the CT system that encloses the x-ray tube and detectors is the _____.
   A. console
   B. gantry
   C. couch
   D. monitor

8. The detector used in CT systems that has an absorption capability of 90 to 100 percent is the _____ detector.
   A. gas
   B. xenon
   C. solid-state
   D. helical

9. The fine beam CT collimator is also termed the _____ collimator.
   A. prepatient
   B. predetector
   C. postpatient
   D. postdetector

10. The operator console controls _____.
    A. kilovolts
    B. milliamperes
    C. slice thickness
    D. all of the above

11. The type of camera used to print CT images that can produce multiple original copies is the _____ camera.
    A. multiformat
    B. matrix
    C. multimatrix
    D. laser

12. Image noise can be controlled by _____.
    A. increasing the radiation exposure
    B. increasing the slice thickness
    C. A and B
    D. none of the above

13. An increase in matrix size represents _____.
    A. an increase in pixel size
    B. a decrease in pixel size
    C. an increase in voxel size
    D. no answer is correct

14. Window settings are adjusted to control the _____ of the image.
    A. size
    B. contrast

C. voxel

D. depth

15. Detail on a CT scan is improved during reconstruction by ____.
    A. increasing pixel size
    B. decreasing matrix size
    C. decreasing voxel size
    D. decreasing scan time

16. Artifacts on a CT image can be caused by ____.
    A. patient motion
    B. metal implants
    C. a malfunctioning detector(s)
    D. all of the above

17. Computed tomography may be preferred over magnetic resonance imaging ____.
    A. in the case of a claustrophobic patient
    B. in patients with metallic implants
    C. for chest scans
    D. all of the above

18. In scanning the head, CT can be used to detect ____.
    A. skull fractures
    B. subdural hematoma
    C. CVA
    D. all of the above

## BIBLIOGRAPHY

Berland, LL: Practical CT Technology and Techniques. Raven Press, New York, 1987.

Bushong, SC: Radiologic Science for Technologists, Physics, Biology Protection. CV Mosby, St Louis, 1988.

Curry III, TS, Dowdey, JE, and Murry, Jr, RC: Christensen's Physics of Diagnostic Radiology, ed 4. Lea and Febiger, Philadelphia, 1990.

GE Medical Systems Program in CT Technology, Milwaukee, WI.

Gedgausdas-McClees, RK and Torres, WE: Essentials of Body Computed Tomography. WB Saunders, Philadelphia, 1990.

Lee, JKT, Sagel, SS, and Stanley, RJ: Computed Body Tomography with MRI Correlation. Raven Press, New York, 1989.

Seeram, E: Computed Tomography Physical Principles, Clinical Applications, and Quality Control. WB Saunders, Philadelphia, 1994.

## PERSONAL COMMUNICATIONS

Askew, MJ (Radiology Manager, Desert Springs Hospital, Las Vegas, Nevada): Interview, January 1991.

Bandt, PD (Administrative Radiologist, Desert Springs Hospital, Las Vegas, Nevada): Interview, January 1991.

Kujath, JL (Service Engineer, Picker International, Inc., CT systems): Interview, November 1990.

Robb, SR (Senior Angiographer, Desert Springs Hospital, Las Vegas, Nevada): Interview, October 1990.

# CHAPTER 33

# MAGNETIC RESONANCE IMAGING

*Kenneth M. Wintch, MEd, ARRT(R)(N), RN*
*Patrick J. Apfel, MEd, ARRT(R)*

Magnetic resonance (MR) is a modality that has created much excitement in the diagnostic imaging community. Magnetic resonance imaging (MRI) has routinely demonstrated its superiority in diagnosing disease and injury, especially in the area of the central nervous system (CNS). The high contrast resolution (as compared to other imaging modalities) results in clearly defined pathologies, including inflammatory lesions, neoplasms, ischemic changes, hemorrhages, degenerative changes, and many other conditions. Because of the ability of MR to differentiate between soft tissues of the brain, which were formerly never visualized, areas such as the substantia nigra, red nucleus, and dentate nucleus are clearly defined. MRI's ability to visualize the CNS in the sagittal, coronal, and transaxial (axial) plane and its superior demonstration of contrast make it the study of choice for most neurologic imaging.

In the short time since its introduction, MR has clearly demonstrated its imaging capability in areas of the body not susceptible to motion, such as the extremities and cranial, facial, and neurologic anatomy. Imaging of the extremities with MR demonstrates soft tissue, bone, and joint abnormalities. The ability to visualize ligamental tears greatly enhances the success of joint surgery. Generally, small ligamental tears can be visualized in all three planes. MR scanning of the major joints, such as the knee, shoulder, hip, and ankle, is routinely performed. Malignant and benign bone tumors and many soft tissue abnormalities are easily differentiated. Although MR does not visualize cortical bone well, the fatty marrow and the adjacent soft tissues allow for excellent detail of the bony structures. To visualize the joints and their working relationship to the surrounding tissue, sequential scans of a joint can be taken. When viewed as a set of cine pictures, joint motion can be readily demonstrated. The motions of the temporomandibular joint and the knee can easily be visualized in this manner.

Initially, imaging of the thorax and abdomen were not possible because of motion artifacts. However, with the aid of respiratory, peripheral, and cardiac gating, and varied pulsing techniques, excellent images of the thorax and abdomen can now be acquired. Also, imaging of the heart using respiratory and cardiac gating has shown promise in detecting cardiac wall motion and ischemia in the heart muscle as well as structural and functional abnormalities. Upper abdominal organs such as the liver, spleen, pancreas, gallbladder, and adrenal glands are clearly defined with the aid of respiratory gating. Structures in the lower abdomen, including the bladder and reproductive organs, are easily visualized with varied pulsing techniques, and when combined with Velcro compression bands placed over the abdomen to decrease motion, the tissue contrast can be superior to computed tomography (CT). Imaging of the head, thorax, and abdomen in the transaxial (axial) plane is generally accepted as the standard viewing method of choice; however, MR's ability to visual-

ize these structures in the sagittal and coronal planes (Fig. 33–1), as well, adds to the reliability of the diagnosis.

Recent advances in MR technology demonstrate the continued potential of MR to noninvasively diagnose abnormalities with precision. Three such areas, magnetic resonance angiography (MRA), cine MR, and spectroscopy MRA, are currently being applied clinically and show great promise in demonstrating vasculature. Cine MR provides clinicians with the ability to visualize organs in relationship to their function in detail never before possible. Spectroscopy on tissues and objects has been in use for 35 years. MR spectroscopy allows for noninvasive direct tissue analysis of living tissue.

Nuclear magnetic resonance (NMR), or magnetic

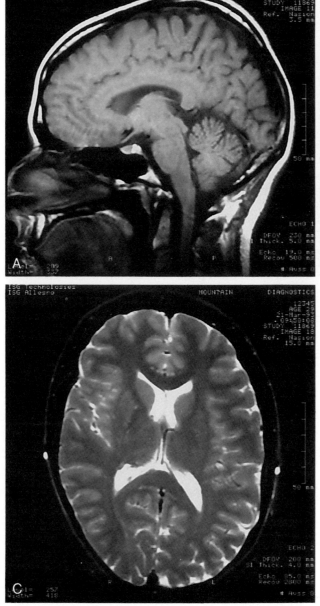

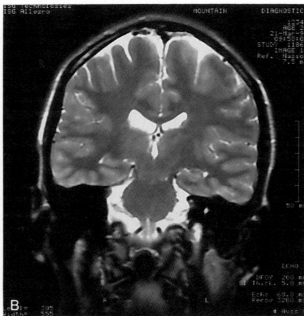

**Figure 33–1.** (A) Sagittal, (B) coronal, and (C) axial MR of the head.

resonance imaging, as it is currently termed, is a modality that uses the basic principles of quantum mechanics. A knowledge of chemistry, biophysics, anatomy, and physiology, and how these interact with normal and pathologic tissue, is necessary for technical proficiency in MR imaging. This chapter presents an introduction to the basic physical principles, imaging aspects, equipment, and future developments in MRI. It should be noted that MR technology is constantly evolving and that at the publication date of this text, new advancements in MR may be evident.

## HISTORY

In 1946, Felix Bloch, a theoretical physicist, published a paper stating that the nucleus of an atom behaved like a small bar magnet. He described this phenomenon as nuclear magnetism and demonstrated this principle mathematically with what are now referred to as Bloch's equations. Bloch's equations demonstrate that a nucleus spins on an imaginary axis and has an associated magnetic field. This magnetic field is known as a magnetic moment.

In the late 1960s, Dr. Raymond Damadian, a physician and engineer, demonstrated that characteristics of malignant tissue measured by NMR were different from those of normal tissue. In 1974, Dr. Damadian produced an NMR image of a rat tumor, which appeared on the cover of Science magazine.

It was in the early 1970s that CT was becoming routine in medicine. The reconstruction techniques used for CT scanning would lend themselves to reconstruction of NMR images. Dr. Paul Lauterbur pioneered reconstruction of NMR images in the 1970s. By this time, large imaging corporations started funding research and production of NMR hardware. The first NMR units were sold commercially in the United States in 1984.

It was during this time, when NMR units were being used clinically, that radiologists deemed it necessary to change the name of NMR to MR technology. It was thought that removing the negative connotation of "nuclear" would lessen patient concerns regarding the procedure.

## NUCLEAR PROPERTIES

The concept of MR technology begins at the atomic structure. The term nuclear magnetic resonance, however, aptly describes the basic components that are the foundation of present-day magnetic resonance imaging.

When the physics of nuclear magnetism is discussed in this chapter, it is important to remember that it refers to the nucleus of an atom. The neutrons and protons of an atom behave like tiny bar magnets known as dipoles. Most neutrons and protons align themselves in such a way as to cancel their magnetic properties (i.e., there are the same number of protons and neutrons).

However, certain elements contain an odd number of protons as compared to neutrons and are unable to cancel out their respective magnetic properties. Hydrogen-1 has only one proton, behaves very predictably, and is also very abundant in the human body. Because of hydrogen's strong magnetic moment and its abundance in the human body, the hydrogen nucleus is the basis of magnetic resonance imaging.

Other elemental isotopes that are medically important (i.e., can be imaged with MR) include fluorine-19, phosphorus-31, sodium-23, carbon-13, hydrogen-2, oxygen-17, and potassium-39. Research centers around the United States are investigating the use of these other isotopes to determine their medical applications. One isotope that has potential in medical applications is fluorine, which is almost completely absent in the human body. Fluorine is, however, a common isotope, has a very stable magnetic moment, and is naturally abundant. If fluorine could be safely introduced into the human body, it would make an ideal tracer of body structures, giving MR the ability to assess body functions similar to nuclear medicine.

## MAGNETIC PROPERTIES

The strength of an artificial magnet usually depends on its type and manufacturer. All artificial magnets produce a magnetic field thousands of times stronger than the earth's own magnetic field. The MR magnet produces a strong external magnetic field known as a static field along an axis designated $B_o$, which is parallel to the patient (Fig. 33–2). The intensity of the $B_o$ axis is measured in tesla (T). One tesla is equal to about 10,000 gauss (G). The magnetic pull on the surface of the earth is about 0.5 G, or about 0.00005 T. Medical imaging magnets have strengths from 0.05 to 2.0 T, with magnets as high as 4 T used in medical research.

On the atomic level, the other magnetic field important to MR is the dipole. A dipole is a magnet that has a north and a south pole, for example, the earth, a bar magnet, or a hydrogen atom. These dipoles are ran-

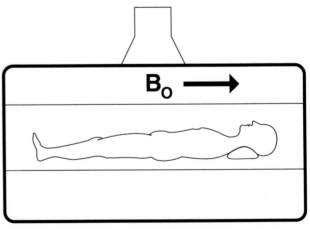

**Figure 33–2.** Depiction of $B_0$ axis.

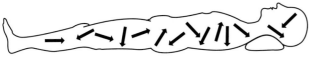

**Figure 33-3.** Random dipoles within the body.

| Table 33-1. **Nuclei and Their Gyromagnetic Ratios for a 1- and 1.5-T Magnet** | | |
|---|---|---|
| **Nucleus** | **1 T** | **1.5 T** |
| Hydrogen-1 | 42.75 | 63.9 |
| Fluorine-19 | 40.05 | 60.1 |
| Phosphorus-31 | 17.23 | 25.1 |
| Sodium-23 | 11.26 | 16.9 |
| Carbon-13 | 10.70 | 16.1 |
| Hydrogen-2 | 6.5 | 9.8 |
| Oxygen-17 | 5.8 | 8.7 |
| Potassium-39 | 2.0 | 3.0 |

domly oriented in the body (Fig. 33-3). When these dipoles are placed in a strong magnetic field, the net magnetizations (sum of all the nuclear moments) tend to align parallel to or antiparallel to the magnetic field. This alignment creates a net magnetization along the axis of the magnet. The body inside the magnetic field now has a north and a south pole (Fig. 33-4). In the presence of the strong magnetic field, the dipoles align along the Z axis and precess. Precession can be compared to a spinning top. When a rotating top's rotation begins to slow down, the top will "wobble," or precess, before it falls. The dipoles in the strong magnetic field precess as well as spin. The precessional frequency can be measured by Larmor's equation:

Precessional frequency =
    gyromagnetic ratio $\times$ magnetic field strength

All elemental species that have a magnetic moment also have what is known as a gyromagnetic ratio. This ratio is analogous to the disintegration constant for a radionuclide. The higher the angulation of the rotation (precession), the higher the gyromagnetic ratio. Hydrogen-1 has the highest gyromagnetic ratio of 42.6 megahertz per tesla (MHz/T).

In accordance with Larmor's equation, a 1-T magnet with a gyromagnetic ratio of 42.6 MHz/T has a precessional frequency of 42.6 MHz/T. Fluorine-19 has a gyromagnetic ratio of 40.1, which is very close to the hydrogen ratio. Fluorine-19 could easily be imaged with present-day imaging magnets. The other medically important elements along with their gyromagnetic ratios for 1- and 1.5-T magnets are listed in Table 33-1.

## RESONANCE

Since a dipole is a magnet, it can interact with an externally applied magnetic field and with the magnetic fields of the surrounding dipoles. The magnetic moments of all dipoles are limited to certain energy levels and orientations. When stimulated to leave these energy levels and orientations, dipoles can store, absorb, and emit electromagnetic radiation in the form of radio waves. For the dipoles to receive and absorb energy, the energy being applied must be at the same frequency as that of the precessing dipole. This phenomenon can easily be demonstrated by using two tuning forks of equal mass and shape. When one tuning fork is struck, with the second tuning fork in close proximity, the second tuning fork resonates at the same frequency as the first. It is the process of stimulating dipoles to change their energy and orientation by absorbing energy and then releasing this energy that is the basis of MR imaging.

## RADIO FREQUENCY

$B_o$ is used to designate the direction of the strength of the external magnetic field commonly called the Z axis in a magnet. $M_o$ is used to designate the amount of net magnetization along this axis. The more nuclei available in a patient for alignment, the higher the $M_o$. A high $M_o$ produces a stronger signal since more nuclei are available. A 1.5-T magnet aligns more nuclei than a 1-T magnet, thus allowing for faster imaging times and higher resolution.

Even if a high $M_o$ is obtained, no signal can be detected because all net magnetizations are in the direction of the external magnetic field, which is designated as $B_o$. The only way that a signal can be detected is to have a net magnetization factor in the XY plane. The axis on which a top is spinning is represented by the Z axis; as the top begins to wobble, it will precess off the Z axis and encompass more and more of the X and Y planes as it slows down. In the presence of a strong magnetic field, the X and Y components of the individual wobbles of a magnetic dipole are canceled, because they are randomly oriented and there is no net magnetization in the XY plane.

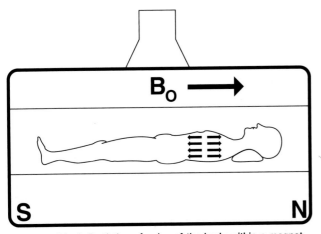

**Figure 33-4.** Depiction of poles of the body within a magnet.

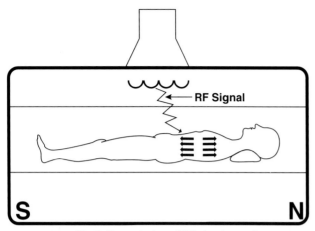

**Figure 33-5.** Transmission of RF signal to patient.

To receive a signal from a patient, there must be an abundance of H nuclei present in the tissue being examined. The net magnetization vector of these nuclei must be tipped away from the Z axis, to some nonzero point of the XY plane. Unless the signal received by the patient is the same frequency as that of its precessing nuclei, no signal is returned. To tip this magnetization factor into the XY plane, a burst of electromagnetic energy (a simple radio frequency wave, RF) is tuned to the same resonant frequency of the patient's own nuclei and transmitted to the patient (Fig. 33-5). Once the patient's nuclei absorb the RF wave, they transmit back an RF wave relative to the amount of mobile hydrogen in the tissue. This transmitted RF wave is returned in the form of a free induction decay (FID) wave or signal (Fig. 33-6). This is the simplest form of an imaging parameter, called partial saturation.

## PULSE SEQUENCES

Pulse sequencing is used to weight the image. In selecting the contrast weighting of an imaging sequence, the MR operator has a range of choices, from the simple technique of partial saturation to the more complex spin echo technique.

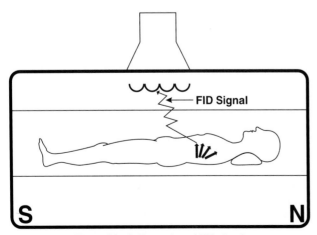

**Figure 33-6.** Reception of FID signal.

## Partial Saturation

Partial saturation uses a series of evenly spaced, 90-degree pulses. These pulses are designed to tip the dipoles' magnetization vectors off the Z axis. As the dipoles or pulses become perpendicular, or approach 90 degrees to the Z axis, they yield the maximum returning RF signal in the form of a FID signal.

To send a burst of a RF wave into a patient and then to receive a corresponding signal, the sending-to-receiving mode must take place very quickly. In most equipment, the main antenna (RF coil) sends the signal and also receives the emitted signal from the patient. No matter how fast the switching electronics are, there is always some signal loss. To compensate for this loss of signal, a spin echo technique is used.

## Spin Echo

To begin a spin echo technique, a resonant RF pulse is sent to tip the net magnetizations off the Z (90 degrees) axis into the XY plane. After some recovery, a second pulse of 180 degrees is applied. This allows some time for the antenna to recover and read the emitted pulse. The time from a 90-degree pulse to the beginning of the spin echo is called the time to echo, or TE. Therefore, sequences that have a 90-degree pulse followed by one or more 180-degree pulses are spin echo pulses (Fig. 33-7).

## Inversion Recovery Pulses

In inversion recovery pulses, the 180-degree pulse is given before the 90-degree pulse. By inverting the

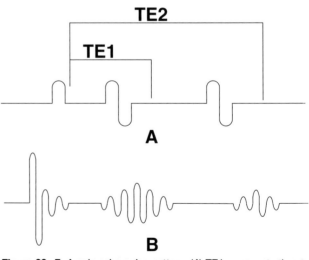

**Figure 33-7.** A spin echo pulse pattern. (*A*) TE1 represents time to echo from the cessation of the 90-degree RF pulse to the middle of the first FID spin echo wave (see *panel B*) created by the first 180-degree RF inversion pulse. TE2 represents the time to echo from the cessation of the 90-degree RF pulse to the middle of the second FID spin echo wave (see *panel B*) created by the second 180-degree RF inversion pulse. (*B*) Spin echo wave created by the RF pulse demonstrated in *panel A*.

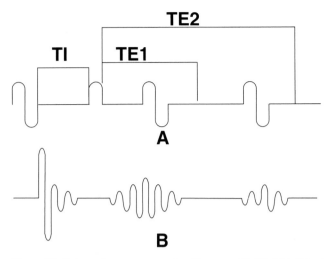

**Figure 33–8.** Inversion recovery pulse. TI represents the time delay from the cessation of the first 180-degree inversion pulse to the beginning of the 90-degree pulse. See Figure 33–7 for explanation of TE1 and TE2.

magnetization 180 degrees, the angle is tipped back to the Z axis. On this axis no signal can be detected. After a small delay called TI, a 90-degree pulse is given to further tip the magnetization vector into the XY plane, to produce a signal. By again adding 180-degree pulses, spin echoes can be created (Fig. 33–8).

## IMAGING CHARACTERISTICS

The ability of MR to distinguish between different types of tissue lends to its application in medical imaging. Hydrogen concentration, velocity artifacts, and T1 and T2 relaxation are major factors that constitute the MR image. Each factor contributes to the brightness of any given image.

To create an image from data obtained from a pulse sequence, multiple sampling of the data is obtained. The samplings are called repetitions. The time from the beginning of one sequence to the start of the next sequence is called repetition time, or TR. The value of the TR may be adjusted to distinguish between tissue characteristics.

### Hydrogen Concentration

Protons of the hydrogen atom are the most predominant in the body. The MR scan demonstrates the concentration of the hydrogen nuclei present in the body. Most organs in the body do not vary by more than 15 percent of hydrogen concentration, except for the lungs, gas, and bone tissue. These areas show up primarily as dark or signal voids on MR scans.

### T1 Relaxation

T1, also called the longitudinal or spin-lattice relaxation time, is the time in milliseconds that the net mag-

netization takes to return to $M_o$ or equilibrium. Nearly all tissues in the body have different T1 values. In a 1-T magnet, the value for fat is 180 milliseconds and water is 2500 milliseconds. A large value for T1 relaxation represents a long, gradual return back to $M_o$, while a small value represents a rapid return. The T1 of diseased and damaged tissue is longer than that of healthy tissue of the same kind. To return to equilibrium, the nuclei must give up their absorbed energy from the RF pulse. The peak of T1 relaxation time toward $M_o$ is demonstrated in Figure 33–9.

The T1 relaxation is the time required for the net magnetic vector to travel 63 percent of the way back to $M_o$. The value of T1 in a tissue is a measure of how efficiently the energy of the resonating photons is absorbed into the surrounding tissue. This surrounding tissue has its own magnetic fields, called lattice. Fats and cholesterol are very efficient in giving up their energy. Their T1 is a fast 180 milliseconds.

Large molecules, like proteins, have a long T1 relaxation time because they have difficulty giving up their energy to surrounding tissue. Therefore, tissue with a short T1 appears bright on an image, while tissue with a long T1 appears dark. T1 is perhaps the most useful in demonstrating the anatomy or pathology of tissue.

## T2 Relaxation

T2 relaxation is a measure of the length of time net magnetization lasts in a perfectly homogeneous magnetic field. T2 relaxation does not involve any energy transfer to surrounding tissue but is a measure of the change of phase of resonating photons. Individual nuclei in tissue stimulated by an RF pulse have the same vector orientation at the cessation of the RF pulse. When the nuclei have the same vector orientation, they are in phase. Over time, the nuclei become out of phase. T2 is the measurement of this loss of phase.

T2 relaxation is known as transverse, or spin-spin, relaxation. The loss of phase in T2 relaxation decreases

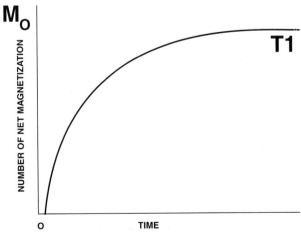

**Figure 33–9.** T1 relaxation.

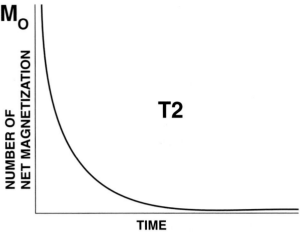

**Figure 33–10.** T2 relaxation.

in time relative to the $M_o$ equilibrium axis. The main reason the nuclei lose their energy is that they give up their energy from one spin to another, thus the name spin-spin. The difference between T1 and T2 relaxation time is as follows: T1 represents an increasing value over time. It represents the increase of net magnetizations of dipoles along the Z axis. T2 represents a decreasing value along the XY axis until it reaches zero (Fig. 33–10 shows T2 decay).

The phase differences in tissue during T2 decay are perhaps the most accurate way to determine the differences in tissue contrast, especially in the detection of pathologic conditions. On T2 weighted images, tissue with a long T2 appears bright and tissue with a short T2 appears dark.

## Velocity Artifacts

Velocity artifacts represent areas of signal void. This occurs when moving nuclei are stimulated by an RF pulse, but move out of the sampling area before their corresponding RF signal can be picked up by receiving antenna. This creates a signal void on the image. This type of artifact is especially noticeable in blood flow.

## HARDWARE

The major components of an MR scanner are the gantry, operator's console, and computer system. These components are essentially the same as those used in CT. Externally, it is not hard to confuse the systems, since they look similar; however, internal components differ significantly.

The gantry consists of a large circular or rectangular structure that houses the main magnet. Three types of magnets can be used in MR: the permanent magnet, the resistive magnet, and the superconductive magnet. Each of these magnets varies in field strength.

Higher field strengths tend to lose some contrast as compared to the lower field strength magnets. Higher

field strength magnets generate increased signal to noise, allowing for expanded imaging parameters and shorter data acquisition sequences. The energy requirements, patient population, sources of funding, and site selection help determine the type of magnet that each facility purchases. The computer and console for these magnets are similar. Differences depend on the type of software packages used and the strength of the magnetic field.

## Permanent Magnet

The permanent magnet (Fig. 33–11) has a field strength that ranges from 0.05 to 0.35 T. This magnet is fairly homogeneous. It requires no electric power or coolant to operate. Because of its low field strength, it requires minimal shielding.

A permanent magnet has several disadvantages. It weighs up to 100 tons, it requires a very strict room temperature to maintain field uniformity, and imaging times are long because of the low field strength.

## Resistive Magnet

The resistive magnet has a field strength of 0.3 T or less. Its field homogeneity is only fair, with a low fringe field. Its major advantages are its low cost and the fact that the magnetic field can be turned on and off, unlike permanent and superconductive magnets.

A resistive magnet's disadvantages are that it has high cooling and the highest electric consumption of the three types of magnets and that it is very sensitive to temperature fluctuations.

## Superconductive Magnet

The superconductive magnet has a field strength that ranges from 0.3 to 2.0 T. A superconductive magnet has excellent field homogeneity (due to software compensation), has very high field strength, requires little electric expense, and is very stable (Fig. 33–12).

In a superconductive magnet there are multiple windings of niobium titanium alloy covered by copper. The niobium titanium functions as a superconductor when cooled by the liquid helium. The outer windings of copper act as an insulator to keep the magnet from overheating.

The major disadvantages of the superconductive magnet are its cost and the fact that it requires expensive cryogens to maintain a temperature of 4°K.

## Coils

The construction and configuration of the coils in the permanent and resistive magnets differ from those used with the superconductive magent. There are two sets of coils inside a typical superconductive magnet, the shim coils and the gradient coils. The shim coils are

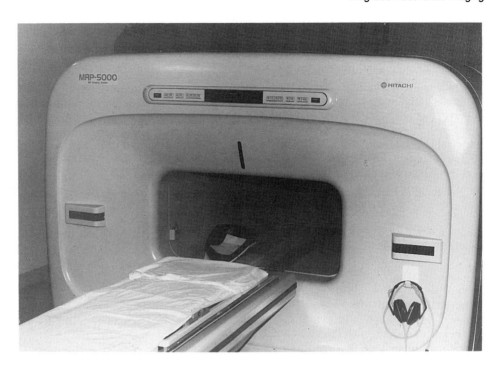

**Figure 33–11.** Gantry housing a permanent magnet.

situated along the bore of the magnet to correct any in-homogeneities of the magnet. The gradient coils are placed in such a way as to superimpose small magnetic fields along the Z, X, and Y axes. By activating these coils at defined intervals during the pulse sequence, transaxial, sagittal, coronal, and oblique slicing can be selected. These coils also provide spatial encoding of the MR signals.

Perhaps the most important part of the magnet is the RF transmitting and receiving coil. During scanning, the RF coil sends a burst of electromagnetic radiation through the patient. The coil then must receive the corresponding signal from the body. The main RF coil, which is both a transmitter and a receiver coil, is commonly called the body coil because its main use is to image large field-of-view areas of the thorax, abdomen,

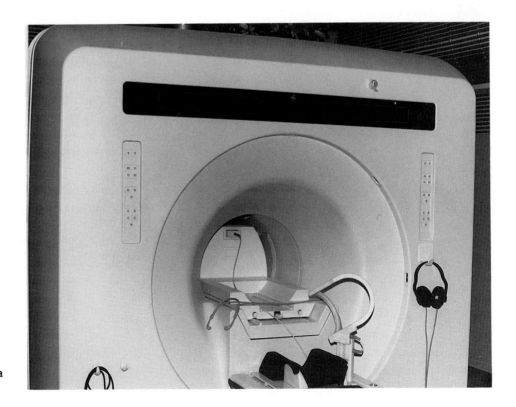

**Figure 33–12.** Gantry housing a superconductive magnet.

and pelvis. Imaging smaller areas of the body can be effectively accomplished by placing a small, interchangeable surface coil next to the body part being imaged. These coils are constructed to allow efficient signal reception. In most systems surface coils are placed close to the body part being imaged. Generally these coils are receivers only, while the main coil inside the magnet remains the sending coil. The surface coils greatly enhance the resolution of an image by decreasing signal drop-off from the body. The disadvantages of surface coils are that they have a limited field of view and that they can be difficult to position. Examples of typical surface coils are demonstrated in Figure 33–13.

## Operating Console

The operating console of an MR scanner is similar to that of a CT scanner. Many modern scanners have screens that are activated by touch. Most sequences are defined by function buttons. Some scanners have a physician's console, interfaced with the main console, which may be located in a reading room, enabling the physician to view images independently. A separate console dedicated for image processing and filming increases productivity.

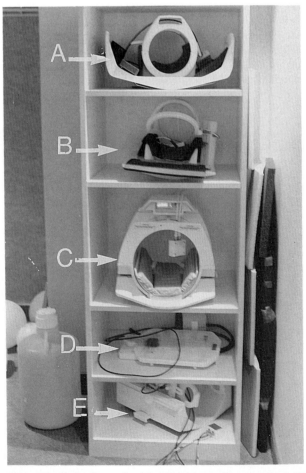

**Figure 33–13.** Surface coils: (A) extremity coil; (B) cervical coil; (C) head coil; (D) Quadrature spine coil; (E) temporomandibular joint coil.

## Computer

The MR computer needs to be powerful and fast. A tremendous amount of data is collected during each scanning sequence. The computer is required to handle several functions at once. These are scanning, archiving, reconstructing, and filming. As software improves, it is anticipated that more functions will become available and scan time will decrease.

## IMAGING PARAMETERS

Imaging parameters are functions that are chosen by the operator to carry out the MR scan and include the imaging plane, slice thickness, number of slices, and matrix size. The parameters chosen directly affect how the image appears.

### Imaging Planes

When performing an MR examination, a technologist must understand the parameters involved in producing the image. Older scanners produced images only in the sagittal, coronal, and axial planes. This was a marked improvement over CT. All three imaging planes were accomplished without moving the patient. Currently, scanners can also produce oblique images.

### Slice Thickness

In selecting the slice thickness of an image, a trade-off exists. An operator can select a slice thickness from 1 to 10 mm. The thinner the slice chosen, the better the anatomic detail of the image. However, a thinner slice generates more noise, unless scan times (averages) are greatly increased. Thicker slices have lower signal-to-noise ratio because the larger volume being sampled produces an image of higher quality.

### Number of Slices

Increasing the number of times a slice is sampled improves the image. Most scanners can select averages from 0.25 to 16.0. The higher the number of averages taken, the better the image quality. Patient motion must be considered when selecting higher averages because there is a limit to the time a patient can hold still. When determining what technique generates the best image data, technologists must weigh the practicality of increasing the scan time against the needs of the patient.

### Matrix Size

The size of a matrix is operator controlled. By adjusting the size of the field of view and the pixel size, the image quality can be directly controlled. Most scanners have matrices of $128 \times 128$ to $256 \times 256$; newer scanners also have $384 \times 384$ and $512 \times 512$ or variations of all four. Selecting a larger matrix can increase the scan time as well as the resolution of an image. Often, with increased matrices, the number of averages must also be increased to produce a good image. A point is reached when the size of the matrix and the number of averages are too great to produce a good examination. A matrix of $512 \times 512$ would be ideal for a scan of the wrist; however, patient comfort and time must be considered. The reader is referred to Chapter 14, Digital Imaging Techniques, for more information on matrices.

## MOTION AND FLOW ARTIFACT COMPENSATION

### Spatial Saturation

Spatial saturation is used to cut down on the flow artifact created by moving nuclei. Simply stated, a saturation pulse is delivered to a volume outside the slice being imaged. Nuclei that are not in the slice receiving a 90-degree RF pulse then receive part of a 180-degree rephasing pulse and give a false signal in the slice being imaged. By adding a presaturation pulse outside the slice, the nuclei are saturated to some degree and are affected by the energy delivered in the slice being imaged.

### Respiratory Compensation

Unlike CT, present MR technology produces pulse sequences that are too long to have a patient suspend respiration while imaging. The body wall and the organs inside move during respiration and create a phase artifact on the image. Some MR scanners use a bellows attached to the patient's chest to track the respiratory movement. The motion of the chest creates air pressure inside the bellows, which is then translated into an electric signal by a transducer. This electric signal is used to correctly map the respiratory movements to produce an image with few motion artifacts.

### Gating

Motion from the heart and pulsating blood in the vessels creates motion throughout the body. In gating, an electric signal is used to trigger slice selection. Gating can be accomplished in two ways, cardiac and peripheral gating. In peripheral gating, a sensor, such as a finger, is placed over a vascular bed and the capillary blood flow is monitored. In cardiac gating, electrodes are placed in specific areas (usually on the posterior chest wall near the left scapula); the electrical activity of the heart is then directly monitored. These signals can be used to produce a gated study of the heart. Often, respiratory compensation and cardiac gating are used in combination to give detailed pictures of the heart

and chest. Cardiac gating can also be used to gate any organ that has vascular flow.

## FAST SCAN

Fast-scan MR is a software application applied to high field strength scanners. Fast scan allows for imaging sequences up to 16 times faster than with conventional pulse sequences. Many of the fast-scan sequences are performed one slice at a time. Fast-scan chest imaging can be accomplished with the patient suspending respiration for each individual slice. As scan times decrease, the ability to do cine MR will become a possibility.

## MAGNETIC RESONANCE ANGIOGRAPHY

Magnetic resonance angiography has the potential to assist present-day invasive angiography procedures for initial diagnosis. The initial application for MRA is to combine MRA with abnormal brain MR images. Cerebrovascular disease is one of the predominant causes of morbidity in the United States. Carotid bifurcation stenosis is one of the areas of concentration for MRA. If this area could be sampled effectively, MRA could evaluate pathology without an invasive procedure.

MRA is not a time-intensive procedure and has few, if any, of the complications of angiography. MRA demonstrates vessels in a three-dimensional format and is an initially simple procedure. MRA application should increase as techniques improve, artifacts are decreased, and clinicians gain confidence in interpreting these scans.

## SUMMARY

In the last several years there has been a proliferation of the number of magnets in the United States. Low field magnets are especially suited for small clinics and as a second magnet for larger facilities. MRA, fast scan, and spectroscopy are facilitated by higher field strength magnets; however, high field strengths have more field uniformity problems than low field magnets. Extensive software is required to compensate for the uniformity problems associated with high field magnets. Low field magnets can cost less and are easier to maintain. With the excellent image contrast provided by MR imaging, coupled with the ability to perform noninvasive angiographic procedures, spectroscopy, and functional cine studies, MRI is truly one of the most valuable imaging tools available to clinicians today.

## REVIEW QUESTIONS

1. MR imaging is superior for neurologic imaging for the following reasons except _____.
   A. superior spatial resolution
   B. visualization in the sagittal, coronal, and axial planes

C. soft tissue visualization

D. superior contrast

2. Motion is the greatest deterrent in which of the following anatomic areas?
   A. neurologic tissue
   B. abdomen
   C. thorax
   D. extremity

3. Select the answer below that represents why hydrogen is the element of choice for MR imaging.
   A. hydrogen behaves very predictably
   B. hydrogen is very abundant in the body
   C. hydrogen has only one neutron
   D. A, B, and C above
   E. A and B above

4. Fluorine would be an excellent imaging element for the following reason(s):
   A. it is abundant in nature
   B. it is abundant in the human body
   C. its magnetic moment is similar to hydrogen's
   D. A, B, and C above
   E. A and C above

5. The MR magnet produces a static magnetic field along the axis of the patient, which is measured in tesla and is called ____.
   A. $B_o$
   B. $M_o$
   C. $N_o$
   D. Z

6. In the presence of the strong magnetic field, the dipoles align along the ____ axis and precess.
   A. X
   B. Y
   C. Z
   D. Q

7. From among the following, select the answer that represents a dipole:
   A. the earth
   B. a bar magnet
   C. hydrogen atom
   D. all of the above

8. Hydrogen will have a precessional frequency of ____ MHz/T in a 0.5-T magnet.
   A. 63.9
   B. 42.6
   C. 29.8
   D. 21.3

9. From the statements below, select the one that is true about dipoles.
   A. dipoles have magnetic moments
   B. dipoles can store and emit electromagnetic radiation
   C. dipoles can interact with externally applied magnetic fields
   D. all of the above

10. What is used to designate the amount (sum) of net magnetizations along the Z axis?
    A. $B_o$
    B. $M_o$
    C. $N_o$
    D. Z

11. To receive a signal, the magnetization factor has to be in the ____ plane.
    A. X
    B. Y
    C. Z
    D. A, B, and C above
    E. A and B above

12. From among the answers below, select the one that represents a pulse sequence of 180 degrees followed by a 90-degree pulse.
    A. partial saturation
    B. spin echo
    C. inversion recovery
    D. A and B above

13. Tissue with a short T1 will be dark.
    A. true
    B. false

14. T2 is a measure of the change of phase of (or loss of) the resonating photons.
    A. true
    B. false

15. From among the answers below, select the one that represents the type of magnet having the highest energy consumption.
    A. resistive
    B. superconductive
    C. permanent
    D. none of the above

16. Select the answer below which represents the type of magnet providing the highest field strength.
    A. resistive
    B. superconductive
    C. permanent
    D. none of the above

17. A surface coil is both a sending and receiving coil.
    A. true
    B. false

18. The thinner the slice, the greater the signal-to-noise artifact.
    A. true
    B. false

19. From among the answers below, select the one that has parameters which the technologist controls.
    A. selection of imaging plane
    B. slice thickness
    C. number of slices
    D. matrix size
    E. all of the above

20. From among the answers below, select the one that compensates for motion.
    A. spatial saturation
    B. respiratory compensation
    C. gating

D. all of the above
E. B and C above

21. Which of the following produces images similar to radiographic angiography?
    A. spectroscopy
    B. fast scan
    C. MRA
    D. gating

## BIBLIOGRAPHY

Bradley, WG, Adey, WR, and Hasso, AN: Magnetic Resonance Imaging. Aspen Systems Corporation, Rockville, MD, 1985.

Bushong, SC: Magnetic Resonance Imaging. CV Mosby Company, St Louis, 1988.

Elster, AD: Magnetic Resonance Imaging. JB Lippincott, Philadelphia, 1986.

Hendee, WR and Hendrick, ER: Fundamentals of Diagnostic Imaging, Vol 1. WB Saunders, Philadelphia, 1988.

# CHAPTER 34

# Multidimensional Imaging

*Kenneth M. Wintch, MA, ARRT(R)(N)RN*

Since 1895, when it was first possible to take anatomic pictures of the human body, the goal has been to visualize the body in its three-dimensional form. The ideal way to demonstrate anatomy and pathology is in its true multidimensional shape in a noninvasive fashion. For example, a typical skull radiograph demonstrates size, shape, and configuration but yields little information about the underlying anatomy (depth). Demonstrating the underlying anatomy is easily accomplished with multislice computed tomography (CT) and magnetic resonance imaging (MRI). These modalities would not be possible without the aid of highly sophisticated computer hardware and software. The images produced by these modalities show anatomy in such detail that diagnosis is now more reliable and definable. Images produced for interpretation are obtained in multiple planes, including sagittal, coronal, axial, and oblique; however, they are only demonstrated in two dimensions. When viewing these multiple slices, the true size, shape, and configuration of the anatomy cannot be appreciated. For this reason, conventional filming (such as x-ray scout films of the imaged area) of the anatomy being scanned is often required for accurate interpretation of the multislice CT and MRI examinations. With multidimensional imaging, highly detailed CT and MR images are rendered to show size, shape, and configuration, with the added ability to visualize underlying anatomy.

## COMPUTER WORKSTATIONS

New developments in computer software and hardware provide for reconstruction techniques to produce multidimensional images from the two-dimensional images obtained by CT and MR. Stand-alone workstations that are dedicated to three-dimensional reconstruction usually have more processing power and software options than those built into the equipment. Three-dimensional workstations that are built into a CT or MRI console often have to share hardware, compromising rapid manipulative and analytic functions. Combined workstations usually are only compatible with the imaging modality with which they are inter-

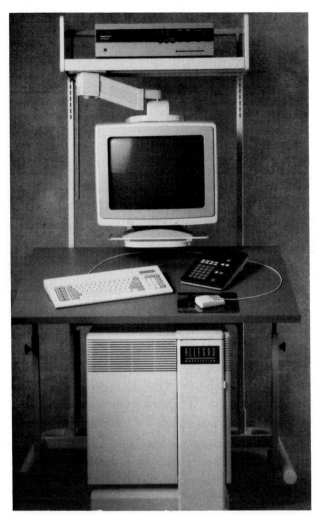

**Figure 34 – 1.** ISG (stand alone) workstation. (Courtesy of ISG Technologies Inc., Toronto, Ontario.)

faced, while stand-alone workstations often are compatible with several imaging modalities (Fig. 34 – 1).

## RECONSTRUCTION TECHNIQUES

High quality, multiple, sequential images are essential to the reconstruction of multidimensional images. Motion and large gaps between slices degrade the resulting image. Most equipment with a magnetic tape storage drive or optical disk can load onto a three-dimensional workstation to perform reconstruction. The best reconstructions are obtained utilizing state-of-the-art MR or CT equipment and software. Some of this equipment can perform reconstruction during the actual scan rather than from stored images after the scan is completed. Standard practice is to load a series of two-dimensional images via magnetic tape into the three-dimensional workstation. The number of images can vary from an average of 10 to 20, to 150 or more.

## Segmentation

CT images of the lumbar spine are excellent for reconstruction. They provide good contrast, and the computer can easily define the edge of the cortical bone from the original images. Generally, the operator selects an area of the two-dimensional images to be reconstructed and manually (or with computer edge detection) "draws," or segments, this same area for all the images in the series of images. Segmentation is defined as separation of an image into its component parts. Usually a computer has set windows for different types of tissue, such as bone, brain, soft tissue, and air. These set windows allow for standard gray-scale assignment to a type of tissue. For a standard three-dimensional reconstruction of the lumbar spine, the vertebral bodies, disks, spinal cord, and nerves are segmented separately (Fig. 34 – 2). When these three areas are segmented, the computer reconstructs all of the segmented areas and displays them multidimensionally (Fig. 34 – 3).

## Postprocessing

The standard way to visualize pathology on CT and MR images is on two-dimensional film. Postprocessing takes these two-dimensional data and downloads them into a data base. There are several advantages of postprocessing image data from CT and MR scanners. Anatomy can be demonstrated at any angle of the three-dimensional plane. The reconstructed image can

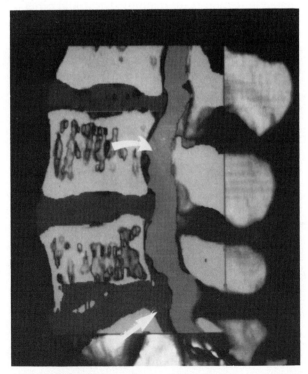

**Figure 34 – 2.** Cross section of vertebral bodies, spinal cord, and disks; *curved arrow* shows postprocessed spinal cord and *straight arrow* shows a herniated disk.

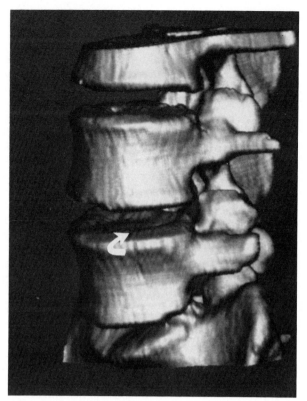

**Figure 34-3.** Three-dimensional reconstruction of Figure 34-2; *curved arrow* shows disk space.

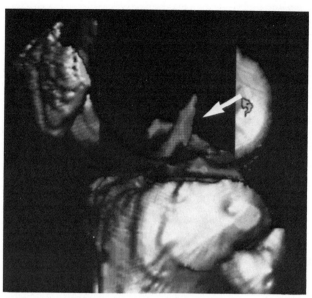

**Figure 34-5.** Translucent femur; *arrow* shows anterior and posterior cruciate ligament projected transparently.

be rotated along any axis in real-time display. This allows the operator to visualize the anatomy as it is physically presented within the body. Joints can be disarticulated to demonstrate anatomy that would otherwise be superimposed. When several structures are seg-

mented individually, one or several can be deleted to expose the superimposed structures. This is very useful, for example, to visualize the anterior and posterior cruciate ligaments of the knee. By deleting the femur and rotating the tibia to visualize the articular surface, the ligaments are easily seen (Fig. 34-4). When the operator needs to visualize a superimposed area in relationship to the surrounding tissue, segmented areas can also be made translucent, which is also very helpful in viewing joints (Fig. 34-5). Tumors of the brain can also be visualized in relationship to surrounding brain

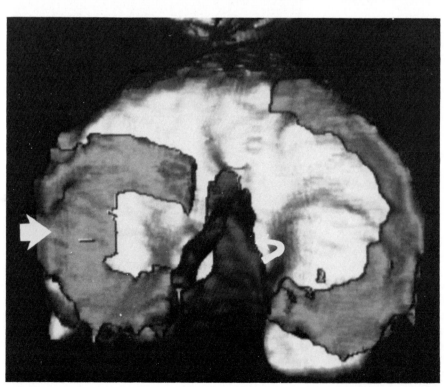

**Figure 34-4.** Articular surface of knee; *straight arrow* shows meniscus, and *curved arrow* shows anterior and posterior cruciate ligament.

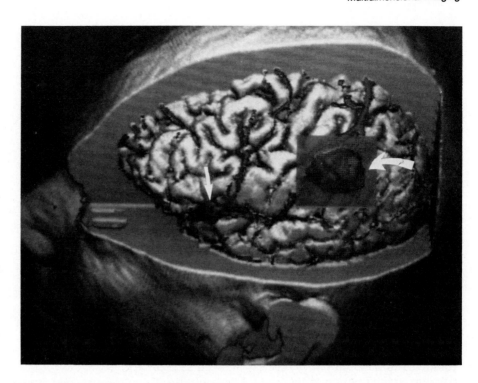

**Figure 34-6.** Brain with tumor; *straight arrow* shows vasculature, and *curved arrow* shows tumor.

tissue. This technique is helpful since the tumor size, shape, and position in the brain is demonstrated (Fig. 34-6).

## SURGICAL APPLICATIONS

### Planning

Multidimensional imaging is perhaps most applicable to planning and guiding surgical procedures. Most surgery is performed without a knowledge of the patient's individual anatomy. Traditionally, during surgery, surgeons obtain visual information from the patient's radiographs, CT, and/or MR images on a view box. These two-dimensional images cannot give precise knowledge of the patient's anatomy. Cranial and facial surgery leaves little, if any, margin for error; thus, prior to surgery, knowledge of the surface anatomy and the underlying structures is critical. By using postprocessed CT and MR images, craniofacial surgery can be precisely planned, thereby avoiding surgical pitfalls. This reduces operating time and patient morbidity. Three-dimensional imaging also aids in detecting facial trauma and temporomandibular joint injuries and in planning dental implants. Typical three-dimensional software tools that aid in craniotomies include cutting planes, depth probes, linear measurements, and volume measurements.

### CUTTING PLANES

Cutting planes remove simulated tissue in wedges similar to that in actual surgery. Real-time viewing can stimulate the actual surgical approach.

### DEPTH PROBES

By using a depth probe on a simulated skull, reconstructed with the patient's actual anatomy, it is possible to simulate the depth and surrounding structures. This tool aids the surgeon in planning the approach, thus preventing unnecessary trauma to the tissues.

### LINEAR AND VOLUME MEASUREMENTS

By using a position of reference, accurate measurements can be obtained in any direction in millimeter increments. When accurate measurements in three-dimensional space can be obtained, the distance, angular correlation between similar structures, and tissue density can be easily measured.

Any structure that is segmented can be measured for its volume. These measurements are useful in determining the response of tumors to therapy. Interstitial fluid can also be measured for its volume, thus facilitating extraction.

### Surgical Guidance

The software planning tools can actually help a surgeon practice surgery as well as determine the accurate size, shape, and configuration of the anatomy in question. Three-dimensional viewing is valuable in planning surgery.

Recent developments even allow three-dimensional viewing to be used in the operating room. New tools being developed are expected to allow the three-dimensional workstation to be taken into the operating room and used as a surgical tool. A "works-in-progress" imaging wand equipped with a 6-degree-of-motion mechanical arm digitizer can be mounted to the side of the operating room table. Together, the wand and the imaging computer provide surgeons with guidance, visualization, and localization of their position intraoperatively. Now, not only will the surgeon be able to visualize the multidimensional data at the operating table, but the surgeon will also be able to use the patient's image data as a guide to his or her individual anatomy. To use the software for a surgical procedure, the patient's presurgical CT or MRI scans are loaded into the system and reconstructed into a three-dimensional presentation. The same landmarks that were placed on the patient when scanned are used to localize the wand to the patient in the operating room. After correlating the patient's anatomy to the computer image, a virtual probe appears on the screen, moving through the image data in correct relationship to the actual probe as it is used by the surgeon. As the surgeon guides the probe, the wand's image is displayed on the computer monitor, mirroring the probe in relationship to its movements. Structures in front of the probe can be "cut away" by using the computer icons. This simulates the anatomy beneath the surgical opening. Also by rotating the wand, any structure can be seen in relationship to the position of the wand. By manipulating the probe, the surgeon is provided with an instant visual feedback to guide the surgical intervention. Being able to view a trajectory through the patient's anatomy and display the image data interactively on the monitor allows the surgeon to accurately intercept the target lesion, thereby minimizing damage to the surrounding tissue.

## DENTAL APPLICATIONS

Dental surgeons also find three-dimensional viewing an accurate tool for planning oral and maxillofacial surgery. Three-dimensional imaging can localize the inferior alveolar nerve (Fig. 34–7) and the maxillary sinus. By visualizing the patient's maxillofacial structure prior to surgery, areas that must be avoided can be localized. Measurement of bone density and volume for implant surgery can also be made. This is helpful for planning endosseous implant positioning. All of the reformatted images can be marked with a millimeter scale to aid in determining the proper fit of a prosthesis.

## FUTURE CONSIDERATIONS

The future is bright for three-dimensional imaging. Complex surgeries for sinusitis may become routine. Obstetricians may use three-dimensional imaging to plan complex abdominal surgery. Medical students of anatomy can use the wand to practice surgery on simulated patients. Heart imaging using three-dimensional techniques helps define wall boundaries and provides a quantitative analysis of the heart wall to show ischemia and damage. The heart and other structures can be visualized with the help of magnetic resonance angiography. Using three-dimensional viewing to manipulate

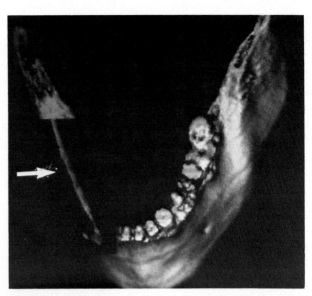

**Figure 34–7.** Dental image transparently projected to localize the inferior alveolar nerve.

these images, a rapid and interactive view can be obtained. By visualizing the vessels in a multidimensional format, there is no limitation to the number of views or projection angles that can be demonstrated. Vasculature can also be seen in relationship to the surrounding anatomy, which is extremely beneficial when performing surgery on hypervascular tumors and areas with (or tumors with) unclear margins.

## EDUCATIONAL APPLICATIONS

Three-dimensional imaging has already demonstrated the capability to speed up the interpretation of images, provide data that would otherwise be hidden, and aid in surgical procedures. There is an increasing demand for three-dimensional images, especially in neurologic, orthopedic, and craniofacial surgery. Oncology and related medical specialties use three-dimensional imaging to aid in the efficient, effective detection and removal of tumors. Educators are now demonstrating how three-dimensional images of the human body in simulated representations of actual anatomy can be visualized from all angles. Many companies see the next step in multidimensional imaging as the combination of virtual-reality technologies with three-dimensional viewing. This would allow visualization of actual human anatomy in its true representation and, through computer manipulation, to the exploration of anatomy from every aspect, both superficially and internally, as if the tissue were being held by the viewer. This can easily be accomplished by using virtual-reality head gear and pressure-sensitive gloves. An excellent teaching application would be to display a total body (patient) in space and have students simulate the injection of the patient with medication and visualize the medication as it interacts with the critical and target organs. With the aid of high speed computers, educational tools that simulate actual minimal invasive instruments, like a laparoscope, will allow physicians to practice surgical procedures on postprocessed data, prior to practicing on real patients. Several companies have already developed, and have available, the software and hardware for these applications.

## CONCLUSION

Multidimensional imaging should be an integral part of a large imaging center, hospital, or teaching institution. General surgical, neurologic, radiographic, and educational applications are already in use. As more applications are developed and the benefits of this imaging are realized, multidimensional imaging is expected to become its own separate discipline.

## REVIEW QUESTIONS

1. From the descriptions below, select the one that does not apply to stand-alone workstations.
   A. generally have less processing power than interfaced workstations
   B. are dedicated to three-dimensional reconstruction
   C. compatibility with several different imaging modalities
   D. have more software options than interfaced workstations

2. The average number of images needed to do three-dimensional reconstruction is ____.
   A. 10 to 20
   B. 20 to 30
   C. 50 to 60
   D. 70 to 100

3. Which of the following is not essential to the reconstruction of multidimensional images?
   A. multiple high quality sequential images
   B. little or no motion on the images
   C. little or no gap between slices
   D. low matrix multiple images

4. Separation of an image into its component parts is defined as ____.
   A. preprocessing
   B. reconstructing
   C. defining
   D. segmentation

5. Postprocessing demonstrates anatomy at any angle in the three-dimensional plane.
   A. true
   B. false

6. Disarticulation means ____.
   A. demonstrating anatomy with a translucent overlay
   B. rotating anatomy to demonstrate the anatomy desired
   C. deleting a segmented section of anatomy and then rotating the anatomy to demonstrate the hidden anatomy
   D. both A and C

7. Which typical software tool allows for viewing an actual surgical approach?
   A. depth probe
   B. cutting planes
   C. linear and volume measurements
   D. high volume lens

8. Which software tool allows for accurate measurements of distance, angle, and density?
   A. depth probe
   B. cutting planes
   C. linear measurements
   D. volume measurements

9. The wand allows the surgeon to do all of the following except ____.
   A. simulate anatomy beneath a surgical opening
   B. visualize multidimensional imaging data at the operating table
   C. provide instant visual feedback to guide surgical intervention
   D. use an 8-degrees-of-motion mechanical arm mounted to the side of the operating table

10. The surgical wand will provide the surgeon with ____, ____, and ____ of their position intraoperatively.

## BIBLIOGRAPHY

ISG Technologies, Inc. Product Information, 3030 Orlando Drive, Toronto, Ontario, Canada L4v 1SB.
Udupa, JK and Herman GT: 3D imaging in Medicine. CRC Press, Boca Raton, 1991.

# CHAPTER 35

# Positron Emission Tomography

*Joan K. MacDonald, MS, ARRT(N)*

Positron emission tomography (PET) is a noninvasive imaging modality that employs tomography to display and quantify various tissue concentrations of internally administered radioactive materials. Those familiar with nuclear medicine may also recognize this as a definition of single photon emission computed tomography (SPECT). The primary difference between positron and single-photon emission imaging is in the type of radionuclide (radioactive atom) administered. This may appear to be a rather small difference that could easily be overcome with simple alterations in the current nuclear medicine detection systems. Unfortunately, new and relatively expensive methods for the detection and production of positron emitters and their subsequent labeling with various chemicals (radiopharmaceuticals) are required.

One may wonder why PET is receiving so much attention since advances in SPECT have provided diagnosticians with greater qualitative and quantitative functional information than ever before. Similar advancements in x-ray computed tomography (CT) and magnetic resonance imaging (MRI) have provided the opportunity to view anatomic structures (morphology) in unparalleled, noninvasive detail. The advantage PET presents over these well-established tomographic modalities is simple. PET offers a greater potential of detecting disease prior to the occurrence of corresponding physical changes, thus allowing for earlier intervention and care.

The effectiveness of PET is directly related to its capability to demonstrate the biodistribution of physiologically important elements, such as carbon, oxygen, nitrogen, and hydrogen. By substituting radioactive elements or compounds for the body's stable ones, the true physiologic response to biologically active compounds may be demonstrated through PET. Although nuclear medicine demonstrates functional responses to various radioactive substances, these materials generally do not contain the natural elements mentioned previously, and, therefore, the physiologic response may not be true to nature.

PET is emerging as a viable clinical modality. Private insurance companies are recognizing the value of this biologic imaging modality and are beginning to reimburse facilities for certain procedures on a case-by-case basis. Prior to a discussion of the clinical role of PET, the basic physics, production, and detection of positron emitters is presented.

## RADIATION PHYSICS OF POSITRON EMISSION

A positron is essentially a positive electron that has been ejected from the nucleus of an unstable or radio-active atom. Being particulate in nature, it can travel a maximum of a few centimeters prior to being captured by an electron of opposite charge (most positron emitters used in PET travel less than 2 mm). Once united, both particles are annihilated, and their masses are converted into energy in the form of two 511-kiloelec-tronvolt (keV) gamma rays, which are emitted in nearly exact opposite directions (180 degrees apart). This "mass-to-energy" conversion is called "annihilation radiation" (Fig. 35-1). It is the two gamma rays that are detected in PET, not the positron. The gamma-ray energy of the most common radionuclide used in nuclear medicine is 140 keV, from the decay of molybdenum-98 to technetium-99m.

Radionuclides that decay by positron emission are attempting to reach stability by increasing their neutron-to-proton ratio. Many of the proton-rich radionuclides are those of lower atomic weights, such as oxygen, carbon, nitrogen, and hydrogen, the primary constituents of virtually all organic molecules. Radioisotopes of oxygen (O-15), carbon (C-11), and nitrogen (N-13) can be directly substituted for their stable counterparts, whereas fluorine (F-18) can be substituted for hydrogen, because the biochemical properties of these two elements are similar.

## PRODUCTION OF POSITRON EMITTERS

The majority of positron emitters used in medicine are produced by bombarding stable nuclei with high-energy beams of charged particles, primarily protons, deuterons, and alpha particles. This generally requires either an electrostatic accelerator or a cyclotron, with cyclotrons being the most common.

A cyclotron and its associated shielding are extremely costly. The fact that many PET centers have their own cyclotrons helps to explain the high cost of PET research and clinical application. The need for in-house cyclotrons is because of the short half-lives of many of the desired positron emitters. A half-life refers to the time it takes for one half of the initial number of radioactive atoms to decay. If, for example, there were 1 million atoms of a positron emitter with a half-life of 5 minutes present initially, only 500,000 atoms would remain after 5 minutes had elapsed. By calculating the exponential decrease of this hypothetical radionuclide, less than 2 percent of the original activity would remain 30 minutes following its production. If this radionu-

**NUCLEUS OF POSITRON EMITTER**

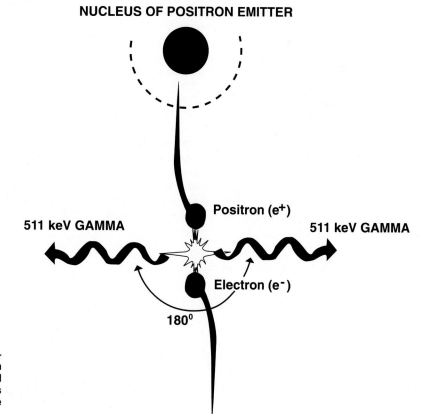

**511 keV GAMMA**      Positron (e⁺)      **511 keV GAMMA**

Electron (e⁻)

180⁰

**Figure 35-1.** Annihilation radiation. Following ejection from the nucleus, a positron (e⁺) unites with an electron (e⁻). These particles are annihilated, and their energies are transformed into two gamma rays of 511 keV each, which are emitted in opposite directions.

clide had to be transported in any major city, its activity would be too low for use by the time it arrived at the clinical location.

Another method of obtaining positron emitters, such as gallium-68 (Ga-68) and rubidium-82 (Rb-82), is by "milking" (drawing off) a radionuclide generator. The basic principle of a generator is that a relatively long-lived radionuclide (the parent) is fixed and contained in a specially shielded column. The parent product decays to a shorter-lived radionuclide (the daughter), which also remains on the column until it is needed. The daughter, having different chemical properties, can easily be separated from the parent by passing fluids or gases over the column. This provides a most convenient and cost-effective method of obtaining radionuclides. The generator-produced positron emitters, however, have limited applications and cannot presently provide for all the radionuclides necessary in a comprehensive PET center.

## DETECTION SYSTEM DESIGN

Conventional nuclear medicine cameras, or "gamma cameras," are designed to capture relatively low gamma rays (140 keV). The detection of the 511-keV gamma rays used in PET has necessitated major changes in the gamma camera design.

Detecting gamma rays is fundamentally the same, regardless of whether they originate from positron decay or from another radioactive process. A relatively high density material capable of absorbing the incoming rays and converting their energy into a measurable form is necessary in any system. Crystals of various compounds generally serve this purpose. Sodium iodide with thallium [NaI(Tl)] is the most commonly used material in nuclear medicine cameras. However, in order to stop the higher energy gamma rays originating from positron emitters, higher density materials such as bismuth germanate oxide (BGO), cesium fluoride ($CsF_2$), or gadolinium orthosilicate (GSO) are more commonly used for PET.

Once a gamma ray interacts in a crystal, its energy is transformed into light photons in proportion to the energy of the incident gamma ray. These photons are then directed toward a photomultiplier tube (PMT), and their energy is converted into electrons (Fig. 35–2). While traversing the PMT, the electrons are greatly

increased in number until the final pulse is large enough for detection. If this pulse corresponds to a preselected range of energies, it, along with the relative positional information of the original gamma ray, is passed through the remaining PET system components to be recorded.

Although there are numerous designs, most modern PET systems contain several rings of detector elements stacked together to permit the simultaneous recording of multiple tomographic sections (Fig. 35–3). Each circular array forms a single image plane, whereas the number of arrays define the number of image planes available (planes 1 through 4 in Fig. 35–3). Within each array of detector elements, individual elements are electronically connected to several opposing elements, creating a "fan-beam"–shaped coincidence detection design.

Since two 511-keV gamma rays are simultaneously emitted in opposing directions following positron emission, the above design is relatively efficient in detecting the two rays when emitted within the detector's field of view. If the electronics verify that two such events have occurred within approximately 5 to 10 nanoseconds (10 to $^-9$ seconds) of each other, an acceptance signal is forwarded through the system. It is assumed that the original activity was located somewhere on a line between the two crystals. This "coincidence detection" defines the basic principle of PET.

The assembly identified above allows for more than 1 million detector pair combinations to simultaneously collect the data. Elements from one detector plane may also be connected to opposing elements of other planes. This permits "cross plane" sampling, which increases the efficiency (sensitivity) of the system.

Occasionally, two unrelated gamma rays may arrive at opposing detection elements within the acceptable coincidence interval. Although they are accepted, the subsequently recorded data point represents a mispositioned event. This negatively affects spatial resolution, or the ability to resolve detail. The likelihood of such "random" events occurring is proportional to the count rate (dose), and it is, therefore, possible to mathematically remove many of these unwanted radiations through computed data manipulation.

Because of the nature of the paired elements coincidence detection design, collimators commonly used in nuclear medicine are unnecessary in PET systems. All off-axis photons (scatter) that are not paired with an

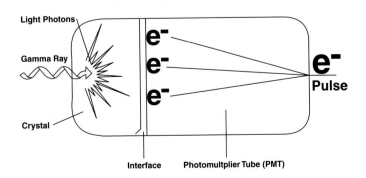

**Figure 35–2.** Detection unit for gamma rays. When a gamma ray interacts within a crystal, its energy is transformed into light photons. These interact at the PMT interface, and their energies are transformed into electrons. The electrons are increased in number manyfold as they traverse the PMT, resulting in a relatively large electron pulse. This terminal pulse is proportional to the energy of the incident gamma ray.

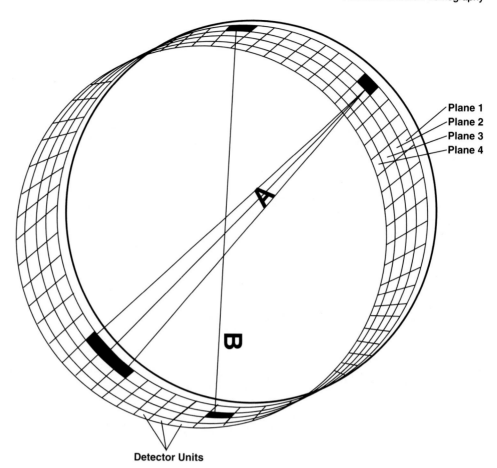

**Figure 35–3.** Modern PET detection design. Circular detector arrays with four imaging "planes." Detection elements within each plane are electronically connected to opposing elements as indicated by lines A. Interplane, or cross-plane, connections such as line B are also possible.

Plane 1
Plane 2
Plane 3
Plane 4

A

B

**Detector Units**

opposing element and/or all paired photons that are not received within the acceptable temporal (time) interval are electronically rejected. The lack of external collimation dramatically increases the sensitivity of these systems. Lead collimation may, however, be placed between the crystal elements within each plane and between each circular array of detectors to further reduce the effects of scatter.

The external packaging of a PET system is similar to CT equipment. A gantry containing the detector system and associated components usually has a 55- to 60-cm opening for whole-body imaging and a smaller opening for dedicated brain imaging. Patient couches also resemble those used for CT. Minicomputers control the system and enable image reconstruction and processing procedures to be performed. Figure 35–4

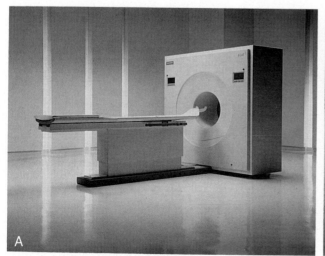

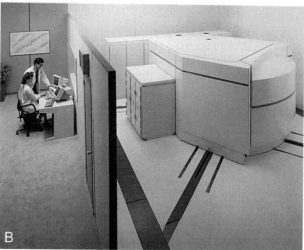

**Figure 35–4.** (*A*) Modern PET system; (*B*) cyclotron (Courtesy of Siemens Medical Systems, Inc., Iselin, NJ.).

shows a modern PET system and the associated cyclotron.

## BASIC PRINCIPLES OF IMAGE RECONSTRUCTION

The principles of image reconstruction for PET are similar to those of CT, MR, and SPECT. Although a comprehensive discussion of reconstruction is beyond the scope of this chapter, the basic principles are presented.

Recall from an earlier discussion that once an event is accepted, it is assumed that the source activity was located somewhere on a line between the two detection elements. In other words, the true location along that projection line is unknown. In order to reconstruct the image for tomographic or sectional display, count profiles or frequency curves are obtained for each detector and then backprojected across an image matrix as a line of activity. For example, assume there is only one point source of activity being imaged and that it is located in the center of the field of view. For simplicity, also assume that there are only four detector pairs and that each detector has accepted its respective coincidence gamma ray (Fig. 35–5*A*). Each detector pair in this example has detected 110 counts, because each pair "sees" the same single point source. Next, a line of activity relative to the count profile and at the same angle as the detector pair combination is projected across an image matrix (Fig. 35–5*B*). The original distribution of the activity can now be approximated from the superimposition of the four summed rays. This "brute-force" backprojection, however, results in considerable blurring around the activity sources, as is evidenced by the "star" effect in the illustration. In order to reduce the blurring and to enhance the contrast, mathematical filters of various types must be applied to the projection images either prior to and/or following backprojection.

Each ring of detectors essentially acquires a transverse image through a particular body part. By stacking all the transverse images together, a composite of the entire area imaged can be displayed. Sagittal, coronal, and oblique sections can then be computer-constructed from the original transverse composite image.

One dilemma shared by several imaging modalities is how to correct for photon attenuation within the body. This unwanted absorption of photon energy is essentially a direct function of the density and thickness of the tissue transversed as well as the energy of the photon. Therefore, those photons that originate in or pass through deeply seated areas and/or those passing through dense material, such as bone, have a greater likelihood of being attenuated prior to reaching the detector. Whenever the true distribution of photons within tissues cannot be correctly reproduced, the degree of certainty of diagnosis is decreased. Additionally, without correction, quantification studies cannot be defined accurately.

The effects of attenuation can be greatly reduced in PET through the use of transmission imaging. Prior to

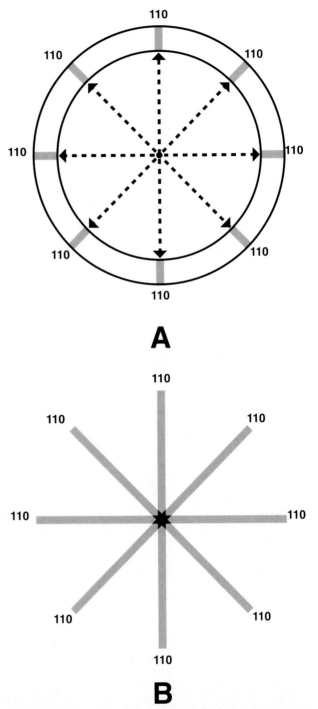

**A**

**B**

**Figure 35–5.** (*A*) A point source in the center of a gantry is detected by four detector pairs. All elements have detected the same number of counts, or intensity. (*B*) The intensity detected by each detector pair is "backprojected" across an image matrix in the same planes as originally detected. Each backprojected line is of uniform density across the entire matrix and, in this example, all four lines are of equal density. Note the increased density at the point of superimposition. This area represents the original point source. With computer filtering, the star effect caused by superimposition can be reduced.

positioning the patient, a "blank" reference scan is obtained and recorded from a positron-emitting source (usually gallium-68 [Ga-68]) placed in the gantry. The patient is then positioned for the study and a second reference scan is obtained using the same Ga-68 source.

During this process, the radiation passes through the patient to the detectors, and all areas of attenuation can be identified. Ratios of the blank to transmission data are calculated, stored, and later used during the reconstruction phase of the patient's study to mathematically correct for attenuation. The PET image, therefore, accurately quantifies the regional distribution of activity. The derived attenuation correction factors will only be accurate if the patient remains in the same position between the transmission scan and the actual procedure. If the patient moves, it may be necessary to apply correction factors or to collect new data.

## CLINICAL APPLICATIONS OF PET

PET imaging and quantification studies presently predominate in the areas of neurology, cardiology, and oncology. A variety of procedures can be performed with one of the more than 500 compounds previously investigated. The majority of these compounds are labeled, with O-15, N-13, C-11, or F-18 with F-18 being the most common. Because the purpose of this chapter is to provide an introduction to PET, only those areas with the greatest clinical utility at this time are presented.

### The Brain

Positron emission tomography has demonstrated considerable diagnostic value in the neurologic disorders of dementia and complex partial epilepsy. Additionally, the assessment of cerebrovascular disease (stroke) and brain tumors has been enhanced with PET.

#### DEMENTIAS

Perhaps the greatest contribution of PET to date has been in the noninvasive differential diagnosis of early symptomatic dementia. In the proper clinical context, PET can provide a specific diagnosis of Alzheimer's, Pick's, Huntington's, Wilson's, and other dementias.

PET currently provides the only noninvasive method of identifying Alzheimer's disease (AD). There are no known biochemical, clinical, or genetic markers for this fatal, and presently untreatable, disease. During PET imaging for AD, the relationship between brain function and glucose metabolism is examined using a radioactive fluorine labeled to deoxyglucose (F-18 FDG). In the normal-brain PET image, FDG reveals symmetrical and relatively uniform uptake throughout the cerebral cortex, cerebellar cortex, basal ganglia, thalami, and other gray cells. In AD, however, a pattern of bilateral, glucose hypometabolism (decreased uptake) appears in the parietal and temporal association areas of the cerebral cortex. As the disease progresses, hypometabolism is likely to be observed in the occipital and frontal cortices as well. Although this pattern may also be present in other disease states, it is pathognomonic for AD in the clinical setting

of a demented patient over 40 years of age with no apparent motor dysfunction, previous trauma, radiation therapy, or sudden neurologic deficits. CT and MR may reveal atrophic structural changes in patients with AD, but this is a nonspecific finding.

The non-Alzheimer's dementias generally reveal glucose hypometabolism in different, but fairly specific areas within the brain. Again, in the proper clinical setting, it is possible to diagnose these diseases. Even though treatment of most dementias presently eludes the medical community, patients and their families can receive tremendous physical, emotional, and financial benefits from an early diagnosis. Additionally, dementias like AD may mask other treatable disease that would benefit greatly by early diagnosis and intervention, such as vascular dementia or depression.

#### COMPLEX PARTIAL EPILEPSY

Thirty to sixty percent of patients with complex partial epilepsy eventually become refractory to medical treatment. Surgical excision of well localized seizure foci, especially in the temporal lobes, may eliminate the seizures or significantly improve the pharmacological control in the majority of these patients. PET imaging may provide the surgical team with a highly sensitive map of the epileptogenic foci noninvasively. CT and MR generally do not show abnormalities, and if they do, they often underestimate the size of the foci.

FDG-PET findings vary with the state of the patient. During seizures (ictal state), all areas of seizure involvement generally show hypermetabolism (increased uptake) of glucose. When the patient is between seizures (interictal state), however, the epileptogenic area is identified as a hypometabolic area.

#### CEREBROVASCULAR DISEASE (STROKE)

A variety of PET studies are performed for the evaluation of cerebrovascular disease. Cerebral blood flow (CBF), cerebral blood volume (CBV), oxygen extraction efficiency (OEF), oxygen and glucose utilization, and pharmacological studies all have proven value. Alone, or in combination, these studies enhance the diagnosis and help assess the prognosis, treatment, and rehabilitation potential of stroke patients.

Although CT is the primary imaging modality for the diagnosis of stroke, PET can provide important functional information that assists in delineating the true extent of impairment. It has been noted that cerebrovascular abnormalities generally appear smaller on CT images than on PET images. This helps to explain the presence of clinical symptoms that have failed to reveal corresponding physical evidence on CT.

#### TUMORS

MR and CT have excellent reputations for delineating brain tumors. In addition, PET can assist in the grading of brain tumors, help to differentiate recurrent tumors from radiation necrosis, and provide a method of monitoring the response to various therapies. Again, these benefits are possible because of PET's ability to identify metabolic activity.

## The Heart

The majority of cardiac diseases are diagnosed only after significant pathologic changes have occurred. PET has the potential to detect disease early in its course, and, consequently, change the current concept of therapy from palliative to curative.

Coronary artery disease (CAD) is a major cause of death in the United States. The "gold standard" for the detection of CAD is contrast medium coronary arteriography. This invasive procedure is currently being questioned by several investigators, as factors other than those assessed by angiography have also been shown to play an important role in determining the hemodynamic significance of this disease. Functional PET studies, such as coronary hyperemic reserve measurements (blood flow) and myocardial viability (myocardial metabolism) imaging offer possible alternatives for the early detection and evaluation of CAD as well as other cardiac diseases.

Diagnosis of CAD by PET is based on the fact that blood flow is generally normal at rest (even in coronary arteries with up to 80% stenosis) but abnormal during exercise (or during vasodilation created by pharmacologic stressing agents). This disparity in regional blood flow can be imaged and/or quantitated with physiologic PET tracers such as rubidium-82 (Rb-82), nitrogen-13 ammonia (N-13), and oxygen-15 water (O-15). For example, a scan may demonstrate the coronary arteries providing sufficient blood flow to the left ventricular myocardium, but upon vasodilation, it may show a diminished capacity to increase flow in the ischemic areas. This hypoperfusion of the myocardium during the hyperemic (high blood flow) phase with an accompanying normal perfusion at rest is diagnostic of CAD.

The above-explained basis for CAD detection with PET is the same as that for SPECT myocardial perfusion imaging. PET, however, with its improvements in attenuation correction, resolution, and quantitative capabilities, offers increased sensitivity and specificity in CAD detection over SPECT.

In addition to the detection of CAD, it is also important to determine those patients who will receive the greatest benefit from revascularization procedures. It is often difficult to differentiate viable (ischemic) myocardial tissue from irreversibly damaged (infarcted) tissue, even with relatively sensitive studies such as the ECG and/or the SPECT myocardial perfusion procedures. With the use of FDG (F-18), a PET glucose metabolic imaging agent, it is possible to map areas of glucose metabolism within the myocardium. Ischemic areas, or areas of viable myocardium, will show uptake of the FDG, whereas irreversibly damaged tissue will not. This ability to map metabolic function noninvasively is currently limited to PET.

A prediction of revascularization benefit can be made by comparing the above two types of PET heart studies. It has been shown that ventricular function improvement is related to the degree of perfusion-metabolism mismatches as indicated by PET blood flow and glucose metabolic studies. Those with the greatest mismatch (greatest degree of hypoperfusion to the greatest metabolic uptake) showed the greatest functional improvement following coronary artery bypass surgery.

## Oncology

Most tumors show biochemical or physiologic changes prior to anatomic changes. It has already been shown how PET tracers such as FDG can provide a map of glucose metabolism in both the brain and the heart. Other functions, such as oxygen metabolism, amino acid uptake, protein synthesis, and DNA replication can also be delineated with PET tracers. The potential of PET to image the whole body and to identify early changes in these, as well as other, functions makes this a promising modality for the diagnosis, staging, and treatment monitoring of many types of cancer.

Currently, FDG is the most commonly used PET agent for cancer studies. It has been used to evaluate brain, head and neck, breast, lung, gastrointestinal tract, and musculoskeletal tumors, and lymphomas. The basis for FDG in these studies is that malignant cells are known to have an increased rate of aerobic glycolysis (increased glucose metabolism in the presence of oxygen). Because of this biochemical characteristic, many neoplasms and metastatic tumors can be detected and quantified by the uptake of FDG. The grading of certain tumors can also be accomplished as the degree of FDG uptake is linearly related to glucose metabolism. High grade astrocytomas (brain tumors), for example, show greater uptake than low grade lesions. Additionally, sequential studies that reveal a decreased uptake of FDG in previously identified malignancies are useful in documenting therapeutic improvement.

## REVIEW QUESTIONS

1. Which of the following imaging modalities is most closely aligned with positron emission tomography (PET)?
   A. transmission computed tomography (TCT or CT)
   B. magnetic resonance (MR)
   C. nuclear medicine
   D. ultrasonography

2. PET's potential as a diagnostic tool lies in its ability to reveal _____.
   A. anatomic structures in unparalleled detail
   B. early morphologic changes associated with disease
   C. early physiologic changes associated with disease
   D. all of the above

3. Which of the following statements is false regarding positron-emitting radionuclides?
   A. positron emission from a nucleus is always followed by a mass-to-energy conversion
   B. positrons generally travel only a short distance prior to being annihilated
   C. they usually contain too many protons in their nuclei
   D. positrons are easily detected in scintillation materials

4. The basic detection design of a PET system is that _____.
   A. one detection element accepts two gamma rays of 511 keV simultaneously
   B. two adjacent detection elements accept a 511-keV gamma ray, simultaneously
   C. two opposing detection elements accept a 511-keV gamma ray, simultaneously
   D. one detection element within each ring of detectors must simultaneously detect a 511-keV gamma ray

5. Collimation in PET systems is primarily accomplished _____.
   A. electronically through coincidence detection
   B. with a circular array of lead placed between the detection elements and the patient
   C. by adjusting the vertical and horizontal lead plates on the detector's head
   D. by shielding the patient

6. Transmission imaging by PET _____.
   A. enables proper filtering of the backprojected image
   B. significantly decreases the amount of scattered radiation
   C. provides for the mathematical correction of attenuation
   D. enables the gamma rays to be more focused

7. Which of the following is not a common method of obtaining positron emitters?
   A. cyclotron
   B. electrostatic accelerator
   C. radionuclide generator
   D. fusion reaction

8. Hypometabolism as evidenced with FDG in Alzheimer's disease will usually _____.
   A. be indistinguishable from normal tissue
   B. be localized in the basal ganglia
   C. be indistinguishable from cerebral vascular disease
   D. appear as areas of decreased activity

9. Alzheimer's disease generally affects the _____.
   A. cerebellar cortex
   B. thalami
   C. parietal and temporal cortex
   D. pituitary gland

10. PET-FDG studies primarily reflect _____ metabolism.
    A. fatty acid
    B. glucose
    C. protein
    D. basal

11. PET-FDG findings of complex partial epilepsy _____.
    A. are dependent upon the clinical presentation of the patient
    B. always appear as areas of increased activity
    C. are less sensitive than CT
    D. always appear as areas of decreased activity

12. The primary imaging modality for diagnosing cerebral vascular disease is _____.
    A. CT
    B. nuclear medicine
    C. PET
    D. ultrasonography

13. Coronary artery disease (CAD) may be diagnosed by PET on the basis of abnormal coronary blood flow at _____.
    A. rest
    B. stress with abnormal blood flow at rest
    C. stress returning to normal at rest
    D. rest, which becomes normal at stress

14. PET for CAD has _____ than does single-photon emission computed tomography (SPECT).
    A. greater sensitivity and less specificity
    B. greater specificity and less sensitivity
    C. less sensitivity and less specificity
    D. greater sensitivity and greater specificity

## BIBLIOGRAPHY

Ahluwalia, BD: Tomographic Methods in Nuclear Medicine: Physical Principles, Instruments, and Clinical Applications. CRC Press, Boca Raton, FL, 1989.

Daghighian, F, Sumida, R, and Phelps, ME: PET imaging: An overview and instrumentation. JNMT 18:5, 1990.

Gottschalk, A (ed): Diagnostic Nuclear Medicine, ed 2. Williams & Wilkins, Baltimore, 1988.

Wagner, HN: Principles and applications of positron emission tomography. In Sharif, NA and Lewis, ME (eds): Brain Imaging Techniques and Applications. Ellis Horwood Limited, New York, 1989, p 280.

# APPENDIX

# Answers to Review Questions

## CHAPTER 1: RADIOLOGY IN MOTION

1. B
2. D
3. A
4. B
5. C
6. D
7. A
8. B
9. C
10. A
11. B
12. B
13. A
14. C
15. D
16. A
17. D
18. B
19. C

## CHAPTER 2: MEDICAL LEGAL IMPLICATIONS

1. B
2. C
3. C
4. A
5. basic patient data
   vital signs (before, during, and after the procedure)
   list of personnel in room
   type and amount of contrast media used
   type and amount of other medications used
   fluoroscopic time
   size and number of films used for each series or run
   techniques used for each series or run
   area for notes and comments
6. B
7. A
8. B
9. D

## CHAPTER 3: CONTRAST MEDIA

1. A
2. B
3. ingestion
   retrograde
   intrathecal
   parenteral

4. C
5. A
6. D
7. B
8. C
9. C
10. A
11. D
12. obtain a thorough patient history
    premedicate the patient
    select the correct contrast agent
    have emergency equipment available
13. A
14. epinephrine
    angiotensin
    vasopressin
15. B
16. D
17. C
18. A

## CHAPTER 4: KNEE ARTHROGRAPHY

1. C
2. B
3. Anterior and posterior ligaments that cross over each other within the joint.
4. C
5. A
6. D
7. C
8. C
9. D
10. D
11. D
12. C
13. D
14. C
15. B
16. C

# CHAPTER 5: ENDOSCOPIC RETROGRADE CHOLANGIOPANCREATOGRAPHY

1. D
2. D
3. D
4. B
5. D
6. B
7. D
8. B
9. C
10. A
11. A
12. B
13. D
14. B
15. D

# CHAPTER 6: HYSTEROSALPINGOGRAPHY

1. D
2. A
3. C
4. C
5. D
6. B
7. B
8. B
9. C
10. B
11. C
12. D
13. A
14. B

# CHAPTER 7: PEDAL LYMPHOGRAPHY

1. D
2. D
3. D
4. C
5. C
6. A
7. B
8. A
9. C
10. D
11. C

# CHAPTER 8: MYELOGRAPHY

1. C
2. A
3. B
4. pia mater
   arachnoid
   dura mater
5. B
6. C
7. C
8. D
9. C
10. D
11. C
12. C
13. D
14. D
15. D
16. D
17. D
18. C

# CHAPTER 9: SIALOGRAPHY

1. parotid, submandibular (submaxillary), and sublingual
2. parotid and Stenson's duct
3. B
4. submandibular and Wharton's
5. A
6. parotitis (mumps)
7. C
8. A secretory stimulant. It causes the salivary gland to contract and expel saliva
9. B
10. Ethiodol (oil-based medium); sinografin (water-soluble medium)
11. true lateral and lateral oblique
12. Calculus, inflammatory lesions (obstructive or nonobstructive), mass lesions (intrinsic or extrinsic). Others include hypertrophy of the masseter muscle and Sjögren's syndrome.

# CHAPTER 10: LOWER EXTREMITY VENOGRAPHY

1. C
2. B
3. C
4. B
5. Anterior and posterior tibial, popliteal, femoral external, and common iliac and tributaries of these vessels. As an option, the inferior vena cava may also be examined.
6. Veins have one-way valves; arteries do not. The walls of veins are thinner than those of arteries.
7. Obstruction and varicose veins or congenital abnormalities exist. Symptoms include pain, swelling, and discoloration of the extremity.
8. D
9. C
10. Normal saline or a 5 percent dextrose solution.
11. The projections and positions include: an AP and lateral of the calf to include the knee; AP and lateral centered at the knee; AP and lateral of the thigh; AP of the pelvis and (optional for the inferior vena cava) AP of the abdomen.
12. 60 degrees, calf to include the knee; 45 degrees, knee area; 20 degrees, thigh; 0 degrees, pelvis. If the inferior vena cava is to be filmed, the table may be angled Trendelenburg, and an abdominal film is taken.

# CHAPTER 11: ANGIOGRAPHIC ROOM FACILITIES

1. C
2. A
3. A
4. C

5. D
6. C
7. B
8. D

9. B
10. D
11. A

5. D
6. A
7. low-pass, high-pass, and band-pass
8. D

# CHAPTER 12: RAPID FILM CHANGERS

1. D
2. C
3. C
4. A
5. C
6. B
7. C
8. A
9. A
10. D
11. B
12. C
13. D
   1000/4 = 250 milliseconds
   0.40 × 250 = 100 milliseconds
   100 − 2.77 = 97.23 milliseconds
14. A

# CHAPTER 13: ELECTROMECHANICAL INJECTORS

1. D
2. B
3. D
4. B
5. B
6. C
7. A fraction of a second was needed to deliver the required pressure.
   Personnel had to be present in the radiographic room to initiate the injection.
   It was impossible to initiate the injection when the heart was in diastole.
   The sryinge was covered in metal and could not be visualized to see if air bubbles were present in the barrel of the syringe.
   Catheter whipping could occur if there was too much pressure.
   Too much pressure could result in vessel dissection.
   The catheter could break if the pressure was set too high.
8. electrocardiogram
   multiple syringes

# CHAPTER 14: DIGITAL IMAGING TECHNIQUES

1. D
2. B
3. D
4. B

# CHAPTER 15: DIGITAL SUBTRACTION ANGIOGRAPHY

1. B
2. D
3. C
4. A
5. C
6. D
7. C
8. D
9. A
10. C
11. A
12. C
13. D
14. C
15. A
16. renal artery stenosis
    large A-V malformations
    abdominal aortic atherosclerosis
    aortic occlusion
    aortic dissection
    intestinal ischemia
17. D
18. D
19. B
20. A
21. C
22. B
23. B
24. B
25. B
26. A
27. C

# CHAPTER 16: GUIDE WIRES AND VASCULAR CATHETERS

1. C
2. A
3. D
4. D
5. B
6. D
7. D
8. B
9. A
10. B
11. A
12. A
13. A
14. B
15. B

16. check for tip flexibility
    inspect the wrapped coils
    inspect the core
17. care in advancing the guide wire in the vessel
    position of the needle bevel relative to the guide
        wire
    cleaning of the guide wire

## CHAPTER 17: SUPPLEMENTARY CATHETERIZATION EQUIPMENT

1. B
2. C
3. A
4. C
5. A
6. A
7. D
8. B
9. C

## CHAPTER 18: STERILE TECHNIQUE

1. C
2. D
3. C
4. D
5. A
6. B
7. D
8. the disposable drape is nonabsorbent
   the disposable drape is self-adhesive
   it prevents slippage
   it is lint free
9. employees
   instruments
   equipment
10. open
    closed

## CHAPTER 19: CATHETERIZATION METHODS AND PATIENT MANAGEMENT

1. B
2. A
3. D
4. B
5. C
6. A
7. B
8. D
9. hypotension
   bradycardia
   nausea and vomiting
   physical dependence
   constipation and paralytic ileus
   dizziness
   blurred vision

10. B
11. D
12. A
13. C
14. B
15. D
16. B
17. D
18. B
19. D
20. C
21. A
22. B
23. D
24. C
25. A
26. B
27. bleeding
    hematoma
    thrombosis
28. pathology of upper extremity
    assessment of cerebral atherosclerosis
    femoral approach is not feasible
    cardiac catheterization
    assessment of internal mammary artery grafts

## CHAPTER 20: CARDIAC CATHETERIZATION

1. C
2. B
3. C
4. B
5. D

6. B
7. C
8. A
9. B
10. D

## CHAPTER 21: THORACIC AORTOGRAPHY

1. C
2. A
3. A
4. B
5. D
6. A
7. D
8. D

9. C
10. B
11. D
12. B
13. D
14. D
15. A

## CHAPTER 22: CEREBRAL ANGIOGRAPHY

1. C
2. D
3. A
4. B
5. A
6. C
7. A
8. C

9. B
10. A
11. A
12. C
13. B
14. C
15. A

# CHAPTER 23: PULMONARY ANGIOGRAPHY

1. B
2. A
3. B
4. B
5. C
6. D
7. C
8. D
9. A
10. A
11. premature ventricular contractions
    perforation of the heart
    arrhythmia
    twisted catheter in the heart
    severe bradycardia
12. pulmonary embolization
    pulmonary stenosis
    pulmonary vascular changes
    coarctation
    patent ductus arteriosus
    tumors

# CHAPTER 24: ANGIOGRAPHY OF LIVER AND SPLEEN

1. B
2. A
3. A
4. D
5. D
6. C
7. B
8. D
9. common hepatic artery
   splenic artery
   left gastric artery
10. portal hypertension
    retroperitoneal tumor
    aneurysm
    cirrhosis of liver
    hepatitis
    vascular narrowing
    bleeding

# CHAPTER 25: RENAL ANGIOGRAPHY

1. E
2. B
3. A
4. B
5. C
6. D
7. A
8. renal vein thrombosis and tumor invasion of the
   renal vein or IVC
9. C
10. C
11. A

# CHAPTER 26: ABDOMEN/LOWER EXTREMITY ANGIOGRAPHY

1. C
2. A
3. A
4. D
5. C
6. B
7. A
8. C
9. A
10. aneurysms
    congenital anomalies
    stenosis or occlusions
    vascular interventional therapy

# CHAPTER 27: UPPER EXTREMITY ANGIOGRAPHY

1. A
2. C
3. C
4. B
5. D
6. C
7. B
8. B
9. D
10. B
11. A
12. C
13. D
14. C
15. A
16. B
17. C
18. A
19. B
20. D

# CHAPTER 28: CARDIAC INTERVENTIONAL ANGIOGRAPHY

1. A
2. C
3. C
4. D
5. C
6. D
7. C
8. A
9. B
10. D

# CHAPTER 29: VASCULAR INTERVENTIONAL RADIOLOGY

1. A
2. C
3. A
4. B
5. D
6. A
7. C
8. D
9. C
10. B
11. D
12. A
13. B
14. loop basket
    balloon-tip retrieval catheter
    hook-shaped catheter
    loop snare

15. D
16. C
17. B
18. C
19. B

17. D
18. B

# CHAPTER 30: NONVASCULAR INTERVENTIONAL RADIOLOGY

1. A
2. C
3. C
4. identifies anatomy
   distends the calyx
5. hematuria
   infection
   hemorrhage
   peritonitis
   pneumothorax
   urine extravasation
   perirenal bleeding
   catheter dislodgment
   catheter obstruction
6. B
7. D
8. C
9. B
10. A
11. C
12. when a major organ, blood vessel, or plural
    space is transgressed
    coagulation deficiency
    intrahepatic echinocococcal cyst
13. B
14. D
15. A
16. to determine if a mass is malignant or benign
17. A
18. D
19. C
20. A

# CHAPTER 31: MAMMOGRAPHY

1. B
2. D
3. C
4. C
5. B
6. D
7. A
8. B
9. B
10. B
11. B
12. The area of the breast and axilla should be clean
    and free from deodorants or powders.
13. B
14. C
15. C
16. D

# CHAPTER 32: FUNDAMENTALS OF COMPUTED TOMOGRAPHY

1. B
2. D
3. C
4. D
5. D
6. C
7. B
8. C
9. A
10. D
11. D
12. C
13. B
14. B
15. C
16. D
17. D
18. D

# CHAPTER 33: MAGNETIC RESONANCE IMAGING

1. A
2. C
3. E
4. E
5. A
6. C
7. D
8. D
9. D
10. B
11. E
12. C
13. B
14. A
15. A
16. B
17. B
18. B
19. E
20. D
21. C

# CHAPTER 34: MULTIDIMENSIONAL IMAGING

1. A
2. A
3. D
4. D
5. A
6. D
7. B
8. C
9. D
10. guidance
    visualization
    localization

# CHAPTER 35: POSITRON EMISSION TOMOGRAPHY

1. C
2. C
3. D
4. C
5. A
6. C
7. D
8. D
9. C
10. B
11. A
12. A
13. C
14. D

# Index

Numbers followed by an "f" indicate figures; numbers followed by a "t" indicate tabular material.